Community-Based Prevention: Programs that Work

Ross C. Brownson, PhD
Professor
School of Public Health
Saint Louis University
St. Louis, Missouri

Elizabeth A. Baker, PhD, MPH
Assistant Professor
School of Public Health
Saint Louis University
St. Louis, Missouri

Lloyd F. Novick, MD, MPH
Commissioner
Onondaga County Department of Health
Professor
Department of Medicine
SUNY Health Science Center at Syracuse
Syracuse, New York

AN ASPEN PUBLICATION®
Aspen Publishers, Inc.
Gaithersburg, Maryland
1999

Library of Congress Cataloging-in-Publication Data

Brownson, Ross C.
Community based prevention: programs that work/Ross C.
Brownson, Elizabeth A. Baker, Lloyd F. Novick.
p. cm.
Includes bibliographical references and index.
ISBN 0-8342-1241-2 (alk. paper)
1. Community health services.   2. Preventive health services.
3. Health promotion.   I. Baker, Elizabeth A.   II. Novick, Lloyd F.
III. Title.
RA425.B7726   1998
362.1'2—dc21
98-43313
CIP

Orders: (800) 638-8437
Customer Service: (800) 234-1660

About Aspen Publishers • For more than 35 years, Aspen has been a leading professional publisher in a variety of disciplines. Aspen's vast information resources are available in both print and electronic formats. We are committed to providing the highest quality information available in the most appropriate format for our customers. Visit Aspen's Internet site for more information resources, directories, articles, and a searchable version of Aspen's full catalog, including the most recent publications: **http://www.aspenpublishers.com**
Aspen Publishers, Inc. • The hallmark of quality in publishing
Member of the worldwide Wolters Kluwer group.

Editorial Services: Stephanie Neuben
Library of Congress Catalog Card Number: 98-43313
ISBN: 0-8342-1241-2

Printed in the United States of America

1   2   3   4   5

Table of Contents

Contributors

Alice Ammerman, DrPH, RD
Assistant Professor of Nutrition
School of Public Health
University of North Carolina at Chapel Hill
Chapel Hill, North Carolina

Elizabeth A. Baker, PhD, MPH
Assistant Professor of Behavioral Science
    and Health Education
Department of Community Health and
    Prevention Research Center
School of Public Health
Saint Louis University
St. Louis, Missouri

Dileep G. Bal, MD, MPH
Chief
Cancer Control Branch
California Department of Health Services
Sacramento, California

N. Warren Bartlett, MDiv
Assistant Director
Maine Bureau of Health
Augusta, Maine

Adam B. Becker, MPH
Professor and Chair
Department of Health Behavior and Health
    Education
School of Public Health
University of Michigan
Ann Arbor, Michigan

Derryl E. Block, PhD, MPH, RN
Assistant Professor
School of Nursing
University of Minnesota
Duluth, Minnesota

Gregory F. Bogdan, DrPH
Director
Division of Disease Control
Maine Bureau of Health
Augusta, Maine

Carol A. Brownson, MSPH
Associate Director of Community Health
Program in Occupational Therapy
Washington University School of
    Medicine
St. Louis, Missouri

Ross C. Brownson, PhD
Professor of Epidemiology
Department of Community Health and
    Prevention Research Center
School of Public Health
Saint Louis University
St. Louis, Missouri

Thomas A. Bruce, MD
Program Director
Kellogg Foundation
Battle Creek, Michigan

Jan K. Carney, MD, MPH
Commissioner
Vermont Department of Health
Clinical Associate Professor of Medicine
College of Medicine
University of Vermont
Burlington, Vermont

M. Elizabeth Carvette, MPH
Planning and Research Associate
Occupational Health Program
Maine Bureau of Health
Augusta, Maine

Daria Chapelsky, MPH
State Coordinator
5 A Day for Better Health Program
National Cancer Institute
National Institutes of Health
Bethesda, Maryland

James Cherveny, MA, FACHE
Executive Vice President
St. Mary's Duluth Clinic Health System
Duluth, Minnesota

Steven Coen, JD
Senior Program Officer
Kansas Health Foundation
Wichita, Kansas

Alan Cross, MD
Professor of Social Medicine and
    Pediatrics
School of Medicine
Director
Center for Health Promotion and Disease
    Prevention
University of North Carolina at Chapel Hill
Chapel Hill, North Carolina

Sue Dabney, MEd, MPH
Health Program Specialist
Psychology Department
University of Missouri
Columbia, Missouri

James D. Davis, MA
Research Analyst III
Bureau of Health Resources Statistics
Missouri Department of Health
Jefferson City, Missouri

Cynthia Dean, BS
Health Program Representative
Division of Chronic Disease Prevention
    and Health Promotion
Missouri Department of Health
Poplar Bluff, Missouri

Janice Dodds, EdD
Associate Professor
Departments of Nutrition and Maternal
    Child Health
School of Public Health
University of North Carolina at Chapel Hill
Chapel Hill, North Carolina

Eugenia Eng, MPH, DrPH
Associate Professor of Health Behavior
    and Health Education
School of Public Health
University of North Carolina at Chapel Hill
Chapel Hill, North Carolina

Caswell Evans, Jr., DDS, MPH
Project Director and Managing Editor
Surgeon General's Report on Oral Health
National Institute on Dental Research
National Institutes of Health
Bethesda, Maryland

Jean F. Ewing, MSW, MSHyg
Chief
Cancer Control Section
Vermont Department of Health
Burlington, Vermont

Gerry Fairbrother, PhD
Associate Professor
Department of Epidemiology and Social
    Medicine
Albert Einstein College of Medicine/
    Montefiore Medical Center
Bronx, New York

Michael Finch, PhD
Associate Professor of Health Services
  Research, Policy, and Administration
School of Public Health
University of Minnesota
Minneapolis, Minnesota

Christine A. Finley, MS, MPH
Nurse Practitioner
University Health Center
University of Vermont
Burlington, Vermont

Susan Foerster, RD, MPH
Chief
Department of Health Services
Nutrition & Cancer Prevention
Sacramento, California

Mary E. Foley, EdD, RN
Assistant Professor
Department of Community and Preventive
  Medicine
Mount Sinai School of Medicine
New York, New York

Julia Francisco
Cancer Control Program Coordinator
Bureau of Chronic Disease and Health
  Promotion
Kansas Department of Health and
  Environment
Wichita, Kansas

Robert M. Goodman, PhD, MPH
Associate Professor
Department of Community Health
  Sciences
School of Public Health and Tropical
  Medicine
Tulane University
New Orleans, Louisiana

Lani B. Graham, MD, MPH
Director
Maine Bureau of Health
Augusta, Maine

Edward B. Hayes, MD
Medical Epidemiologist
Division of Health Promotion Statistics
National Center for Health Statistics
Maine Bureau of Health
Augusta, Maine

Jerianne Heimendinger, ScD, RD, MPH
Acting Director
AMC Cancer Research Center
Denver, Colorado

Rosemarie M. Henson, MPH, MSSW
Chief
Program Services Branch
Division of Cancer Prevention and Control
Centers for Disease Control and
  Prevention
Atlanta, Georgia

Rose Hollis, BA
Community Health Coordinator
Detroit Health Department
Detroit, Michigan

David R. Holtgrave, PhD
Director, Division of HIV/AIDS
  Prevention
Centers for Disease Control and
  Prevention
Atlanta, Georgia

Barbara S. Hoskins, AB
Chief
Bureau of Health Resources Statistics
Missouri Department of Health
Jefferson City, Missouri

Barbara A. Israel, DrPH
Professor and Chair
Department of Health Behavior and Health
  Education
School of Public Health
University of Michigan
Ann Arbor, Michigan

Larry Jecha, MD, MPH
Director
Wichita-Sedgwick County Health
    Department
Wichita, Kansas

Ann M. Kinney, PhD
Research Scientist
Minnesota Center of Health Statistics
Minnesota Department of Health
Minnesota Health Care Commission
Minneapolis, Minnesota

Pierre Kory, MPA
Project Director
Epidemiology and Social Medicine
Albert Einstein College of Medicine/
    Montefiore Medical Center
Bronx, New York

Garland H. Land, MPH
Director
Center for Health Information
    Management and Epidemiology
Missouri Department of Health
Jefferson City, Missouri

Barbara Laraia, MPH, RD
Doctoral Student in Nutrition
School of Public Health
University of North Carolina at
    Chapel Hill
Chapel Hill, North Carolina

Nancy C. Lee, MD
Associate Director for Science
Division of Cancer Prevention Control
Centers for Disease Control and
    Prevention
Atlanta, Georgia

Patricia MacDonald
Supervisor of Health Education
Wichita-Sedgwick County Health
    Department
Wichita, Kansas

Barbara J. Maciak, PhD
Health Scientist
Urban Research Centers
Epidemiology Program Office
Centers for Disease Control and
    Prevention
Atlanta, Georgia

Nilsa E. Mack, MPH
Epidemiology Specialist
Office of Epidemiology
Missouri Department of Health
Jefferson City, Missouri

Lewis Margolis, MD, MPH
Associate Professor of Maternal and Child
    Health
School of Public Health
University of North Carolina at
    Chapel Hill
Chapel Hill, North Carolina

Tim McAfee, MD, MPH
Associate Director
Department of Preventive Care
Medical Director
Center for Health Promotion/Health at
    Work
Group Health Cooperative of Puget Sound
Seattle, Washington

Paul Miller
Marketing Research Manager
St. Mary's Duluth Clinic Health System
Duluth, Minnesota

Nancy Milio, PhD
Professor of Health Policy and
    Administration, and Nursing
School of Public Health
University of North Carolina at
    Chapel Hill
Chapel Hill, North Carolina

Robert L. Muelleman, MD, FACEP
Emergency Physician and Associate
   Professor
Truman Medical Center and School of
   Medicine
University of Missouri-Kansas City
Kansas City, Missouri

Lloyd F. Novick, MD, MPH
Commissioner
Onondaga County Department of Health
Professor
Department of Medicine
SUNY Health Science Center
   at Syracuse
Syracuse, New York

Marguerite Pappaioanou, DVM, PhD
Chief
Community Preventive Services Guide
   Development Activity
Division of Prevention Research and
   Analytic Methods
Epidemiology Program Offices
Centers for Disease Control and
   Prevention
Atlanta, Georgia

Edith A. Parker, DrPH
Assistant Professor of Health Behavior and
   Health Education
School of Public Health
University of Michigan
Ann Arbor, Michigan

Jennifer Peterson, MSW
Coordinator
Health Quest Program
St. Mary's Duluth Clinic Health System
Duluth, Minnesota

Stephen Pickard, MD
Epidemiologist
Bureau of Chronic Disease and Health
   Promotion
Kansas Department of Health and
   Environment
Topeka, Kansas

Karen Pippert
Coordinator
Behavior Risk Factor Surveillance Unit
Bureau of Chronic Disease and Health
   Promotion
Kansas Department of Health and
   Environment
Topeka, Kansas

Michael Pratt, MD, MPH
Professor of Epidemiology
Department of Community Health and
   Prevention Research Center
School of Public Health
St. Louis University
St. Louis, Missouri

Patricia Riley, CNM, MPH
Program Director
Health Promotion and Disease Prevention
   Research Center Program
National Center for Chronic Disease
   Prevention and Health Promotion
Centers for Disease Control and
   Prevention
Atlanta, Georgia

Amy J. Schulz, PhD
Assistant Research Scientist
School of Public Health
University of Michigan
Ann Arbor, Michigan

Randy H. Schwartz, MSPH
Director
Division of Health Promotion
Maine Bureau of Health
Augusta, Maine

Gloria Stables, RD, MS
Director
5 A Day for Better Health Program
National Cancer Institute
National Institutes of Health
Bethesda, Maryland

Robert S. Thompson, MD
Director
Department of Preventive Care
Group Health Cooperative of Puget Sound
Seattle, Washington

Susan J. True, MEd
Cancer Services Program
Bureau of Adult and Gerontological
    Health
New York State Department of Health
Albany, New York

Ronald O. Valdiserri, MD, MPH
Acting Deputy Director
Division of HIV/AIDS Prevention
Centers for Disease Control and
    Prevention
Atlanta, Georgia

Mary Ann Van Duyn, RD, MPH
Nutrition Consultant
Row Sciences, Inc.
Rockville, Maryland

William A. Watson, PharmD, ABAT
Managing Director
South Texas Poison Center
The University of Texas Health Science
    Center at San Antonio
San Antonio, Texas

Stephen W. Wyatt, DDM, MPH
Director
Division of Cancer Prevention and Control
Centers for Disease Control and
    Prevention
Atlanta, Georgia

Foreword

As has been recently reviewed elsewhere,[1] the field of public health has a long history of examining environmental, social, and economic determinants of health status and of involving community members themselves in the identification and resolution of public health problems. More recently, however, public health research and interventions have tended to emphasize individual risk factors and behavior change, and public health practitioners and researchers have been viewed as the "experts" guiding prevention efforts. This emphasis on individual behavior and the role of the health professional has served to undervalue the contributions of environmental and social factors in understanding health and disease, and the expertise of community members in improving the public's health. This change in focus is particularly problematic given the growing evidence of the inequities in health status associated with, for example, poverty, poor housing conditions, inadequate job opportunities, powerlessness, and racism. This situation has given rise to renewed interest in community-based approaches to prevention and research.[1]

Practitioners and researchers alike have called for a more comprehensive and integrated approach to prevention that includes: greater attention to the complex set of factors (e.g., social, economic, political) that impact on health status at multiple levels (e.g., individual, family, interpersonal, community, policy); increased community involvement in and control over the design, implementation, and evaluation of interventions; enhanced competence in working with diverse cultures; and expanded use of both qualitative and quantitative methods in conducting formative and summative evaluations.[1] There has also been a growing number of funding initiatives by the federal government and private foundations that require community-based prevention approaches.[1] This has been accompanied by an increasing number of community-based prevention interventions, with varying degrees of success, and a wealth of lessons learned that need to be gleaned and disseminated.

With the introduction of *Community-Based Prevention: Programs that Work,* a timely resource is available that will be valuable to academicians, practitioners, and community members alike. The editors present a useful outline of three key characteristics of community-based prevention programs: (1) the use of an ecological approach that involves multiple levels of practice; (2) the tailoring of interventions to meet the needs of individuals and communities; and (3) the involvement and influence by those affected by the programs in designing, implementing, and evaluating them. The editors provide a well-organized framework for presenting the experiences of the authors involved that explicates: the fundamental concepts and approaches of community-based prevention; how data can be collected, analyzed, and applied; the development and implementation of interventions; the use of coalition building; evaluation considerations; and opportunities and future challenges. The chapters in the book make important contributions through their description and analysis of specific examples of community-based prevention efforts. Included in these pages is a rich array of strategies, techniques, methods, and skills needed to successfully conduct community-based prevention programs. The authors also provide a critical perspective on the challenges and limitations involved. The editors include a very helpful synthesis across the chapters in their introductory remarks to each section of the book, along with a set of questions for consideration that makes this a useful tool for instructional purposes.

The resurgence of interest in community-based prevention and research, with its emphasis on more comprehensive approaches and community involvement and control, has the potential to successfully address the growing inequities in health status that exist in communities throughout this country and the world. This book provides a much-needed compendium of examples and suggestions that will enable others to learn from and build upon the authors' experiences. It is an excellent resource that once again places community-based prevention approaches at the forefront in public health, a perspective worthy of remaining as a valued component of public health practice and research.

Barbara A. Israel, DrPH
Professor and Chair
Department of Health Behavior
and Health Education
School of Public Health
University of Michigan
Ann Arbor, Michigan

REFERENCE

1. Israel, B.A., et al. "Review of Community-Based Research: Assessing Partnership Approaches to Improve Public Health." *Annual Review of Public Health* 19 (1998): 173–202.

1

Challenges in Community-Based Prevention

Ross C. Brownson, Elizabeth A. Baker, and Lloyd F. Novick

"Without health there is no happiness. An attention to health, then, should take the place of every other object."
—Thomas Jefferson, 1787

Community-Based Prevention: Programs that Work is devoted to the exciting and rapidly evolving area of community-based prevention. The goals of this bridging of research and practice are to determine the underlying causes of death, injury, and disability and to apply research discoveries at the community level through focused interventions (i.e., policies or programs).

Chapters in this book have been compiled from recent issues of the *Journal of Public Health Management and Practice*. Because community-based prevention is so broad and can be defined in several contexts, these chapters are not intended to cover the entire range of issues. Rather, topics are highlighted that we believe are most relevant for practitioners in the current era of rapidly evolving public health and health care systems. Some chapters present methods or approaches that are essential for effective communitywide intervention. Others show the application of these methods by describing specific interventions (i.e., case studies). Examples selected often illustrate the actual development of programs by federal, state, or local health agencies. The broad areas of importance are highlighted in six sections: (1) fundamental concepts and approaches, (2) data-based assessment, (3) intervention development and implementation, (4) coalition-building, (5) evaluation, and (6) opportunities and future challenges. To assist persons using the book in teaching, each section has an introductory summary along with an initial set of study/discussion questions. This compilation of experiences is intended to stimulate and assist practitioners, academics, and students in applying this rewarding public health model.

Although approaches and methods in community-based prevention have gained in comprehensiveness and sophistication over the past few decades, we are confronted by many important challenges. Among these are the need for:

- **Recognizing the community as the focal point for intervention**

For practitioners working on community health issues, the most important consideration is often the effectiveness of the *application* of the intervention to the general population and the adaptation of the intervention to population subgroups at highest risk. This series of chapters emphasizes applications at the *community* level. This focus on the community has been reflected in regional and national health plans and is recognized as perhaps having the greatest potential for affecting overall health status. The community refers to a group of persons with one or more common characteristics, that have a shared sense of belonging, and may involve a geographically coherent place such as a neighborhood. Wallack and Dorfman define the community as ". . . not just the sum of its citizens, but rather the web of relationships between people and institutions that hold communities together."[1] Community-based interventions may therefore address individual behavior, the relationship among individuals, institutions or organizations, and policies that affect any of these. The notion of community "empowerment" (tapping into and building community competence) is often essential.[2,3]

- **Increasing community involvement in research**

Intervention specialists have increasingly recognized the opportunities presented by community-based prevention including what these interventions can bring to our current understanding of the complex factors that influence health on a population basis. One of the most critical lessons learned from community-based interventions is the importance of *community involvement* in the design and conduct of public health research—sometimes called participatory research.[4] It helps make research questions more relevant to the community, methods more acceptable and appropriate, and results more meaningful. In a variety of current public health interventions, participation of the community through coalitions or advisory boards is mandated by funding agencies.[5]

- **Utilizing partnerships to improve health**

"Partnerships" of multidisciplinary teams from multiple settings including public health agencies, academicians, health care providers, private business, and community members can enhance the sharing of information and therefore prevention efforts. Despite the relative lack of research on long-term predictors of successful partnerships, future partnerships in community-based prevention are likely to benefit from mutual goal setting and effective communication.

- **Public health leaders and policy makers taking a "long view" of health**

Such a vision is needed because many of the "modern epidemics" such as cancer and HIV/AIDS are manifested over years and decades. Moreover, working in partnership requires a substantial commitment of time and energy to build the necessary trust among academics, public health practitioners, and community members.

- **Recognizing multiple indicators of success in community-based interventions**

In addition to typical outcome evaluations, other approaches to determining the "success" of community interventions are needed. For example, setting out an evaluation "road map" early in the life of a project is beneficial in focusing the team on collecting data that are key for answering project evaluation questions.[6] This approach allows collection of process and impact evaluation data to measure health-related changes prior to long-term outcomes.

- **Focusing on health improvement in the highest-risk communities**

In some populations (e.g., low-income groups and some racial/ethnic minority groups) health indicators have remained level or declined over the past decade while indicators in the overall population have improved. A renewed commitment to eliminating these health disparities through focused and tailored interventions is essential.[7]

- **Increasing evidence-based approaches in communitywide prevention**

Unlike biomedical applications (e.g., studying a new type of heart bypass surgery), public health practitioners often rely on intervention designs lacking randomization.[8] Hence, the evidence base for many public health interventions is insufficient or widely dispersed in the public health and social sciences literature. A stronger focus on the conduct and dissemination of applied prevention research is needed to expand the scientific basis for many communitywide interventions.

- **Making better use of data and information technologies**

The ability to use new and existing data is enhanced by unprecedented new tools and opportunities that are available to practitioners working at the community level. Modern information technologies make timely collection and analysis of data more feasible. Access to multiple public health databases (national, state, and local) through the World Wide Web will increase capacity in the future. Even with the unparalleled advances in information technologies noted earlier, in many areas of public health, information systems have been created that cannot "talk" to each other, making their use less than optimal. In addition, with the growth of managed care and its overlap with traditional public health, data systems have sometimes become more proprietary with less likelihood for sharing of information due to fears of regulation or competition.

- **Improved skills in working in multidisciplinary teams**

While the changes in the health care system and increases in managed care enrollment have brought about increased interest in community-based interventions, professionals from governmental public health and medical care sectors may have differing views on the best ways to improve health. It is critical that everyone involved in health care make a commitment to understand and respect each other's perspectives in order for the skills of each group to be brought together to create positive change.

• **Attention on how best to apply discoveries from the basic sciences**

As findings from the laboratory are available on a population basis, some profound questions and ethical quandaries will emerge. For example, if a simple and affordable genetic test becomes available to test for presence of the breast cancer gene (BRCA1 or BRCA2),[9] how will use of this test in the community affect the employability and insurability of women?

It is our hope and belief that public health practitioners will respond to these and other challenges of the new millennium with an increasing focus on community-based prevention. The approaches outlined in this book will help make this vision a reality.

REFERENCES

1. Wallack, L., and Dorfman, L. "Media Advocacy: A Strategy for Advancing Policy and Promoting Health." *Health Education Quarterly* 23 (1996): 293–317.

2. Eng, E., and Parker, E. "Measuring Community Competence in the Mississippi Delta: The Interface between Program Evaluation and Empowerment." *Health Education Quarterly* 21 (1994): 199–220.

3. Israel, B.A., Checkoway, G., Schulz, A., and Zimmerman, M. "Health Education and Community Empowerment: Conceptualizing and Measuring Perceptions of Individual Organizational and Community Control." *Health Education Quarterly* 21, no. 2 (1994): 149–170.

4. Institute of Health Promotion Research, University of British Columbia, and B.C. Consortium for Health Promotion Research. *Study of Participatory Research in Health Promotion. Review and Recommendations for the Development of Participatory Research in Health Promotion in Canada.* Vancouver, British Columbia: The Royal Society of Canada, 1995.

5. Institute of Medicine, Committee on Public Health. Stoto, M.A., Abel, C., and Dievler, A., eds. *Healthy Communities: New Partnerships for the Future of Public Health.* Washington, D.C.: National Academy Press, 1996.

6. Brownson, R.C., Mayer, J.P., Desseault, P.G., Dabney, S., Wright, K.S., Jackson-Thompson, J., Malone, B.R., and Goodman, R.M. "Developing and Evaluating a Cardiovascular Risk Reduction Project." *American Journal of Health Behavior* 21 (1997): 333–344.

7. Aday, L.A. "Health Status of Vulnerable Populations." *Annual Review of Public Health* 15 (1994): 487–509.

8. Brownson, R.C., Gurney, J.G., and Land, G. "Evidence-Based Decision Making in Public Health." *Public Health Reports* (in editorial review).

9. Hill, J.M., Lee, M.K., and Newman, B., et al. "Linkage of Early Onset Breast Cancer to Chromosome 17q21." *Science* 250 (1990): 1,684–1,689.

PART I

Fundamental Concepts and Approaches

The two chapters in this section review some of the fundamental concepts within community-based health promotion and prevention and some common approaches used when working within a community-based framework.

In the first chapter, Baker and Brownson present definitions of community and health promotion that have guided community-based efforts. They then discuss some of the defining characteristics of community-based health promotion and prevention including the use of ecological frameworks, the tailoring of programs to meet the needs of individuals and communities, and the inclusion of those affected by programs in the development, implementation, and evaluation activities. Lastly, they discuss some of the challenges faced by practitioners who wish to engage in community-based health promotion and prevention.

In the next chapter in this section, Milio highlights how policy decisions have affected community health. Because of the significant impact of policies, it is important for health practitioners and communities to be involved in the policy arena. In order to facilitate this involvement, Milio presents a framework for gathering information and presents a number of skills that are important for those who wish to take part in policy development and change.

As you read these chapters, consider the following set of questions:

Objectives and Data Sources

1. How do the objectives of community-based health promotion programs differ from other health promotion activities?
2. How can data be used to influence policy decisions?
3. What sources of data could you draw upon to bolster your position on a particular policy initiative?

Methods and Strategies

4. What specific methods and strategies might be appropriate to use when trying to influence change at the various levels of the ecological framework?
5. What are some ways you could communicate your position on policies to the
   various stakeholders of interest?

Dissemination and Implications for Public Health Practice

6. How might local health departments use community-based health promotion
   programs to reach their goals?
7. What are some potential advantages and disadvantages to using community-
   based health promotion approaches?
8. What can health practitioners and community members do to increase their
   role in health policy development?
9. What are the potential effects of increased practitioner and community participation in the health policy arena?

Defining Characteristics of Community-Based Health Promotion Programs

Elizabeth A. Baker and Carol A. Brownson

Since the 1970s, community-based health promotion programs have been viewed as a potentially viable public health approach to disease prevention and health promotion. However, the definitions of health promotion and community have differed according to who is asked to define these terms and the purpose for which the terms are being defined. Not surprisingly, community-based health promotion programs have varied accordingly. It could be argued, however, that if *every* health promotion program is called community-based then the concept becomes so diluted that the label is meaningless. Moreover, it becomes difficult to determine if these approaches are more effective than other approaches. While it is important to elucidate some of the general characteristics of community-based health promotion, it is also important to acknowledge that these programs do not conform rigidly to a set of predefined criteria. Rather, each of these programs share characteristics, and each characteristic has within it a continuum, or set of stages. Community-based health promotion programs may fall anywhere along these continua and still be defined as community-based health promotion programs.

This chapter will first review the different definitions of health and community, and then describe the defining characteristics of community-based health promotion programs and the stages through which programs progress with regard to each characteristic. It is not intended as an exhaustive review of the broad field of community-based health promotion; rather it is intended as a brief overview of key concepts with links to other literature and chapters in this book. Some of the challenges faced in conducting this work will also be discussed.

HEALTH PROMOTION

According to a recent review, the major contributors to mortality in the United States in 1990 were: tobacco use, poor diet and physical inactivity, microbial

J Public Health Management Practice, 1998, 4(2), 1–9

agents, toxins, firearms, sexual behaviors, motor vehicle accidents, illicit drug use, poverty, and lack of access to medical care.[1] While some of these causes of death are the result of individual behavior, our current understanding suggests that these behaviors are influenced by broader social and economic factors.[2] Moreover, as this review and other researchers have indicated, social and economic factors are also directly associated with health and illness.[1,3] A definition of health (and the scope of community-based health promotion programs) must, therefore, include individual behaviors as well as broader social and economic factors. The Ottawa Charter for Health Promotion states that

> To reach a state of complete physical, mental and social well-being, an individual or group must be able to identify and realize aspirations, to satisfy needs, and to change or cope with the environment. Health is a positive concept emphasizing social and personal resources, as well as physical capacities. . . . The fundamental conditions and resources for health are peace, shelter, education, food, income, a stable ecosystem, sustainable resources, social justice and equity. Improvement in health requires a secure foundation in these basic prerequisites.[4]

DEFINITION OF COMMUNITY

Many programs purport to be community-based or to be working with "the community." However, programs vary widely as to who is included in the definition of community. For some, a community may be defined as a geographic area or neighborhood. For others, in order to be considered a community, members of the community must have a sense of shared identity with other members of the community; a sense of belonging and emotional connection to the community; and a set of shared values and norms.[3] Lastly, some consider communities to be defined by formal and informal collective associations or organizations.[5] Therefore, many practitioners consider themselves to be working with the community when they are working with community-based organizations or associations.

COMMUNITY-BASED HEALTH PROMOTION PROGRAMS

Given these definitions of health and community, it is clear that community-based health promotion programs may be conducted with any one of a number of defined communities (e.g., a geographically bound area, a group with a sense of shared belonging, or a collective association or community-based organization), with the purpose of acting to change individual or social determinants of disease. In doing so, community-based health promotion programs may use a variety of strategies and approaches. Community-based health promotion programs may focus on changing individual behaviors; modifying community structures, processes, and policies; or some combination of these, and what is most effective will depend on the definition of community and the changes desired.

With such broad definitions, one is left questioning how community-based health promotion programs differ from other programs or classes offered in community settings; that is, what are the defining characteristics of these programs. While community-based health promotion programs may take place *in the community* (e.g., in community centers, churches, managed care settings, schools, or work places), they are not defined by their location. Rather, it is the *philosophy* or *characteristics* of the programs that defines community-based health promotion programs.[5] Specifically, these programs: (1) use ecological frameworks that attend to individual, interpersonal, community (including social and economic factors), organizational, and governmental factors, (2) are tailored to meet the needs of individuals and communities, and (3) provide the opportunity for those affected by programs to participate in (and influence) program development, implementation, and evaluation.

Use of ecological frameworks

Many community-based health promotion programs use ecological frameworks to guide the development of their program activities. Ecological frameworks suggest that it is important to incorporate efforts to address individual, interpersonal, community (including social and economic factors), organizational, and governmental factors because of the effect these factors have on individual behavior change, and because of their direct effect on health (see Table 1 for descriptions and possible interventions at each level).[2,3,6]

Programs focused on changing individual behavior may provide information and/or teach skills to enable individuals to change their behaviors. These programs may focus on changing knowledge, attitudes, beliefs, and/or behaviors. Stages of change theory (as will be described below) suggests that different approaches are likely to be more or less useful depending on the individual's readiness for change.[7,8]

To address interpersonal factors, many programs include strategies to strengthen social support. As described by Israel, these programs may act to strengthen existing networks or develop new network ties; however, the building of social ties may be a secondary aim of programs focusing on other types of community-based activities.[9] For example, a program aimed at strengthening existing networks to enhance individual behavior change might invite family members to join fitness facilities or take cooking classes together. Programs may also seek to enhance the total network through lay health advisors.[9] Lay health advisors

Table 1 Interventions at each level of the ecological framework

Target	Individual	Interpersonal	Community	Organizational	Governmental
Objectives	knowledge attitudes behavior physiology abilities	practices social support social network reinforcement	programs practices policies resources facilities norms	programs practices policies resources facilities	programs practices policies legislation ordinances resource allocation regulation enforcement
Approaches	education training counseling self regulation	develop new social ties strengthen existing ties lay health advisors peer support groups	social change media advocacy community development resource development education environmental change	organizational change consulting networking organizational development	political action lobbying policy advocacy

Source: Data from B.G. Simons-Morton, et al., *Introduction to Health Education and Health Promotion,* Prospect Heights, IL: Waveland Press, 1995.

are "lay people to whom others normally turn to for advice, emotional support and tangible aid."[10(p.8)] Lay health advisors may provide specific health information and information about services available to address different health needs, assist clients in improving their communication skills, or establish linkages with health and human service agencies for efficient and appropriate referral.[11,12]

In addition to addressing interpersonal factors, community-based health promotion programs may attempt to create changes in community factors including social and economic factors. These efforts often focus on creating changes in community structures, processes, and policies. In terms of policy changes these programs may, for example, focus on creating worksite smoking policies or smoke-free restaurants to support changes in individual smoking behavior and attempt to alter community norms around smoking. Alternately, efforts may be focused on creating policy changes in other social, community, or economic factors such as housing, jobs, education, and the environment.[13]

Ecological frameworks suggest that because these factors (intrapersonal, interpersonal, organizational, social, and economic) are interrelated, programs that address one level are likely to enhance outcomes at the other levels. It is important to note that ecological frameworks are useful whether the program is categorical (e.g., focused on a particular disease process) or a broadly defined community program (e.g., community development). For example, programs that focus on a disease category (e.g., breast cancer), and receive categorical funding to change individual behavior (e.g., mammography), will enhance their ability to influence this behavior if they consider the impact of other factors (e.g., interpersonal, economic), and intervene accordingly. This may entail providing low or no cost mammograms, changing the policy in the state so that more women are eligible for low or no cost mammograms, or developing a lay health advisor approach to enhance breast cancer screening. These different programmatic activities may occur simultaneously or sequentially.

The Healthy Cities/Healthy Communities program is an example of a broadly defined community-based health promotion program that addresses individual, community, social, and economic factors. Healthy Cities/Healthy Communities programs began in response to the World Health Organization's *Global Strategies for Health for all by the Year 2000*.[14] Toronto, Canada, is one city that has worked extensively on their Healthy Cities/Healthy Communities program. This program has the goal of establishing partnerships between community members and governmental and community organizations to ensure that "everyone has access to the basics needed for health; the physical environment supports healthy living; and communities control, define and direct action for health."[15(p.37)] This approach resulted in efforts to address jobs, housing, air quality, smoking, AIDS, hunger, transportation, safety, and physical activity (i.e., individual, social, community, and economic factors).

Tailored approaches

Whether one is working to change individual behaviors or working to change broader community structures, processes, and policies, it is essential to tailor the program to meet the current needs of individuals and communities or to "start where the people are."[16-18] The specific strategies and tools for assessing the current needs depend on the focus of the program activities, or the level of the ecological framework one is hoping to affect.

In terms of programs working to create individual behavior change, recent work suggests that individuals may go through various stages in attempting to change their behavior (i.e., precontemplation, contemplation, preparation, action, and maintenance) (Table 2).[7,8]

According to stages of change theory, different strategies will be more useful at certain stages than others. For example, broad-based community messages such as bulletin boards and messages on buses (information) are more likely to help someone move from precontemplation to contemplation than to help individuals move from contemplation (through preparation) to action. In order to influence action and maintenance it may be more important to use other methods, such as self-regulation, modeling, and skill development.[19] One example of how this has been translated to a specific methodology is the use of tailored messages. This methodology entails designing a health assessment for the specific population of interest. Each individual completes a health assessment and is provided with a personalized health message or tailored message. These tailored messages provide individuals with information about their health status and health behaviors, as well as their readiness to make behavior changes.[20]

It is also important to start where people are when working to create changes in community structures, processes, and policies. For example, in order to be successful, community development and empowerment approaches require community members to have a shared sense of belonging, mutual support, and common goals. If community members do not have this "sense of community," then programs may need to focus on building this prior to engaging in more task-oriented activities.[3]

Community coalitions are frequently being used to create changes in community structures, programs, and policies. However, while community coalitions are growing in popularity, their ability to create healthful changes depends in part on the coalition's ability to move through various stages of development (Table 3). There are many recent efforts to define and describe these various stages.[19,21-24] Most generally, in order for these groups to be effective, it is essential that they begin by developing a common vision of what they want to do, and a common set of skills to engage in the change process together. In addition, it is important that the individuals involved in the coalition build relationships as individuals and as representatives of their respective community organizations. One important element of these relationships is "social capital," that is, a sense of trust and long-term reciprocity, and the common good. It has been suggested that coalitions that have developed social capital are more likely to be effective than those that have not.[25] As with other types of community-based health promotion programs, in order to be effective coalitions may need to focus on different things (developing a common set of skills or building trust) at different stages of development.

Community participation and influence

Community participation and influence have been cited as defining characteristics of community-based health promotion programs.[3,26] Participation and influence are considered essential for developing effective programs, and more importantly are considered health promoting in and of themselves.[18,26] As such, one of the key roles of health practitioners is to build the capacity of communities to

Table 2 Stages of change

Stage	Description	Strategies for change
Precontemplation	No intention to take action within next 6 months	Information Role models
Contemplation	Intends to take action in next 6 months	Information Role models Weighing pros and cons
Preparation	Intends to take action in next 30 days and has taken some behavioral steps in this direction	Social support Goal setting Contracts/commitments Preparatory behaviors
Action	Made behavior change and has sustained it for less than 6 months	Social support Cues Self regulation Development of new skills (replace old habits with new health behaviors)
Maintenance	Changed behavior and maintained change for greater than 6 months	Rewards Development of new coping skills

Source: Data from J.O. Prochaska and C.C. DiClemonte. "Stages and Processes of Self-Change of Smoking: Toward an Integrative Model of Change." *Journal of Consulting and Clinical Psychology* 51, no. 3 (1983): 390–395, and J.O. Prochaska et al. "Patterns of Change: Dynamic Typology Applied to Smoking Cessation." *Multivariate Behavioral Research* 26 (1991): 83–107.

engage in the processes associated with participation and influence. As with the previous characteristics, communities may participate in and influence community-based health programs in a number of ways. This may range from requests from program managers for input regarding design and implementation, to community members taking an active role in the design, implementation, and evaluation of program activities.

In terms of input, community members may be helpful in designing and implementing community-based health promotion programs. Any one of a number of programs (e.g., to reduce the rate of smoking in a community, to provide breast cancer screening, or to provide prenatal care) can benefit by asking the intended participants what types of programs they would like, what barriers they face in trying to change their behaviors, and what would enhance their ability to change. This information can be collected through both qualitative (e.g., interviews, focus groups) and quantitative (e.g., surveys) methods. It is, however, crucial to go beyond the mere collection of data. The findings from these data must be reported back to those from whom the data was collected and must also be used to modify

---

Table 3 Stages of coalition development

Stage of coalition development	Examples of tasks associated with each stage
Initial mobilization	Recruit participants including formal and informal leaders, ensure linkages with appropriate related community agencies
Establish organizational structure	Establish roles, decision making structures, group process
Build capacity and plan for action	Orient members to processes used in assessment procedures, prioritization mechanisms, and intervention development
Implementation	Develop specific work plan with roles, responsibilities, timeline, and allocation of resources
Evaluation	Process evaluation to identify gaps in programming and modify activities accordingly
Institutionalization	Develop plans for recruiting new members, assess alternative program strategies, develop outcome evaluation

Source: Reprinted with permission from P. Florin et al., "Identifying Training and Technical Assistance Needs in Community Coalitions: A Developmental Approach," *Health Education Research: Theory and Practice* 8, no. 3, p. 419, © 1993, Oxford University Press.

program activities as appropriate. When feedback is not provided, or it appears to be ignored, trust is eroded and it lessens individuals' willingness to provide information in the future.

On the other end of the continuum, community members may take part in all aspects of program activities. One approach to engaging the community in this way is participatory action research. Participatory action research is a problem solving process that includes community members in diagnosing the community's strengths and problems, planning interventions, implementing interventions, and evaluating program activities. Using this approach, community members decide what interventions to develop (rather than having the program imposed by categorical funding opportunities), and decide how to implement and evaluate these programs.

CHALLENGES

While we are aware of many different models, strategies, and methods that will enhance community-based health promotion programs, we must also acknowledge the limits in our knowledge and the challenges we face in implementing these strategies. These limits are most notable in an examination of our methodologies and professional roles.

Acknowledge limitations in methodologies

"We have to learn to work within the community frame of reference, with people who represent the authentic voice of the community, who are from the start committed to some kind of problem solution as active participants and even initiators. More specialized procedures, including refined survey tools, need to emerge from this, not precede it."[26(p.156)]

The review of the defining characteristics assumes that practitioners have the methods, skills, and resources necessary to work at multiple levels of the ecological framework; engage the community members in a process where they can take part in (and influence) program activities; and ensure that program activities will be tailored to community needs. However, most practitioners do not have all of the skills necessary to engage in all of these processes. While some practitioners are skilled at individual behavior change, others are more skilled at creating changes in policy. Therefore, one of our challenges is to work in multidisciplinary teams through which we look for outside resources and partners with complementary skills.

The above review also implies that community-based health promotion may have advantages over other methods of creating changes in health, and that it is therefore something to strive toward. However, health practitioners often do not have a full range of options for how to conduct their work. For many practitioners, work is determined by the organizations they work for and/or the organizations funding their projects. It is, therefore, important that we come to see how we can incorporate these characteristics into programs in multiple ways rather than seeing them as rigid rules. Moreover, it is critical that we begin to educate those who fund programs about the benefits of community-based health promotion programs. One of the most effective means of doing this is through evaluation activities.

While evaluation is an essential tool, we need to examine the strategies we use to evaluate what are often very complex community-based health promotion program activities, and acknowledge our limitations in this area as well.[28] A few examples will serve to illustrate this point. We have few rigorously evaluated quantitative tools that can measure important characteristics such as coalition effectiveness, social capital, and community competence. Even when these scales are available, it is often difficult to reach many community members through traditional survey techniques such as mail or telephone surveys. Including members of the community in the implementation of door-to-door surveys is a viable alternative, but is itself a formidable task.[29] Similarly, including community members in the collection and analysis of qualitative data (e.g., interviews and focus groups) presents its own set of challenges. For example, some community members may be less comfortable working with the written word than the spoken word. While audio and videotapes can be used for data collection, jointly analyzing the data in this form requires modifying existing, and creating new, techniques.[30]

Professional roles: Are health practitioners part of "the community"?

While some health practitioners work within what could be considered their "own" communities, many health practitioners do not live in, nor are they considered part of, the communities in which they conduct interventions. For those of us who work in our "own" community, it is important to acknowledge that the very fact of being in the role of health practitioner is likely to distinguish us from our peers even if we are similar in other ways. In other words, while we may share one characteristic (e.g., gender, race/ethnicity, class, age, religion, sexual orientation, abilities, personal history, etc.) our experiences may still be very different from other's experiences. Within our role as a professional we must strive to offer our expertise (both in terms of professional skills and personal experience) while acknowledging the limitations of our expertise. We must remember to see our similarities, while acknowledging our differences. One way to capture the breadth of experiences within a community is to build in mechanisms to ensure community input. This may entail surveys or focus groups, or it may involve representatives from different identified constituencies jointly taking part in the initiation, development, implementation, and evaluation of program activities (e.g., development of coalitions).

For those who are not part of the community in which they work, it is important to recognize that the factors that influence health (e.g., job opportunities, income, housing, education, and social justice) affect us all.[31] Even if we are not part of the particular community in which we are working, we are not immune from the factors that affect community health. As individuals, and as professionals, we must begin to question how we fit into, affect, and are affected by, community health and its determinants. The appropriateness of our engagement in community-based health promotion programs may well be determined by our answer. As stated by Lily Walker of Australia, "If you are here to help me, then you are wasting your time. But if you come because your liberation is bound up in mine, then let us begin."[32(p.148)]

●   ●   ●

Recent work in the field suggests that the factors that influence many of the major causes of death in the United States, and factors that facilitate community health, are both behavioral and social in nature.[1,33] Health practitioners need to begin to see that individual lifestyle behaviors, the environment, socioeconomic factors, and local, state, and federal regulations and policies are all within the purview of public health, yet not be overwhelmed by the numerous intervention options. It is important to coordinate community-based efforts and utilize multiple skills and disciplines to understand and act upon the complexity of factors that influence health, and to maintain momentum for change. While some programs may focus on multiple levels of the ecological framework simultaneously, others may use a more sequential approach, addressing one level and then another. Alternately, community-based health promotion programs may involve building coalitions or alliances of organizations, each of which address different aspects of a community health issue.

Regardless of the approach, community-based health promotion programs need to be tailored to the needs of specific individuals and communities. In addition, research suggests that programs that build community capacity (e.g., enhance community member involvement, skills, and control over programs) and build community infrastructures are more likely to have long-term impacts.[18] In order to accomplish this, it is essential that community members themselves take an active role in the planning, implementation, and evaluation of such efforts.

REFERENCES

1. J.M. McGinnis and W.H. Foege. "Actual Causes of Death in the United States." *Journal of the American Medical Association* 270, no. 18 (1993): 2207–2212.

2. K.R. McLeroy et al. "An Ecological Perspective on Health Promotion Programs." *Health Education Quarterly* 15, no. 4 (1988): 351–377.

3. B.A. Israel et al. "Health Education and Community Empowerment: Conceptualizing and Measuring Perceptions of Individual, Organizational and Community Control." *Health Education Quarterly* 21, no. 2 (1994): 149–170.

4. World Health Organization, Health and Welfare Canada, and Canadian Public Health Association. Ottawa Charter for Health Promotion. (Paper presented at the International Conference on Health Promotion, Ottawa, ON, Canada, 1986.)

5. J.L. McKnight. "Redefining Community." *Social Policy* (Fall and Winter): 56–63.

6. B.G. Simons-Morton et al. *Introduction to Health Education and Health Promotion.* Prospect Heights, Ill.: Waveland Press, 1995.

7. J.O. Prochaska and C.C. DiClemente. "Stages and Processes of Self-Change of Smoking: Toward an Integrative Model of Change." *Journal of Consulting and Clinical Psychology* 51, no. 3 (1983): 390–395.

8. J.O. Prochaska et al. "Patterns of Change: Dynamic Typology Applied to Smoking Cessation." *Multivariate Behavioral Research* 26 (1991): 83–107.

9. B.A. Israel. "Social Networks and Health Status: Linking Theory, Research and Practice." *Patient Counseling and Health Education* 4, no. 2 (1982): 65–79.

10. B.A. Israel. "Social Networks and Social Support: Implications for Natural Helper and Community Level Interventions." *Health Education Quarterly* 12, no. 1 (1985): 65–80.

11. E. Eng and R. Young. "Lay Health Advisors as Community Change Agents." *Family and Community Health* 151 (1992): 24–40.

12. E. Eng and J.W. Hatch. "Networking Between Agencies and Black Churches: The Lay Health Advisor Model." *Prevention in Human Services* 10, no. 1 (1991): 123–146.

13. N. Milio. "Priorities and Strategies for Promoting Community-Based Prevention Policies." *Journal of Public Health Management and Practice,* in press.

14. D.L. Patrick and T.M. Wickizer. "Community and Health." In *Society and Health,* eds. B. Amick et al. New York: Oxford University Press, 1995: 46–92.

15. City of Toronto. *Toronto's First State of the City Report.* Produced for Healthy City Toronto. City Clerk, Communication Services Division, Toronto, ON, Canada, 1993.

16. D. Nyswander. "Education for Health: Some Principles and Their Applications." *Health Education Monographs* 14 (1956): 65–70.

17. M. Minkler. "Ten Commitments for Community Health Education." *Health Education Research: Theory and Practice* 9, no. 4 (1994): 527–534.

18. N. Freudenberg et al. "Strengthening Individual and Community Capacity to Prevent Disease and Promote Health: In Search of Relevant Theories and Principles." *Health Education Quarterly* 22, no. 3 (1995): 290–306.

19. D.J. Bowen et al. "Preliminary Evaluation of the Processes of Changing to a Low Fat Diet." *Health Education Research: Theory and Practice* 9, no. 1 (1994): 85–94.

20. V.J. Strecher et al. "The Effects of Computer-Tailored Smoking Cessation Messages in Family Practice Settings." *Journal of Family Practice* 30, no. 3 (1994): 262–269.

21. E.A. Parker et al. "Coalition Building for Prevention: Lessons Learned From the North Carolina Community-Based Public Health Initiative." *Journal of Public Health Management and Practice* 4, no. 2 (1997): 25–36.

22. F.D. Butterfoss et al. "Community Coalitions for Prevention and Health Promotion." *Health Education Research* 8, no. 3 (1993): 315–330.

23. P. Florin et al. "Identifying Training and Technical Assistance Needs in Community Coalitions: A Developmental Approach." *Health Education Research: Theory and Practice* 8, no. 3 (1993): 417–432.

24. C. Alter and J. Hage. *Organizations Working Together: Coordination in Interorganizational Networks.* Newbury Park, Calif.: Sage Publications, 1992.

25. M. Kreuter, N.A. Lezin, and A.N. Kaplan. Social Capital: Evaluation Implications for Community Health Promotion. Working Paper prepared for WHO/EURO Working Group on Evaluating Health Promotion Approaches and Division of Adult and Community Health, National Center for Chronic Disease Prevention and Health Promotion, Centers for Disease Control and Prevention, 1997.

26. G. Steuart. Social and Cultural Perspectives: Community Intervention and Mental Health. (Paper presented at the Fourteenth Annual John W. Umstead Series of Distinguished Lectures. Raleigh, N.C., 1978.)

27. L.W. Green et al. *Study of Participatory Research in Health Promotion.* Institute of Health Promotion Research, The University of British Columbia and the British Columbia Consortium for Health Promotion Research, The Royal Society of Canada, 1995.

28. R.M. Goodman. "Principles and Tools for Evaluating Community-Based Prevention and Health Promotion Programs." *Journal of Public Health Management and Practice,* in press.

29. A.J. Schulz et al. "Conducting a Participatory Community-Based Survey for a Community Health Intervention on Detroit's East Side." *Journal of Public Health Management and Practice* 4, no. 2 (1997): 10–24.

30. E.A. Baker et al. "Latino Health Advocacy Program: A Collaborative Lay Health Advisor Approach." *Health Education Quarterly* 24, no. 4 (1997): 495–509.

31. R.C. Brownson and M.W. Kreuter. "Future Trends Affecting Public Health: Challenges and Opportunities." *Journal of Public Health Management and Practice* 3, no. 2 (1997): 71–77.

32. N. Wallerstein and E. Bernstein. "Introduction to Community Empowerment, Participatory Education, and Health." *Health Education Quarterly* 21, no. 2 (1994): 141–149.

33. M. Feinleib. "New Directions for Community Intervention Studies." *American Journal of Public Health* 86, no. 12 (1996): 1696–1697.

3

Priorities and Strategies for Promoting Community-Based Prevention Policies

Nancy Milio

Public health involves promoting and protecting health, preventing disease, and enhancing quality of life through policies that assure equitable access to the conditions under which people can be healthy. These conditions involve places to live, work, learn, obtain health and supportive services and information, and participate in public life in safe, sustainable environments.[1] Accordingly, public health requires organizational and collaborative action directed toward several entities, including policy bodies, the press, and the public.[2] Through these actions, public health attempts to influence organizational changes that in turn impact the individual, resulting in a healthy population living to a healthy late life, with health equality among all social groupings.[3]

As a core public health function, *policy development* is consistent with public health responsibility for assessing and assuring the public interest in health. Providing for more than specific benefits to particular individuals, which is the domain of clinical services, it includes population health planning, constituency mobilization, and policy advocacy.[4] The federal and state agencies have a mandate to assure the capacity and accountability in carrying out the public health mission through core funding of health departments, technical assistance, regulation, evaluation, and direct policy action.[5]

An understanding of policy development is especially important now as public health issues move to local and state jurisdictions. Public health workers must be able to recognize when community health might be affected by policy choices and find ways to initiate and influence policies to promote and protect health; assess tradeoffs, make judgments, and enhance the feasibility of healthy policy options.[6,7]

A framework for gathering relevant information and guiding strategic action is a useful tool to support this core function. Such a framework is provided below.

The author is grateful for the clerical assistance of Carolyn Williams and Marie Buzzetta.

J Public Health Management Practice, 1998, 4(3), 14–28
© 1998 Aspen Publishers, Inc.

Following its overview, strategic issues are discussed, including a summary of lessons learned. Examples of processes and activities are drawn from the literature. The chapter concludes by noting the need for building the public health community's capacity to pursue policy development.

AN OVERALL FRAMEWORK FOR PUBLIC HEALTH POLICY DEVELOPMENT

This framework is among several others[8–10] that have described health policy development and enactment. It is noteworthy that no single framework is all-encompassing or applicable in every situation. Rather, it is useful for conceptualizing the overall environment, inputs, and outputs.

Public policy may be thought of as a guide to government action at any jurisdictional level to alter what would otherwise occur. The intent is to achieve a more acceptable state of affairs, and, from a public health perspective, a more health promoting society. Policies usually indicate a direction toward broad goals, operate across one or more types of organization, and affect large populations. They may focus on ends (goals) or means (e.g., participatory processes or taxation). Organization policy is that of a single agency (e.g., health department) or type of organization (e.g., public schools), either public or private, and is often tied to governmental policy changes. Some key settings and processes for health policy making are discussed in this section.

Health-related organizations: Settings and processes

Governmental policies affect the policies of health and related organizations by mandates, or enable change through incentives or deregulation (Figure 1). Such policies are directed to specific types of organizations, such as health departments or housing agencies, or to the environments in which they operate, i.e., other organizations and client groups with whom they work, such as voluntary and managed care organizations (MCOs), third-party payers, beneficiaries, and poor families. In this way, government policies trigger policy action in an organization and feed into a group's own self-starting initiatives. External policy shifts may also spur organizational efforts to amend or rescind government policies. Health and health-related organizations are a subset of the organizational universe, all of which is affected by tax, monetary, employment, and environmental policies.

The new policy environment for public health involves the rapid transition to managed care health services, decentralization of federal policy and control to the states through block grants and deregulation, continued efforts at deficit and income tax reduction, and a growing gap in wealth and health between disadvantaged people and communities compared with their better-off counterparts.

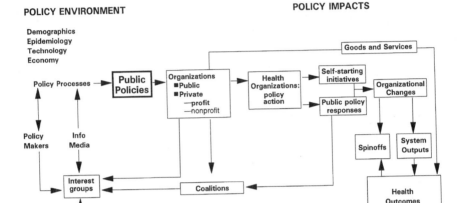

© Copyright 1997, Nancy Milio

Figure 1. Framework for the interactions between the policy environment and policy impacts.

Health-related organizations respond to policy shifts by examining their fiscal, administrative, program operations, and, more rarely, their mission. Consequent internal actions may then affect collaborating organizations, clients, and community populations. These agency, individual, and population outcomes, when monitored and fed back into the political policy process, can impact policy change.

The changing health care marketplace

Due to the emphasis on cost control and changing state and federal policies, MCOs are now receiving funds previously provided to health departments for Medicaid and Medicare patients. One estimate suggests that almost half (46%) of state public health spending went to the delivery of personal health services.[11] The overall effect will be that MCOs will deliver contract-explicit services, avoiding costly support services often needed by disadvantaged groups, such as outreach, transportation, translation, food stamps, and other family services.[12] At the same time, state health insurance reforms have had minor impact for the uninsured working poor, while fewer than 54 percent of workers (two-thirds of Americans) now have employer-based coverage.[13] These groups will be forced to turn to the public health system for basic services.[14]

The foreseeable shape of the MCO delivery system remains unclear and uncertain. Although profitmaking MCOs are the fastest growing systems, only about one-third were profitable in 1996 compared with 90 percent in 1993. In addition, early Medicaid contracts have not been very profitable, with some entrepreneurs preferring to leave the market rather than reduce their profit margins and stock value. A third source of uncertainty is continuing consolidation of companies, leading to predictions of an eventual 40–50 managed care firms covering the entire country.[15] The prospective loosening of federal Medicaid waiver-process, which served to guarantee a national standard of prevention and treatment for eligible people, will mean an increased variety of Medicaid programs in the states, adding further to uncertainties for public health planning.[16]

Early evidence suggests that the economic pressures and privatization of health care for the poor and elderly are resulting in a drop in some clinical primary preventive services and related family/environmental services.[17–20] Community-based prevention may become relegated to peripheral, public relations activities by private provider systems; monitoring and quality assurance data are being inadequately reported or kept controlled by private holders for the proprietary value; health departments are being sidestepped in health services planning by private systems; and nurses and other hospital personnel are moving into community-based services without public health training.

Welfare reform and Medicaid eligibility

Another critical facet of the public health environment, the Welfare Reform Act, may have further adverse effects on health and health services delivery in poor communities. Many welfare-eligible families may no longer be automatically enrolled in Medicaid. Others may lose their welfare benefits because of new time limited eligibility. Cuts in job training and education, school breakfast and lunch programs, food stamps, Supplemental Security Income benefits, and immigrant eligibility will limit health services for large numbers of disadvantaged families, children, and elders. Separate application for Medicaid is likely to deter the use of health care until sickness compels it, discouraging access to clinical prevention and early treatment, in turn requiring more costly care. This will raise per capita costs for MCOs and ultimately for state payments, placing further demands on state budgets.[21]

Public health problems and policy

Federal decentralization and deregulation has given states gains in power and in larger fiscal and ethical burdens to support vulnerable people in addition to the poorest. Congressional and state budget cuts in health, housing, education, social, and environmental programs, and enforcement capacity, accompanied by growing gaps in income and health, foreshadow a smaller, weaker safety net and growing health risks among many social groupings.[13,22]

Although public health has had notable successes[23] and life expectancy continues to rise in the United States and other westernized societies, patterns in the general population, such as the widening extent of excessive dietary intake and declining physical activity especially among younger people, augurs future chronic disease, disability, and related social and economic costs.[24–26] At the same time, gaps in disease, disability, and death between disadvantaged and other populations are increasing.[27]

Health gaps, not explainable solely by typical biomedical and behavioral risk factors,[28] are mediated by a complex web of linked living conditions shaped by policy action or inaction regarding jobs and workplaces, homes, and communities.[29] These inequalities are related not only to poverty, but also to income inequality.[30,31] The U.S. wealth gap is now largest since the 1920s.[32] Children in low-income single parent families, especially blacks, are the most likely to feel the adverse impacts of reforms first.[13,33] Lack of adequate food, poor housing in poor neighborhoods, and lack of prenatal care may increase risks to health and longevity of low-income adults and children[34,35] (Figure 2). These living conditions are closely tied to the nature of public policies.[36] Much has been written about the need for broad policies to promote health.[2,31,37,38]

Policy processes and stakeholder interests

Policy processes encompass initiation, adoption, implementation, assessment, and reformulation or repeal. They are not linear, and are often punctuated by legal or social challenges, retrenchment, or rescissions. They are always embedded in historical and current social contexts. Policy-making processes shape content as interested parties attempt to direct the course and pace of policy development to their own needs and priorities.[39] The results often have indirect and direct impacts on population health. Indirect effects involve access to housing, jobs, information and education, health insurance, protective environments, tax burden, and civil rights.[40–42] More direct effects include the scope, quality, and availability of primary and secondary preventive, and rehabilitation services.

The ability to influence policy development is more likely when organized interest (stakeholders) groups, including legislative committees, public agencies, and professional groups, press the issue and strategically use the mass media and other channels to promote their views.[43] All of this policy activity occurs in an environment of demographic, epidemiological, economic, political, and technological change. Strategists scan this environment for opportunities and threats to their aims and actions.

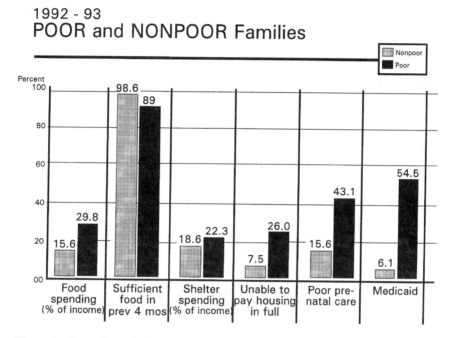

Figure 2. Comparison of selected indicators for nonpoor and poor families, United States, 1992–93. *Source:* Data from U.S. national survey data in M. Federman, Monthly Labor Review, May 1996.

Strategic choices

The emerging political, fiscal, organizational, and health situation presents a major choice in policy direction for public health systems. One option is to give priority to providing clinical health services, directly or through state Medicaid contracts or subcontracts for "carve-out" services with managed care networks.[44,45] Another option would place priority on policy development and advocacy to promote the conditions for health, including assuring the arrangements for, but not health department delivery of, adequate managed care services to low-income and uninsured populations.[6,46] All proposed options stress leadership and cooperative initiatives. Local and state health department decisions are being made on both sides of this strategic issue.[46] The policy development option is the focus here.

A policy-focused strategy aimed at organizational or system change (e.g., water supply, housing) has been the historic approach to achieve population health during much of its first century.[47] However, in more recent decades, as federal funds for health care for the poor became available, public health agencies directed more of their attention to the direct delivery of personal health services. As a result, the practice of policy development in political arenas has declined in priority, re-source commitment, skills, training, and effectiveness.[2,48,49] The range of strategic options for the future can be framed in the context of a population-based view of health.

Population health and its meanings

While the public health community agrees that its appropriate goal is popula-tion health, the population focus itself can have different meanings and be pursued in basically different yet complementary ways. The conception of a "population focus" and the chosen strategic approach to address health needs have different potential health effects and resource costs.[50,51] It can mean a policy development, organization-directed approach or an individual-oriented, information driven ap-proach directed toward total geographic or more limited high-risk populations, attempting to change individual behavior (Figure 3). Priority-setting and re-sources necessarily will produce a shift in one direction or the other in public health organizations.

Population change and public health policy

To have important health effects, programs require community-wide applica-tion, so that even modest individual improvements can shift the total population average to lower levels.[52,53] A community-wide approach to population health, such as community health promotion campaigns, usually focus on *individuals* in defined populations to produce behavior change. They often use mass media, and are sometimes supported by small group work or clinical services (Figure 3). However, the cost of an effective media program can be high; a sustainable down-ward curve requires costly re-injections of funds, and may succeed mainly in im-proving knowledge and attitudes rather than behavior.[54]

The shift from individual-level interventions to changing the overall policy-related environment can have a larger beneficial effect.[38] For example, policy changes affecting smoking in public places or raising tobacco taxes are as or more effective than individual-change strategies.[52,55] The most complex commu-nity-based trials that focused on an individual-information-driven model have had some disappointing long-term impacts, achieving little beyond secular changes, usually within chance limits.[50,56] Conclusions from program reviews suggest that institutionalization of health promoting programs had failed and that future efforts should target and evaluate organizational change.[57–60]

A policy change strategy can achieve long-term population-wide impacts by changing the conditions under which people live by providing incentives and re-

Strategies for PREVENTION

Intervention Strategy	Focus	
Individual information-mediated change	**Homes and communities** (e.g., computers, TV, campaigns, health fairs)	**Organization settings** (e.g., counseling, computers, print, small group training of patients, clients, customers, healthcare practitioners, librarians, teachers, employers, clergy)
Organization-mediated policy change	**Congress, legislatures, independent agencies** (e.g., EPA, FDA) **Government administration** (rule-making, executive order)	**Government health and other organizations** (e.g., health departments, housing education) **Non-government organizations** (e.g., managed-care organizations, community health centers, medical centers, schools, companies, food manufacturers, retailers)

Copyright 1996, Nancy Milio

Figure 3. Comparison of individual vs. organizational intervention strategies.

---

quirements for changes in organizational decisions about products, services, information, and environmental conditions. It makes for a more effective population approach than an attempt to change individuals' behavioral or biomedical risk factors.[38,61,62] But it can also carry administrative, social, and political costs to which some public health professionals are risk adverse.[6,49]

Prevention strategies directed at the overall environment that mediates the living conditions require work with organizations and communities on a variety of public, institutional, or corporate policies. For example:

- To address the interests of commercial establishments in safe and expanding markets, local governments and community organizations (led by health departments) can use their market power to influence the macronutrient shape of the local food supply and limit access to tobacco.[63] They could require that vending machines in their facilities contain low fat, high fiber food choices and no tobacco products. This would encourage vending companies to change their supplier contracts in order to retain their own vending contracts, with ripple effects on food processing corporations. The new options in these facilities would result in changes in eating and smoking habits for clients and employees as well as suggesting a "healthy practices" model for the public and the media.

- Prevention policy development can involve neighborhoods with high rates of unemployment, poverty, high rent, and crowded housing. These conditions are associated with the high incidence of low birth weight babies.[35] Local policies affecting housing and industry siting, transportation infrastructure, and environment controls, have both individual and community-wide health impacts.[64,65] While not under the direct control of health departments, they can be addressed through defining the type and scope of health issues, the necessary changes in policy to support health, and working with the local and state organizations in housing, economic development, land use, and the environment to advise on and advocate changes.[37,66]

POLICY DEVELOPMENT ACTIVITIES: STRATEGIC ACTION AND MANAGEMENT

Policy development based on the strategic choices in the preceding section requires strategic planning and action and is more effective when it includes an organizational unit to manage monitoring, tactics, and coordination. Essential ingredients for effective action include continuous monitoring and assessment of the policy environment; favorably framing the terms of debate; collaborative policy design, presentation, and communication that is sensitive to the interests of stakeholder groups and audiences; committed coalitions with resources that are adequate to the task, and alliances with key policy makers.[67]

Strategic action

A descriptive study of antismoking policy development in several states illustrates some critical elements for public health policy making.[43] Analysis showed important differences in strategic action in successful states where strong laws were passed (e.g., bans on smoking in public places and private worksites and large penalties) compared with states enacting weaker legislation (e.g., narrow restrictions, smokers' rights clauses, minor penalties). These factors included assertive legislative leadership backed by determined coalitions and persistent lobbying by either the top public health official and/or governor's office. In most cases, however, neither state health departments, public health associations, medical societies, nor large voluntary health organizations did more than lend their names to the coalitions.

Each of these mainline organizations had competing priorities. Examples include the fear of budget cuts from opposition lawmakers, lack of staff, or legal restrictions in some local health departments. The medical societies chose to use their political capital to seek better clinical payment rates, and the large not-for-profit groups feared a backlash from some donors. These organizational decisions about public health advocacy were strategic choices made by each organization that, as always, took into account tradeoffs in resources for the group and its purposes. Alternatively, a case could have been made whereby visible and active support of strong antismoking laws could have enhanced future public support for these organizations concerning other issues on their agendas.

The five following "lessons learned" for policy action were gleaned from the above report and others cited, and filtered through the policy-making frame represented in Figure 1. They may be regarded as working hypotheses to be refined with each experience in the policy arena.

1. Monitoring the policy environment

Organized activity surrounding the policy-making process on any given issue is set in a historical context derived from past experience with similar issues and current constraining circumstances that affect all interested parties. Constraints include the demographic and epidemiologic nature of the population, the economy and distribution of resources, political party agendas, and organizational hierarchies.[68] All these can affect whether and how policy making will proceed and must to some extent be taken into account in the strategic plans of the players.[69]

In the antismoking case, the relevant policy environment included the decline in U.S. tobacco sales, the rising costs of domestic production, and the costs of increased legal challenges made the tobacco industry somewhat less politically threatening than in the past.

2. Choosing frame, forums, and channels for debate

An important early step in policy initiation is to get the debate framed in the public's health interests while being sensitive to the current environment. The place of tobacco control on policy agendas, for example, will differ depending on how proponents frame the issue, especially when advocates are aware of government budget constraints and conservative political priorities. The issue could be framed as a problem in health insurance and public health care cost control versus a free market; or, as an environmental and child health issue whose control can help make healthier children more ready-to-learn and parents more ready-to-work versus smokers' right to take personal risks with a legal product.

Another strategically useful step is to attempt to use forums and communication channels that are favorable to public health proponents but not to their rivals. Tobacco control advocates, for example, tried to use the open arenas of legislatures and to seek news media coverage, in contrast to the highly paid, behind-the-scenes lobbying and television advertising of the tobacco industry. In addition, again depending on the environment, local ordinances rather than state law may be more readily enacted, in spite of the narrower public health impact. Sufficient community-level action can be a learning laboratory and create political conditions for stronger statewide policy action.

3. Designing policy proposals

The actual design of a public health policy, if it eventually requires some health tradeoffs with collaborating groups and policy makers, should nonetheless offer clear public health gains and prospects for steady incremental policy progress. Back-up compromise positions should be explored and assessed in advance, held in reserve, and be based on a feasibility analysis.[70]

Apart from information on the overall policy environment, the kinds of local data that are useful for health-supporting policy development, whether tobacco control or better housing, define the geographic community in ways that measure and monitor relevant trends. These involve environmental and personal measures from organization-level, individual-specific, and aggregated data sources. For example, there are environmental measures, such as numbers of workplaces and schools with smoking-control policies or the adequacy of housing requiring organization-specific data, and the size of tobacco sales requiring individual-level, aggregated data. More traditional individual-specific, personal smoking behavior is also useful. Much of this may be secondary data and is readily available.

The choice of *policy instruments* is critical in policy design. They determine, along with funding authorization, appropriation, and allocation, a policy's effectiveness in reaching stated goals. Legislative, executive, and regulatory policy makers have numerous instruments and mechanisms:

- economic and in-kind incentives
- regulation and enforcement
- research and development
- information development (educational and strategic)
- information transfer (via old and new media)
- education and training
- administrative and participatory mandates/rights
- organization development, collaboration, cooperation, and coordination
- direct service provision
- government, voluntary agency, and corporate modeling
- market management and marketpower
- investment in organizational and physical infrastructure

Inflation-adjusted tobacco taxes are an obvious example of an economic disincentive to smoking, especially for young people. Prohibition of smoking in public places is an example of a low cost use of regulation. Market management and market power are used when, as noted above, organizations redesign vending machine policies around health promotion goals (or when state health agencies develop MCO Medicaid contract criteria to obtain a particular direction in personal health services for the poor).

4. Negotiating with allies and opponents

Identifying relevant players in the specific policymaking arena is another important step in policy development. Targeted groups are those that have a stake in the outcome of a policy. They include elected and appointed officials, commercial, scientific, medical, and voluntary not-for-profit entities and public interest groups.[71,72] The policy message must be tailored to the interests of each group in ways that attempt to obtain their support or neutralize their opposition, offering some short- or longer-term gain (or non-loss) for self-perceived risk. Elected and other officials are wary of political risk and so, want assurances of political support; voluntary organizations must please their boards and donors; commercial groups seek safe and expanding markets.[73] The light involvement of certain professional groups and large voluntary organizations in the antismoking policy study noted above illustrates typical risk-benefit calculations of organizations.[43,67]

Successful coalition formation requires addressing the interests, rather than simply appealing to the short-term goodwill, of target organizations. It means forging links with those who can speak for the policy and resource interests of the organization, who can influence the direction of its resources toward specific purposes.[58,68] Effective collaboration is more likely when all parties benefit from an alliance, when their core missions are protected, or when the relationship helps them gain resources and legitimacy. Collaboration can be distinguished from cooperation by the exchange of tangible assets as contrasted with more peripheral and verbal support in cooperative ties, which augur a shorter-term or less-effective relationship, as was apparent in antismoking policy processes.[43,74]

The types of strategies that organizations can undertake to pursue their policy interests often depend on their size and resources, as well as depth of interest. The most effective strategies, demanding the most resources, include lobbying legislators or appointees directly, through influential parties, or through their constituents (e.g., clients, donors, voters); election of sympathetic political leaders, litigation, community group mobilization, private debriefing meetings; and press conferences as part of a wider media program. Less-effective means, often used by small groups, involve developing publicity through the media, demonstrations, conferences, and public education programs.[75]

5. Influencing the social climate: public opinion and the media

Most people base their beliefs and opinions, of necessity, on what they directly experience and what they learn through other channels of information (i.e., other persons or some form of media). All such conduits select and shape the information they pass on, according to their own priorities. Most Americans get most of their information or news through the mass media, primarily television. The mass media thus provide much of the basis on which public opinion is formed. The new media-electronic reality has implications for the policy development tasks of public health proponents.[7,76]

Although public opinion can form a supportive backdrop for public health policy action, it is not sufficient to ensure policy makers' assent to new policies, especially when there are strongly opposed interest groups. To impact policy, as suggested in the policy successes of the antitobacco case, public opinion must be mobilized into organized local group support, contacts by district constituents to key legislators, and visibility of supporters in the mass media. Taken together, these elements spurred governmental action and neutralized the campaign financing, organized lobbies, and longtime ties between policy makers and protobacco forces.[43]

Although personal access to policy makers remains perhaps the most effective, yet select, path, the networking of old and new information and communication technologies presents new ways to reach policy makers. Studies covering the introduction and demise of the Clinton Health Care Plan (September 1993–July 1994) demonstrate how the mass media are woven into policy-making processes and so must be taken into account in public health policy strategies.[77-79]

- Two-thirds of all coverage was on political strategy, not content or the pros and cons of each major proposal.
- Coverage focused on the President's plan while others, like the single payer bill, had almost no public airing.
- Random samples of viewers participating in controlled screenings of strategy-based versus issue-centered coverage revealed that they saw policy makers as posturing, deceptive, self-interested, and unconcerned with the welfare of citizens. Groups viewing only issue-centered stories were less cynical.
- News coverage of political advertising emphasized the attack and controversial nature of the ads, dramatically enlarging the ads' audiences, and reached legislators on key committees and their media markets.
- The public was generally poorly informed; less than half had heard of the single payer bill; they wanted much more information and blamed the media for not providing it.
- Reportage of opinion polls was uncritical, magnifying the impact of uninformed opinion, and influencing the actions of leading members of Congress.
- Media coverage ultimately had an impact on Congress's rejection of major reform. Leaders said that Congress was influenced by public opinion and interest group advertising, while acknowledging that the public was not well informed and that the media had done little public issue education. Yet lead-

ers' "main sources of information about public opinion"[79,p.21] were the polls, the trade group lobbies, and the media.

Strategic management

In a study of the 1993 national health care reform, failure was attributed to the Clinton administration's inadequate strategic *management* of the policy-making process.[80] The principal errors included an overemphasis on the technical nature of the policy and the predominance of health policy experts, the closed nature of the design process and limited attempts to involve allies in Congress and voluntary groups, vague and tenuous efforts to educate the public, delays in activating the formal Congressional process, and inconsistency in tactics.

This and other studies suggest that ongoing strategic management throughout all phases of policy making, including implementation, is essential to policy success.[39,43,48,67,69] This organized, proactive process is largely underdeveloped in the public health community.[49,81] Its purposes, noted earlier, are to monitor and guide policy planning and action. It must remain sensitive to changing environments and adjust tactics and timing accordingly in pursuit of sustained political and public support.

The task requires that policy proponents set up an organizational unit with operating resources (e.g., funds, staff, site, equipment, and access to information) for guiding policy development. Such a unit may be institutionalized in a department, an office of strategic planning or legislative liaison, or a professional society. It may be a joint venture by a coalition, or a subcontracted service from an appropriate public interest group (e.g., an antismoking or an affordable housing group). The unit's actions attempt to propel movement from the initial policy idea to on-the-ground reality by enhancing policy feasibility, using an array of types of information to establish and gain support for public health claims. A proposed policy must be made economically feasible to its supporters and users; politically acceptable to the more powerful groups affected by it; socially acceptable within the milieu in which it is to operate; and administratively and technologically possible.[82]

Environmental scanning is basic to strategic management. The purpose of this continuous information-seeking activity is to anticipate and identify bottlenecks, determine the causes, and adjust tactics accordingly. It involves gathering, interpreting, and reporting to policy proponents progress in every phase of policy development, from design and initiation (to support framing, debating, and support-seeking) through implementation and reformulation. It includes tracking the resource investment and tactics of opposition groups. The depth of commitment to policy advocacy by any group is readily measured by the share of its resources that it allocates to the task.

Using information for substantive and strategic ends in policy making

Policy processes, both formal and nonformal, are driven by the interplay of stakeholder interests. Information is the basic medium of exchange in that interplay, conveyed face-to-face or through various channels.

Information used in policy making may be thought of as two types, each having two main purposes. *Science-based* information is mainly used for substantive policy purposes—e.g., identifying problems and solutions, including the efficacy, effectiveness, and economic costs of a policy or of potential policy instruments, as in strong or weak clean indoor air policies. Science information is most often and readily used in the early design phases of policy development.[83] The traditional scientific ideal is to use knowledge to educate policy constituencies.

Substantive policy issues are also influenced in policy arenas by the opposite type of information, *nonscience-based* and less verifiable information. The main sources are stakeholders in and out of government who offer their informed judgments and personal experience. The purpose is to promote the legitimacy of an issue to justify a place on the policy agenda.[70]

These two types of information (science- and nonscience-based) are intended to educate about and legitimize the substantive aspects of a policy. In addition, they have additional critical purposes, which are strategic—to promote action on proponents' preferred policy choices. Here, both science-based and other information is used to persuade publics, potential allied groups, and policy makers. From the viewpoint of policy makers who cite scientific findings, the purpose is to justify choices that may be determined on a political, negotiated basis as trade-offs are made between the major stakeholders in a particular situation or policy domain.[67,69] In health-related policy making, strategic information comes from non-biomedical sources, i.e., economic and political knowledgebases used to demonstrate acceptable costs or gains and external organized, and public opinion support, which are relevant to policy-makers' interests.

In other words, the task is not to win a science battle, as has long been done. It is rather to develop a wide range of scientific and other knowledge to win the social, economic, and political battle that has not yet been conclusive. The strategic purpose is to persuade groups by lowering the political costs of their support, showing how they will not lose, and may gain in status or resources in any or all phases of the policy process, including implementation and reauthorization.[39,82]

Formats and sources

Any type of information that is used in a strategically effective way will be audience-specific and interest-sensitive. It will be presented in ways that take account of the desired image, resource needs, purposes, and future prospects for the targeted group or organization. These targets range from defined publics and media gatekeepers to stakeholders such as key elected, appointed, or career officials and specific public interest, voluntary, or proprietary groups in a given policy domain. The choice of content, format, and media mix are matters of strategic planning for policy proponents; the information needed to survey this organizational and policy universe is a form of strategic information.

Other forms of strategic information include material denoting other supporters. This is available, for example from opinion polls, editorials, evidence of unanimity among advocacy groups, endorsements by prestigious organizations or individuals, reports on comparable policies in other jurisdictions. Additional information that can enhance the political feasibility of a policy proposal includes demonstrating its administrative simplicity, and clearance of any legal challenges or other counterarguments by opposition groups.[43]

Identifying, gathering, assessing, formatting, and communicating such information is a task for strategic management. Major sources of this kind of information are in the "fugitive" literature, material outside the traditional refereed journals, statistical databases, and legal documents used by health professionals. This strategic information pool includes policy reports and statements, articles, and newsletters from governments, commissions, task forces, think tanks, academia, foundations, professional and industry associations; the industry and public press; and a wide array of electronic media, including the Internet.

Science-based information—whether for substantive or strategic purposes—tends to be narrow, not policy-focused, and often not user-friendly.[82,84] In addition to audience-appropriate selection and packaging of usable information, its effectiveness for policy purposes also depends on proponents' previous links to policy makers, the competition of other information used in the policy arena, and the political (risk-control) value of the information.[73,85,86] These rules of thumb apply in national and community jurisdictions, in governmental and nongovernmental arenas.

The incremental nature of science knowledge usually limits its immediate impact on policy. In the longer term, it can affect policy perspectives and influence development to some degree, depending upon changing conditions, "retranslation" of the information to make it relevant to the time, and the persistence of proponents.[83] However, it need not be limited in the midterm, if public health policy proponents plan its use strategically.

CONCLUSIONS

Essential public health services, including policy development activities, are available to only 40 percent of Americans, while the national goal is to have 90 percent so served by the turn of the century.[87] Little more than one-fourth of estimated state public health spending is invested in such core functions.[11] In recent decades public health agencies have not been as active in policy development as earlier, but rather have been reactive to short-term public pressure.[49] Many have rarely had the strategic capacity to carry out a policy agenda.[49] Recent studies show that health departments are weak in performing policy development activities, have limited capacity to build support for policy changes, and rarely monitor broader health-related policy issues, such as community poverty levels.[5,81,88,89]

Public health capacity-building to support core functions with an emphasis on policy issues, whether tobacco control, housing development, or Medicaid managed care contracting, requires a number of competencies in health departments beyond those of current individual incumbents. These skills include:

- Political: to mobilize prime constituencies, including government officials, voluntary, health, welfare, and economic development organizations, and the public through face-to-face and media techniques[7]
- Managerial: to provide organizational leadership, planned resource use, implementation, organizational evaluation, and change in response to changing environments[57]
- Programmatic: to develop broader approaches than individual change in population health through improvements in the social, economic, physical, and political conditions that shape behavior, using legal and policy strategies[38]
- Technical: to ensure adequate data collection for assessment and evaluation; and information development and dissemination that is usable by constituencies, using a variety of media, including electronic networks[90,91]
- Fiscal: to develop new sources and ways to fund core functions[46]

•   •   •

As the public health community faces major and historical choices in priorities for its mission, it has the option of placing greater emphasis on public health policy development for prevention and health promotion. Public health policy making requires a grasp of the interplay among stakeholders, policy makers, the press, and the public. Strategic management of policy participation in community, state, and national arenas is essential to success in the promotion of health and prevention of disease in our populations. A focus on organized and organization-targeted approaches in the policy sectors that support health can make policy advocacy, community mobilization, and public education about policy issues more widespread and effective. The capacity to use these skills requires the investment and reallocation of resources in much of the public health community.

REFERENCES

1. Canadian Public Health Association. *Health Impacts of Social and Economic Conditions: Implications for Public Policy.* Ottawa: CPHA, 1997.

2. Institute of Medicine. *The Future of Public Health.* Washington, D.C.: National Academy Press, 1988.

3. Office of Disease Prevention and Health Promotion. *Healthy People 2000. National Health Promotion and Disease Prevention.* Public Health Service Pub. No. 91-50212. Washington, D.C.: U.S. Dept. of Health and Human Services; DHHS Publications, 1991.

4. Public Health Functions Steering Committee. *Core Functions Project.* American Public Health Association, September 1994.

5. Miller, C., et al. "A Proposed Method for Assessing the Performance of Local Public Health Functions and Practices." *American Journal of Public Health* 84 (1994): 1743–1749.

6. Brown, R. "Leadership to Meet the Challenges to the Public's Health." *American Journal of Public Health* 87 (1997): 554–557.

7. Baker, E.L., et al. "Health Reform and the Health of the Public: Forging Community Health Partnerships." *Journal of the American Medical Association* 272 (1993): 1275–1276.

8. Tugwell, P., et al. "The Measurement Iterative Loop: A Framework for the Critical Appraisal of Need, Benefits and Costs of Health Interventions." *Journal of Chronic Diseases* 38 (1985): 339–351.

9. Shapiro, S. "Epidemiology and Public Policy." *American Journal of Epidemiology* 134 (1991): 1057–1061.

10. Brownson, R.C., et al. "Policy Research for Disease Prevention: Challenges and Practical Recommendations." *American Journal of Public Health* 87 (1997): 735–739.

11. Public Health Foundation. *Measuring State Expenditures for Core Public Health Functions.* Washington, D.C.: September 1994.

12. General Accounting Office. *Medicaid: Factors To Consider in Managed Care Programs.* Washington, D.C.: U.S. Congress, June 1992.

13. General Accounting Office. *Family Health Insurance.* Washington, D.C.: U.S. Congress, February 1997.

14. Lipson, D., and Schrodel, S. *State-Subsidized Insurance Programs for Low-Income People.* Washington, D.C.: Alpha Center, 1996.

15. Darby, M. "Trajectory of Managed Care." *Center for Studying Health System Change Issue Brief* 9 (1997): 1–4.

16. Reichart, R. "Budget Agreement." *Medical & Health Perspectives* (May 19, 1997): 5–6.

17. Kaiser Commission on the Future of Medicaid. *Medicaid and Managed Care: Lessons from the Literature.* Menlo Park, Calif.: KFF, 1995.

18. Chapel, T. *Medicaid Managed Care and Childhood Lead Poisoning Prevention Programs.* A Report Prepared for the National Center for Environmental Health, Centers for Disease Control and Prevention. Atlanta, Ga.: Macro International, Inc., 1995.

19. Chapel, T. *Working with Community-Based Organizations To Advance the Childhood Lead Poisoning Prevention Agenda.* A Report Prepared for the National Center for Environmental Health and Prevention. Atlanta, Ga.: Macro International, Inc., 1995.

20. Macro International, Inc. *Private Sector Health Care Organizations and Public Health: Potential Effects on the Practice of Local Public Health.* Final Report to the Centers for Disease Control and Prevention. Atlanta, Ga.: Macro International, Inc., March 1996.

21. Rosenbaum, S., and Darnell, J. "An Analysis of the Medicaid and Health-Related Provisions of the Personal Responsibility Act of 1996." *Health Policy and Child Health* 3 (1996): 1–6.

22. Service Employees International Union. *Block Grants: A State-by-State Analysis of the Fiscal Impacts of Program Consolidation.* Washington, D.C.: SEIU, 1995.

23. Office of Disease Prevention and Health Promotion and Centers for Disease Prevention and Control. *For A Healthy Nation. Returns on Investment in Public Health*. Washington, D.C.: DHHS, Public Health Service, 1993.

24. Centers for Disease Control and Prevention. "Daily Dietary Fat and Total Food-Energy Intakes—Third National Health and Nutrition Examination Survey. Phase 1, 1988–1991." *Morbidity and Mortality Weekly Report* 43 (1994): 116–125.

25. Kuczmarski, R., et al. "Increasing Prevalence of Overweight among U.S. Adults." *Journal of the American Medical Association* 272 (1994): 205–211.

26. Hoffman, C., et al. "Persons with Chronic Conditions: Their Prevalence and Costs." *Journal of the American Medical Association* 276 (1996): 1473–1479.

27. Clark, D. "U.S. Trends in Disability and Institutionalization among Older Blacks and Whites." *American Journal of Public Health* 87 (1997): 438–440.

28. Krieger, N. "Epidemiology and the Web of Causation." *Social Science and Medicine* (1994): 887–903.

29. Link, B., and Phelan, J. "Social Conditions: A Fundamental Cause of Disease." *Journal of Health and Social Behavior* 2 (special issue) (1995): 80–94.

30. Kaplan, H. "Inequality in Income and Mortality in the U.S.: Analysis of Mortality and Potential Pathways." *British Medical Journal* 312 (1996): 999–1003.

31. Duleep, H. "Mortality and Income Inequality." *Social Security Bulletin* 58 (1995): 34–50.

32. Montgomery, L., et al. "Effects of Poverty, Race, and Family Structure of U.S. Children's Health: Data from the NHIS, 1978 through 1980 and 1989 through 1991." *American Journal of Public Health* 86 (1996): 1401–1405.

33. Wolff, E. *Top Heavy: A Study of The Increasing Inequality of Wealth in America*. New York: Twentieth Century Fund, 1995.

34. Lynch, J., et al. "Workplace Conditions, Socioeconomic Status, and the Risk of Mortality and Acute Myocardial Infarction: The Kuopio Ischemic Health Disease Risk Factor Study." *American Journal of Public Health* 87 (1997): 616–622.

35. Roberts, E. "Neighborhood Social Environments and the Distribution of Low Birth Weights in Chicago." *American Journal of Public Health* 87 (1997): 597–603.

36. Federman, M., et al. "What Does It Mean To Be Poor in America?" *Monthly Labor Review* (May 1996): 3–10.

37. Slater, C., and Carlton, B. "Behavior, Lifestyle, and Socioeconomic Variables as Determinants of Health Status: Implications for Health Policy Development." *American Journal of Preventive Medicine* 1 (1985): 25–33.

38. Schmid, T., et al. "Policy as Intervention: Environmental and Policy Approaches to the Prevention of Cardiovascular Disease." *American Journal of Public Health* 85 (1995): 1207–1211.

39. Milio, N. "Nutrition Policymaking: How Process Shapes Product." In *Beyond Nutrition Information,* edited by B. Garza. Ithaca, N.Y.: Cornell University Press, 1997: 275–290.

40. Office of Technology Assessment. *An Inconsistent Picture: A Compilation of Analyses of Economic Impacts of Competing Approaches to Health Care Reform by Experts and Stockholders.* Washington, D.C.: Government Printing Office, June 1994.

41. Flynn, P. *State Health Reform: Effects on Employment and Economic Activity*. Washington, D.C.: Urban Institute, 1993.

42. Milio, N. *Promoting Health through Public Policy*. Philadelphia: F.A. Davis, 1981.

43. Jacobson, P., et al. "Politics of Antismoking Legislation." *Journal of Health Policy, Policy Law* 18 (1993): 787–818.

44. Agency for Health Care Policy Research. *Roles, Responsibilities, and Activities in a Managed Care Environment. A Workbook for Local Health Organizations.* Washington, D.C.: DHHS, Public Health Service and AHCPR, 1995.

45. Centers for Disease Control and Prevention. "Prevention and Managed Care: Opportunities for Managed Care Organizations, Purchasers, and Public Health Agencies." *Journal of the American Medical Association* 275 (1996): 2628–2631.

46. Association of State and Territorial Health Officers. *Introduction To Managed Care For State Health Agencies.* Washington, D.C.: ASTHO, 1995.

47. Frazer, W. *Duncan of Liverpool.* London: Hamish Hamilton, 1947.

48. Williams-Crowe, S., and Aultman, T. "State Health Agencies and the Legislative Policymaking Process." *Public Health Reports* 109 (1994): 361–366.

49. Stivers, C. "The Politics of Public Health: The Dilemma of a Public Profession." In *Health Politics and Policy*, edited by T. Litman and S. Robins. Albany, N.Y.: Delmar Publications, 1991: 356–369.

50. Winkleby, M. "The Future of Community-Based Cardiovascular Disease Intervention Studies." *American Journal of Public Health* 84 (1994): 1369–1371.

51. National Cancer Institute. *Strategies to Control Tobacco Use in the United States: A Blueprint for Public Health Action in the 1990s.* Smoking and Tobacco Control Monographs 1 (NIH Pub. No. 92-3316). Bethesda, Md.: National Cancer Institute, U.S. Dept. of Health and Human Services, 1991.

52. Rose, G. "Future of Disease Prevention: British Perspectives on the U.S. Preventive Services Task for Guidelines." *Journal of General Internal Medicine* 5 suppl. (1990): S128–132.

53. Rose, G. "Sick Individual and Sick Populations." *International Journal of Epidemiology* 14 (1995): 32–38.

54. Rice, R., and Atkin, C. "Principles of Successful Public Communication Campaigns." In *Media Effects: Advances in Theory and Research*, edited by J. Bryant, and D. Zillman. Hillsdale, N.J.: Lawrence Erlbaum, 1994: 365–387.

55. Teh-Wei, H., et al. "Reducing Cigarette Consumption in California: Tobacco Taxes vs. an Anti-Smoking Media Campaign." *American Journal of Public Health* 85 (1995): 1218–1222.

56. Koepsell, T., et al. "Commentary: Symposium on Community Intervention Trials." *American Journal of Epidemiology* 142 (1995): 594–599.

57. Fortmann, S., et al. "Community Intervention Trials: Reflections on the Stanford Five-City Project." *American Journal of Epidemiology* 142 (1995): 576–586.

58. Schwartz, R., et al. "Introduction: Policy Advocacy Interventions for Health Promotion and Education: Advancing the State of Practice." *Health Education Quarterly* 22 (1995): 421–426.

59. Lanvin, A., et al. *Creating an Agenda for School-Based Health Promotion: A Review of Selected Reports.* Cambridge, Mass.: Harvard School of Public Health, 1992.

60. Office of Technology Assessment. *Adolescent Health,* Vol. 1. Washington, D.C.: U.S. Congress, 1991.

61. Susser, M. "Tribulations or Trials—Intervention in Communities." *American Journal of Public Health* 85 (1995): 1568–1571.

62. Goodman, R., et al. "A Critique of Contemporary Community Health Promotion Approaches: Based on a Qualitative Review of Six Programs in Maine." *American Journal of Health Promotion* 7 (1993): 208–220.

63. Association of State and Territorial Health Officers and Association of State and Territorial Public Health Nutrition Directors. *The National Project to Develop a Strategic Plan for Changing the*

American Diet to Prevent Cancer, Heart Disease, and Other Chronic Diseases. Atlanta, Ga.: Centers for Disease Control and Prevention, 1993.

64. Martin, A. *Health Aspects of Human Settlements: A Review.* Geneva: World Health Organization, 1977.

65. General Accounting Office. *Housing Issues.* Washington, D.C.: U.S. Congress, December 1993.

66. Hardy, J., and Satterthwaite, D. "Housing and Health." *Cities* 4 (1987): 221–235.

67. Brewer, G., and de Leon, P. *Foundations of Policy Analysis.* Homewood, Ill.: Dorsey, 1983.

68. Milio, N. "Making Healthy Public Policy: Developing The Science By Learning The Art: An Ecological Framework for Policy Studies." *Health Promotion International* 2 (1987): reprinted in *Health Promotion Research,* edited by B. Badura and I. Kickbusch. London: Oxford University Press,1992, 28–46.

69. Laumann, E., and Knoke, D. *The Organizational State.* Madison: University of Wisconsin Press, 1987.

70. Rochefort, D., and Cobb, R. "Problem Definition, Agenda Access, and Policy Choice." *Policy Studies Journal* 21 (1993): 56–71.

71. Feldstein, P. *The Politics of Health Legislation. An Economic Perspective.* Chicago, Ill.: Health Administration Press, 1996.

72. Jasanoff, S. *The Fifth Branch: Science Advisors as Policymakers.* Cambridge, Mass.: Harvard University Press, 1993.

73. Benjamin, K., et al. "Public Policy and the Application of Outcomes Assessments: Paradigms vs. Politics." *Medical Care* 33, suppl. (1995): AS299–306.

74. Hord, S.M. "A Synthesis of Research on Organizational Collaboration." *Educational Leadership* (February 1986): 22–26.

75. Walker, J. *Mobilizing Interest Groups In America: Patrons, Professions, and Social Movements.* Ann Arbor: University of Michigan Press, 1991.

76. Cohen, L. "Managing the Managed Care Environment." *Center for Studying Health Systems Change Issue Brief* (April 1997): 1–4.

77. Cappella, J., and Jamieson, K. *Public Cynicism and News Coverage in Campaigns and Policy Debates: 3 Field Experiments. Research Report.* Philadelphia: Annenberg School for Communication, 1994.

78. Braun, S. "Media Coverage Of Health Care Reform. A Content Analysis." *Columbia Journalism Review* 3 suppl. (March/April 1995): 1–8.

79. Columbia Institute. *What Shapes Lawmakers' Views? A Survey Of Members Of Congress And Key Staff On Health Care Reform.* Washington, D.C.: CI, May 1995.

80. Aaron, H. *The Problem That Won't Go Away: Reforming US Health Care Financing.* Washington, D.C.: Brookings Institution, 1995.

81. Halverson, P., et al. "Performing Public Health Functions: The Perceived Contribution of Public Health and Other Community Agencies." *Journal of Health and Human Service* 18 (1996): 288–302.

82. Alderman, H., and Rogers, B. "Science and the Policy Process: Does Economics Differ from Nutrition?" In *Beyond Nutrition Information,* edited by B. Garza. Ithaca, N.Y.: Cornell University Press, 1997, 291–307.

83. Brint, S. "Rethinking the Policy Influence of Experts: From General Characterizations To Analysis of Variation." *Sociological Forum* 5 (1990): 361–385.

84. King, L., et al. *A Review of the Literature on Dissemination and Uptake of New Information and Research Related to Health Promotion and Illness Prevention.* Canberra, Australia: Commonwealth Department of Health and Family Services, 1996.

85. Office of Technology Assessment. *Researching Health Risks.* Washington, D.C.: U.S. Congress, 1993.

86. General Accounting Office. *Improving the Flow of Information to the Congress.* Washington, D.C.: U.S. Congress, January 1995.

87. Turnock, B., et al. "Local Health Department Effectiveness in Addressing the Core Functions of Public Health." *Public Health Reports* 109 (1994): 653–658.

88. Studnicki, J., et al. "Analyzing Organizational Practices in Local Health Departments." *Public Health Reports* 109 (1994): 485–488.

89. Zucconi, S.L., and Carson, C.A. "CDC's Consensus Set of Health Status Indicators: Monitoring and Prioritization by State Health Departments." *American Journal of Public Health* 84 (1994): 1643–1644.

90. Milio, N. "Beyond Informatics: An Electronic Community Infrastructure for Public Health." *Journal of Public Health Management Practice* 1 (1995): 35–43.

91. Lasker, R., et al. *Making a Powerful Connection: The Health of the Public and the National Information Infrastructure.* Report of the Public Health Data Policy Coordinating Committee U.S. Public Health Service. Washington, D.C.: July 7, 1995.

PART II

Data-Based Assessment

This section of *Community-Based Prevention: Programs that Work* highlights the scope and power of public health data. Public health agencies and health care organizations collect a wealth of valuable information on various health conditions, risk factors, and prevention options. In many cases, these data are vastly underutilized in developing public health programs and policies. Some of the chapters in this section are based on routinely-collected surveillance data. Others rely on specialized surveys to collect much-needed information. Although five chapters cannot begin to show the full range of data-based opportunities, these do give excellent illustrations of how data can be collected, analyzed, and used by public health practitioners.

The first two chapters in this series rely on information regularly reported to state health departments. Carvette et al. used mortality data for the state of Maine to determine excess deaths due to nine preventable chronic diseases. This analysis not only shows the overall burden of chronic diseases in Maine, but also allows county-specific estimates that are critical in targeting local efforts. Similarly, the chapter by Muelleman et al. provides a descriptive analysis of external cause of injury (E-code) data that were reported to the Missouri Department of Health. State statutes passed in 1992 required these data to be reported by all Missouri hospitals and ambulatory surgical centers. The analysis of E-code data allows a comprehensive review of injury-related deaths, hospitalizations, and outpatient visits, as well as hospital charges due to injuries. As with the Maine data on chronic diseases, these injury statistics are extremely valuable in assisting communities in quantifying the impact of injuries.

The next chapter in this section describes baseline and follow-up survey data on cardiovascular disease (CVD) control efforts among local health agencies in Missouri. The surveys were brief and inexpensive and yielded high response rates

(95% in 1990 and 92% in 1994). These data showed that while local health administrators recognize the overall importance of CVD, prevention practices ranked lower than those for many other public health issues. From 1990 to 1994, there was little improvement in prevention activities related to CVD. These results suggest several priority areas for working with local health agencies.

Pippert et al. describe the use of methods from the Behavioral Risk Factor Surveillance System (BRFSS) to conduct a local risk factor survey on tobacco control in Sedgwick County, Kansas. Their survey found that the vast majority of local residents were aware of the detrimental health effects of exposure to environmental tobacco smoke. Wide support was shown for health policies to discourage tobacco use by children and adolescents. In part due to the use of these local data, policies to restrict tobacco vending machines and smoking in public places were passed. Their study illustrates the powerful effect of local data and their use by coalitions to promote better health.

In the final chapter in this section, Schulz et al. report on their experience and lessons learned in conducting a participatory survey in Detroit, Michigan. There are several important concepts contained in this chapter. First, it describes the process of participatory, community-based research—in which community members are actively involved in the research process. By engaging community members, a greater potential for empowerment can be realized. Second, it highlights the importance of working with high-risk, traditionally underserved populations, such as Detroit's East Side African American community. And finally, the chapter provides a step-by-step account of how the survey was conducted. This information is valuable for others undertaking similar efforts.

As you read these chapters, consider the following set of study questions:

Objectives and Data Sources

1. For each of the studies described, are the objectives and research questions well described?
2. What are sources of routinely available data that would allow you to conduct studies such as those by Carvette et al. and Muelleman et al.?
3. Are such data available via the WWW, for example through WONDER (http://www.cdc.gov)?

Methods and Strategies

4. How would you define "community-based research"?
5. What are some strengths and weaknesses of a participatory approach to community-based research?

6. Do local risk factor data such as those collected by Pippert et al. exist for a variety of health conditions? What are some of the limitations of such data?

Dissemination and Implications for Public Health Practice

7. How best might you communicate public health surveillance data (such as those contained in these chapters) to policy makers?
8. What are the implications of the findings of Mack et al. in shaping the priorities of local health agencies in Missouri?

4

Assessing the Targets for Prevention of Chronic Diseases

*M. Elizabeth Carvette, Edward B. Hayes, Randy H. Schwartz,
Gregory F. Bogdan, N. Warren Bartlett, and Lani B. Graham*

From 1982 through 1991, 111,249 Maine residents died. The leading causes of death were heart disease, cancer, stroke, chronic obstructive pulmonary disease (COPD), unintentional injuries, pneumonia and influenza, diabetes, suicide, and chronic liver disease and cirrhosis. On a national level, McGinnis and Foege have argued that these "causes" are in fact only the pathophysiologic conditions identified at the time of death, and that the actual leading causes of death are tobacco use, unhealthy diet and activity patterns, alcohol consumption, microbial and toxic agents, firearms, risky sexual behavior, motor vehicle crashes, and illicit drug use.[1] They estimated that half of the deaths that occurred in the United States in 1990 were attributable to these causes, all of which can be controlled or reduced through public health efforts.

Hahn et al. noted that nine chronic diseases—stroke, heart disease, diabetes, COPD, lung cancer, female breast cancer, cervical cancer, colorectal cancer, and cirrhosis—accounted for 52 percent of all U.S. deaths in 1986.[2] They estimated the proportion of these deaths that was preventable using three methods. Similar methods have been applied at a state level.[3] We set out to determine the proportion of excess deaths from the nine diseases in Maine and the proportion of deaths from each disease attributable to "actual" preventable causes. Such estimates can be used to help target resources and in determining the potential impact of state and local prevention programs.

The authors acknowledge the help of Ken Keppel in reviewing the manuscript and providing the focus on the core public health function of assessment. In addition, we thank Robert Hahn, Steve Teutsch, and Richard Rothenberg for their suggestions and comments during the initiation of this work.

J Public Health Management Practice, 1996, 2(3), 25–31

METHODS

Following the methods described by McGown et al., we searched the national compressed mortality files using CDC WONDER to obtain underlying cause mortality rates for nine chronic diseases by county in Maine from 1982 through 1991 (Table 1).[3,4] Previous investigators have estimated excess deaths by taking the lowest age-adjusted county rate as the minimum achievable rate and multiplying each county's excess rate percent by the number of deaths in that county.[3] However, since age-adjusted rates only estimate the mortality that would have occurred if that county had had the same age distribution as the standard used for age-adjustment, this does not provide a true estimate of the actual number of excess deaths in a county.

We attempted to estimate the actual number of excess deaths using age-specific rates for the nine diseases for each county to obtain a lowest theoretically achievable rate for each age group. For each age group we used the lowest county rate that did not include zero in the 95 percent confidence limits as the lowest theoretically achievable rate. While this does not eliminate unstable rates, it helps to avoid using a very low and unstable rate as the minimum achievable rate, and incorporates into the calculations the conservative assumption that some mortality will occur in every age group even with optimal public health prevention strategies. The excess mortality rates for each county in each age group were then calculated by subtracting this lowest rate from each county's rate. The excess rate percent for each county was obtained by dividing the excess rate by the county rate. The number of excess deaths for each county in each age group was then calculated by multiplying the excess rate percent by the actual number of deaths. Excess deaths

---

Table 1 Deaths from nine chronic diseases in Maine, 1982–1991

Disease	ICD-9 codes	Deaths
Ischemic heart disease	410–414, 429.2	32,890
Cerebrovascular disease	430–438	7,592
Lung cancer	162	7,213
Chronic obstructive pulmonary disease	491–496	4,869
Colorectal cancer	153–154	3,290
Diabetes	250	2,201
Breast cancer	174	2,115
Chronic liver disease, cirrhosis	571	1,331
Cervical cancer	180	260
Total		61,761

in each age group were summed across counties to get total excess deaths in the state for each age group.

We examined the contribution of actual causes to each disease category using estimates of population attributable risk (PAR). Estimates of preventable deaths were limited to those causes, or risk factors, which are both widely accepted as important from a public health standpoint and amenable to intervention. The following risk factors were considered: cigarette smoking, high blood pressure, physical inactivity, diet, alcohol abuse, residential radon, failure to screen, and high-risk sexual behavior. Using available local data, PAR for Maine was calculated using estimates of the prevalence (p) of the risk factor in Maine for the midpoint year 1987 and published estimates of relative risk (RR) as $PAR = p(RR-1)/[p(RR-1)+1]$. When local data were not available, PAR estimates were obtained from a nationally recognized review of chronic disease epidemiology.[5] If estimates were not available from this source, additional references were consulted.[1,6]

PAR represents the proportion of deaths in a population attributable to a particular risk factor, or the proportion of deaths that would not have occurred if the risk factor had not been present. When more than one risk factor for a disease is considered, any deaths that are associated with more than one risk factor are independently attributed to each of the risk factors, under the assumption that the death would not have occurred in the absence of any one of the risk factors. Thus, the sum of deaths attributed to each risk factor can easily add up to more than the total number of deaths. To conservatively estimate the total number of chronic disease deaths caused by preventable risk factors, we summed the greatest number of deaths for each disease that were attributed to any single risk factor. The less important risk factors for each disease may have contributed to some of the same deaths attributed to the single most important risk factor, but may also have independently caused deaths that will not be included in this sum.

RESULTS

Based on the underlying cause of death, the nine chronic diseases accounted for 61,761, or 55.5 percent of Maine deaths occurring from 1982 to 1991. Table 1 shows the number of deaths for each disease. Table 2 shows the total number of deaths and excess deaths for each county. If all counties in the state had achieved the lowest theoretically achievable county rate for each age group, the number of deaths credited to these nine chronic diseases over the 10-year period would have been reduced by more than 8,000 (Table 2).

The age distribution of deaths from the nine diseases over the 10-year period is shown in Figure 1. The greatest proportion of excess deaths occurred among adults in the age groups 25 to 34 and 45 to 54. However, the greatest number of

Table 2 Excess deaths from nine chronic diseases in Maine, by county, 1982–1991

County	Deaths	Excess deaths	Excess (%)
Franklin	1,288	75	6
Cumberland	11,316	862	8
Piscataquis	1,041	84	8
Lincoln	1,727	158	9
Knox	2,253	232	10
York	7,605	917	12
Washington	2,174	320	15
Hancock	2,802	430	15
Penobscot	6,602	1,083	16
Kennebec	6,075	996	16
Oxford	3,065	502	16
Androscoggin	5,629	949	17
Waldo	1,588	273	17
Somerset	2,603	456	18
Sagadahoc	1,516	288	19
Aroostook	4,477	847	19
Maine Total	61,761	8,472	14

excess deaths occurred in those 65 years and older, paralleling the age distribution of total deaths from the nine chronic diseases.

PREVENTABLE CAUSES AND DEATHS FOR THE NINE DISEASES

A summary of the number of deaths attributable to various causes is shown in Table 3. Since deaths associated with multiple risk factors are attributed independently to each of the risk factors, the sum of PARs across risk factors for a given disease may exceed 100 percent. Summing the deaths attributed to the one risk factor accounting for the greatest proportion of deaths for each disease results in a total of 25,388 deaths that can be attributed to preventable causes. This represents 41 percent of the 61,761 deaths from the nine diseases over the 10-year period. Since this assumes that none of the other risk factors for each disease caused deaths independently of the most important risk factor, it probably underestimates the proportion of preventable deaths.

Over the 10-year period, cigarette smoking contributed to 17,688 deaths, physical inactivity contributed to 13,479 deaths, high blood pressure contributed to 10,197 deaths, diet contributed to 9,830 deaths, alcohol abuse contributed to 865

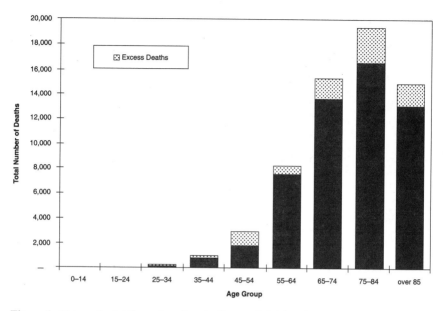

Figure 1. Excess deaths from nine chronic diseases in Maine, by age group (1982–1991).

deaths, failure to screen contributed to 592 deaths, residential radon contributed to 361 deaths, and high-risk sexual behavior contributed to 99 deaths.

DISCUSSION

Over the 10-year period from 1982 to 1991, more than 25,000 or 40 percent of the deaths from nine chronic diseases in Maine can be attributed to preventable causes. This is a conservative estimate based on the assumption that all deaths attributed to lesser risk factors are included in the sum of deaths attributed to the most important risk factor for each disease. Since it is likely that at least some of the lesser risk factors caused deaths independently of the major risk factors, the true number of deaths attributable to preventable causes is probably higher. A more precise estimate could only be obtained with information on the relative risk of death associated with combinations of risk factors, and the prevalence of various combinations of risk factors in the population.

The number of deaths that could actually have been prevented over the 10-year period is more difficult to estimate. In order to have prevented all of the 25,000 deaths attributed to preventable causes here, the most important risk factors for each disease would have had to have been completely absent, and the prevalence

Table 3 Proportion of deaths in Maine attributable to preventable causes, 1982–1991

Diagnostic category	Actual deaths total	Cigarette smoking	Physical inactivity	High blood pressure	Diet	Alcohol abuse	Failure to screen	Residential radon	High risk sex
Ischemic heart disease	32,890	(22%)* 7,236	(35%)* 11,512	(25%)[5] 8,223	(21.5%)[†] 7,071				
Stroke	7,592	(22%)* 1,670		(26%)[5] 1,974	(10%)[‡] 759				
Lung cancer	7,213	(72%[§]) 5,193						(5%)[||] 361	
COPD	4,869	(72%)* 3,506							
Colorectal cancer	3,290		(32%)[5] 1,053		(33%)[5,6] 1,086				
Diabetes	2,201		(30%)** 660		(30%)** 660				
Female breast cancer	2,115		(12%)[††] 254		(12%)[††] 254		(22%)[5] 465		
Chronic liver disease	1,331					(65%)[5] 865			
Cervical cancer	260	(32%)[5] 83					(49%)[5] 127		(38%)[5] 99
Total	61,761	17,688	13,479	10,197	9,830	865	592	361	99

Population attributable risks (PAR) appear in parentheses and represent the proportion of total deaths attributable to each risk factor. Numbers can be added for each risk factor across disease categories, but not across risk factors.

*Based on Maine prevalence data and conservative estimates of relative risk.[5,7]

[†]Conservatively assuming only half of the 43 percent of CHD deaths attributed to high blood cholesterol are due to modifiable dietary factors.[5]

[‡]Conservatively assuming only half of the up to 20 percent of stroke deaths attributed to high blood cholesterol are due to diet.[5]

[§]Based on a relative risk of 10 and Maine prevalence data.[6,7]

[||]Conservatively taking half of the estimate that up to 10 percent of lung cancer deaths are attributed to radon.[5]

**30 percent of diabetes deaths could be related to diet or physical inactivity.[1]

[††]For postmenopausal obesity.[5]

of other risk factors could not have increased. Nevertheless, the figure provides an indication of the size of the preventable disease target at which prevention programs could take aim.

Any estimation of the number of deaths that could actually be prevented by such programs would have to take into account the proportion of the population that could be reached by the programs, the efficacy of interventions in reducing the prevalence of risk factors, and the effect of residual risk from past exposure among individuals for whom the risk factor is eliminated. In the case of smoking and lung cancer, for example, it is unlikely that any intervention would reach all smokers and that all those who were reached would stop smoking. Even those who did quit would have some residual risk of lung cancer from their previous smoking. Nor is it likely that a campaign to prevent people from starting to smoke will be completely successful. Thus, it is unlikely that *all* of the deaths attributed to smoking could be prevented by public health campaigns directed against smoking. Nevertheless, programs that seek to prevent the acquisition of risk factors are likely to have a greater impact than those that seek to reduce the prevalence of risk factors that have already been acquired.

The calculation of excess deaths using county and age-specific rates for the nine chronic diseases is an alternative approach to estimating the target for prevention programs. It is based on the premise that if some county in the state were able to realize a low age-specific death rate for these diseases, all counties within the state should be able to achieve at least the same low rate. This reasoning has a certain practical appeal, since it does not require the hypothetical elimination of existing risk factors, but simply achieving a reduction of risk to levels that presumably already exist for a portion of the general population within the state. If uniformly low age-specific chronic disease rates had occurred, at least 8,000 Maine residents either would not have died or would have died from causes other than these chronic diseases over the 10-year period. On the one hand, this number may more closely approximate what could realistically be achieved by prevention programs for these chronic diseases. However, the difference between the estimates of 25,000 deaths attributed to preventable causes and 8,000 excess observed deaths suggests that even the lowest age-specific rates could be further decreased by reducing the prevalence of the risk factors considered in this chapter.

The calculation of excess deaths using age-specific rates provides an assessment of the potential impact of prevention programs on mortality at different ages. The age distribution of excess deaths suggests that by achieving the theoretically achievable lowest rates, the greatest proportional reduction in deaths could be achieved among those aged 25 to 34 and 45 to 54, but the greatest reduction in number of deaths would be among those aged 65 and older. These results support the importance of primary prevention to avoid acquiring risk factors at young ages. Programs aimed at reduction of risk factors among those over 34 years of age might prevent a large number of deaths, but most of these will be toward the end of the average life span. Such late interventions will miss the age groups with the greatest proportion of excess mortality. Further, early primary prevention programs would presumably have a greater impact on morbidity from chronic diseases.

Cigarette smoking was the single largest contributor to chronic disease mortality in Maine over the 10-year period. Physical inactivity, high blood pressure, and diet were also major contributors to mortality. The contributions of alcohol abuse, failure to screen, residential radon, and high-risk sexual behavior to these nine chronic diseases were in order of magnitude less than the four leading causes. These results suggest that Maine should place extra effort in the prevention programs that address the four leading causes of chronic disease mortality. However, the efficacy of prevention programs directed at different risk factors may vary greatly, and it is possible that a highly effective program directed at a lesser contributing cause of mortality may save more lives than an ineffective one directed at a leading cause. In addition, the results presented here do not address the impact that reduction of a given risk factor might have on acute or other chronic diseases that were not included in the analysis, nor do they address the impact on morbidity. Decisions about the relative emphasis placed on different prevention programs should be based on prevention effectiveness analyses that define the desired outcome (for example, whether the program is intended to reduce mortality or morbidity), and that consider the efficacy of the interventions and the proportion of the population that will be affected by the interventions.

The results presented here have several limitations. First, the analysis included only risk factors believed to be well-established and modifiable from a public health standpoint. Including more risk factors would increase the proportion of deaths that could be attributed to preventable causes. Second, we used estimates of PAR and RR from the cited references rather than conducting an extensive literature review. Third, these analyses were based on deaths where one of the nine chronic diseases was listed as the underlying cause of death. While errors or inconsistencies in assigning the underlying cause could change the numbers of deaths due to these diseases, we believe such errors would not occur frequently enough to substantially alter the conclusions of this chapter. Finally, when estimating excess deaths, we accounted for age differences but did not account for possible effects of gender or socioeconomic differences on the age-specific rates for each county.

The type of assessment can help identify the most important preventable risk factors within a state or local area, provide a measure of the size of the prevention target, and may help identify counties or other subdivisions with the most room for lowering disease rates. It represents a first step in assessing the potential impact of chronic disease prevention programs.

REFERENCES

1. McGinnis, J.M., and Foege, W.H. "Actual Causes of Death in the United States." *Journal of the American Medical Association* 270 (1993): 2207–2212.

2. Hahn, R.A., et al. "Excess Deaths from Nine Chronic Diseases in the United States, 1986." *Journal of the American Medical Association* 264 (1990): 2654–2659.

3. McGown, R., Remington, P.L., and Chudy, N. "Deaths from Nine Major Chronic Diseases, Wisconsin, 1979–1988." *Wisconsin Medical Journal* 92 (1993): 524–530.

4. U.S. Dept. of Health and Human Services, Public Health Service. CDC Wide-ranging ONLine Data for Epidemiologic Research (WONDER). Centers for Disease Control and Prevention, June 1992.

5. Brownson, R.C., Remington, P.L., and Davis, J.R., eds. *Chronic Disease Epidemiology and Control.* Washington, D.C.: American Public Health Association, 1993.

6. Tomatis, L., ed. *Cancer: Causes, Occurrence and Control.* Lyon, France: International Agency for Research on Cancer, 1990.

7. Division of Health Promotion and Education. *Behavioral Risk Factor Surveillance System.* Augusta, Me.: Maine Department of Human Services, 1990.

5

Emergency Department E-Code Data Reporting: A New Level of Data Resource for Injury Prevention and Control

Robert L. Muelleman, William A. Watson, Garland H. Land,
James D. Davis, and Barbara S. Hoskins

With the growing awareness of injury as a major public health problem, there is a need for surveillance of the various causes of fatal and nonfatal injuries.[1] Descriptions of the prevalence of injury types, causes, and patient outcomes are necessary to develop the most appropriate injury control programs and evaluate their efficacy.[2] Comprehensive information regarding the causes of injury that result in emergency department (ED) evaluation and treatment of the patient has not been available. Current estimates of nonhospitalized injuries, including ED visits, are based on self-reported patient data reported by the National Health Interview Survey.[3]

To improve our understanding of the causes of nonfatal injury that do not require hospitalization, standardized coding of the external cause of injury (E-code) should be applied to the health care records of injured patients who receive ED care.[4,5] The International Classification of Diseases, 9th Revision, Clinical Modification (ICD-9-CM) has been supported as the universal method of defining and classifying this information, and endorsed by the National Committee on Vital and Health Statistics, American Health Information Management Association, and the American Public Health Association.[6,7]

Comprehensive E-code reporting from the health care records of hospitalized patients is currently required by 15 states. Two states, Nebraska and Missouri, have legislated E-code assignment to the medical records of patients evaluated, treated, and discharged from EDs. This information provides an accurate description of the different injury causes; quantifies the nonfatal, nonhospitalized level of the injury pyramid; and allows measurement of the impact of various injury causes on public health and health care resources.

J Public Health Management Practice, 1997, 3(6), 8–16

The Missouri Department of Health had been collecting information on deaths due to injury since 1977, but information on nonfatal injuries was submitted on a voluntary basis and for inpatient records only. In 1989, the department received a capacity building grant for injury control from the Centers for Disease Control and Prevention. During the early planning for grant activity, staff members from the Division of Health Resources recognized the importance of collecting information from all hospitals and from EDs as well as inpatient records. At the same time, the Missouri legislature was considering legislation that would mandate reporting of certain information from all ED and inpatient records from all hospitals in a patient abstract system. Because of the work with the capacity building grant for injury control, the staff of the Division of Health Resources recognized this opportunity to require E-codes on all patient records with an injury diagnosis. The legislation passed in 1992 and was enacted in 1993.

The purpose of this study was to describe the results of the first year of statewide reporting of injury type and external cause of injury for the state of Missouri and to demonstrate the ability of utilizing the statewide database to determine local injury information in a selected metropolitan statistical area. The results demonstrate the feasibility of requiring injury cause reporting at a statewide level using ICD-9-CM criteria.

METHODS

The 1993 injury data were reported to the Missouri Center for Health Statistics, Missouri Department of Health, by EDs in the state. The requirement for data reporting was the result of HB1574, SB721, and SB796, which were passed by the Missouri legislature during the 1992 session. The bills established data reporting requirements for hospitals and ambulatory surgical centers. Sections 192.665 and 192.667 RS MO (Cum. Supp. 1992) require hospitals to provide to the Department of Health inpatient and ED data beginning with the calendar year 1993. The reporting requirements apply to all inpatient admissions and outpatient visits to all Missouri EDs. Effective January 1, 1994, ambulatory and surgical departments were also required to report.

The requirements for reporting included at least the following data for each patient visit: date of birth, sex, race, Zip code, county of residence, admission date, procedures, total billed charges, and expected source of payment. The principal and other diagnoses and external cause of injury were required to be coded using ICD-9-CM definitions.

Fatality data were obtained from death certificates maintained by the Missouri Center for Health Statistics. Data from these records include cause of death and E-codes.

For this study, all health care encounters that involved an injury were defined as medical records that included an ICD-9-CM diagnosis from 800 to 995.9. This was not required to be the principal diagnosis. The frequency of E-codes was determined for all records of injured patients that resulted in death, hospitalization, or ED encounter.

The frequency of injury with an associated external cause of injury for falls (E880–E888), motor vehicle crashes (E800–E848), poisonings (E850–E869), burns and scalds (E890–E899, E924–E924.9), drowning (E910–E910.9), and firearms (E922.0–922.9, E955.0–955.4, E965.0–965.4, E970, E985.0–985.4) was determined separately from other external causes of injury. Cause of injury rates per 100,000 population per year were determined for hospitalized patients and outpatient visits. These results were determined for the state (1993 population 5,234,000) and for the Springfield, Missouri, metropolitan statistical area (MSA) (1993 population 282,300). The Springfield MSA data consisted of reports from the hospitals in Green, Webster, and Christian counties in the southwestern portion of the state.

RESULTS

In 1993, injury was the fourth most common cause of hospitalization and the leading cause of ED encounters in Missouri. There were 3,415 deaths, 67,552 hospitalizations, and 592,902 ED visits for injuries reported for 1993 to the Missouri Department of Health. These results indicate that for every injury death there were 19.7 reported hospitalizations and 173.6 reported ED visits in Missouri (Figure 1). The annual crude rates were 65/100,000 injury deaths, 1,291/100,000 injuries resulting in patient hospitalization, and 11,328/100,000 injuries resulting in ED health care. E-coding was reported on 84 percent of hospitalized and outpatient patient visits statewide and 95 percent of reported data from the Springfield MSA.

The ratio of overall injury-associated deaths, hospitalizations, and ED visits were compared for six different causes of injury (Figure 1). Falls were the most commonly reported cause of injury; however, falls infrequently resulted in death. In contrast, firearms and drowning were less common causes of injury, but relatively more frequently fatal events.

The contribution of the six different causes of injury for injury-associated deaths, hospitalizations, and ED visits were different (Table 1). Firearms and motor vehicle crashes were the leading causes of injury death. In contrast, falls and motor vehicle crashes were the leading causes of injury hospitalizations and ED visits.

Comparison of statewide data to the Springfield MSA was undertaken using raw data, and corrected for the relative difference in E-code reporting rates (84% statewide and 95% Springfield MSA). This correction of multiplying statewide rates by 1.19 and Springfield MSA rates by 1.05 assumes that the injury records

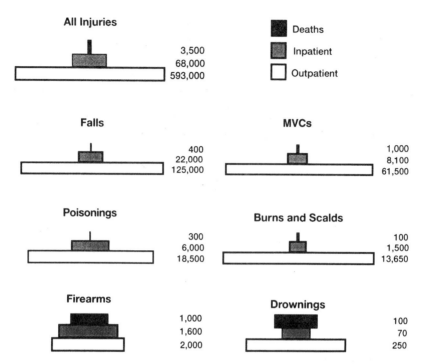

Figure 1. Relative relationship of deaths, inpatient, and outpatient dispositions for all injuries and six causes of injury (numbers rounded).

without an E-code had the same injury types, causes, and frequency as the reported data. Comparisons of the annual injury rate for Missouri and the Springfield MSA used combined hospitalization and ED visit data (Figures 2–7). The relative shapes of the curves for Missouri and the Springfield MSA are similar for falls, motor vehicle crashes, poisonings, burns, and drownings. The Springfield MSA rates are higher for these injury causes. The firearms rates have different shapes, indicating that firearm injuries are more frequent in older populations and less frequent in younger populations in the Springfield MSA when compared to the overall statewide data.

Comparison of total and per capita direct medical charges associated with injuries in the state and the Springfield MSA demonstrates that hospital charges for injuries were more than $1 billion in Missouri in 1993. Although there were nine times more ED visits than hospitalizations, the charges for inpatient visits were nearly three times higher than ED visits. The per capita hospital charges for injury visits were more than $200. The Springfield MSA per capita charges were higher, and may reflect the higher injury rates (Table 2). Statewide, approximately 18

Table 1 Injury causes of outpatient visits, hospitalizations, and deaths

	Outpatient (n = 592,902) (%)	Hospitalizations (n = 67,552) (%)	Deaths (n = 3,415) (%)
Falls	21.1	33.3	11.7
MVCs*	10.4	12.0	29.3
Poisonings	3.1	8.7	8.8
Burns	2.3	2.2	2.9
Firearms	0.3	2.4	29.3
Drownings	0.04	0.1	2.9
Other	47.1	25.4	18.0
Unknown	15.8	15.9	0.0

*MVCs, motor vehicle crashes.

percent of hospitalized and ED visits for injuries were uninsured, accounting for $100 million. An additional 15 percent of the charges were for Medicaid recipients and accounted for $130 million.

DISCUSSION

The implementation of statewide requirements for reporting injury data from ED records provides the first comprehensive description of the external causes of injury associated with patient presentation to the ED. The relative frequency of injury related deaths, hospitalizations, and ED care also provides an understanding of the outcome of injuries associated with certain causes in Missouri as well as for specific areas of the state. This information eliminates the requirements for assumptions and potential biases associated with different sampling strategies.

Table 2 Hospital charges

	State ($)		Springfield MSA ($)	
Total hospitalized	791,850,432	(73%)	64,020,066	(81%)
Total outpatient	296,672,564	(27%)	14,555,484	(19%)
TOTAL	1,088,522,996		78,575,550	
Per capita hospitalized	151		227	
Per capita outpatient	57		52	
TOTAL per capita	208		278	

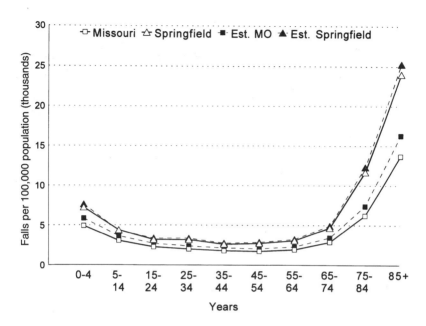

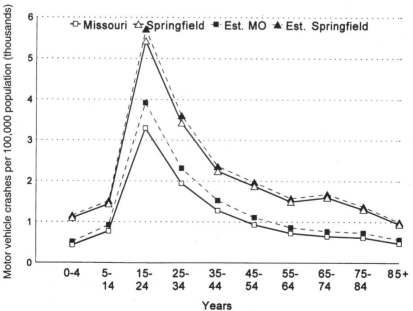

Figures 2–7. Comparison of age-specific injury rates in Missouri and the Springfield MSA for six causes of injury.

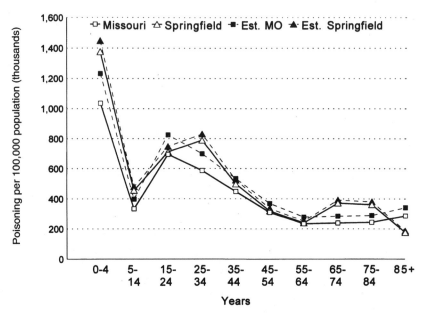

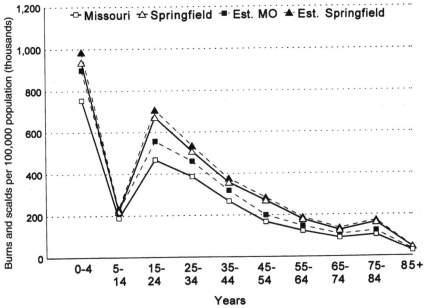

Figures 2–7. Continued

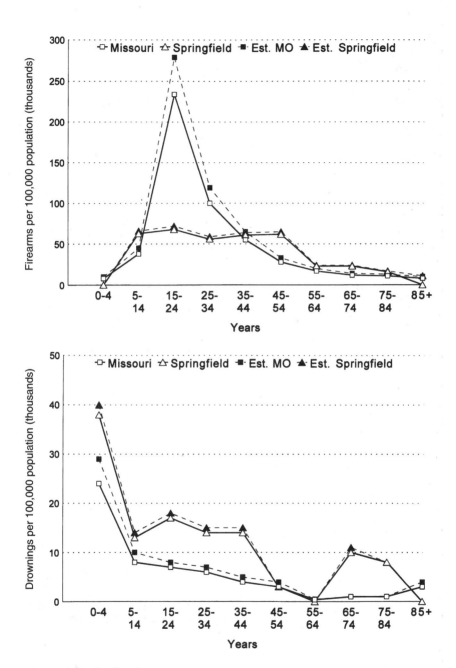

Figures 2–7. Continued

The collection of these data became possible secondary to legislation requiring E-code reporting for hospitalized patients, and those treated by EDs. Missouri is the first state that mandated reporting of these data. In 1993, 84 percent of hospital and ED records with the required data were provided to the Missouri Center for Health Statistics. The reporting rate increased to 94 percent for hospitalized and 91 percent for ED patients in 1994.

The impact of injury on public health and health care resources is generally estimated using the ratio of hospitalizations and nonhospitalized injuries to injury-associated deaths. National estimates are 16 hospitalizations and 377 nonhospitalized injuries (including those that did not require medical attention) for every injury death.[8] The Missouri data are 20 injury hospitalizations and 173 injury-related ED visits for each death.

The estimates of national injury hospitalizations estimates were developed from the National Hospital Discharge Survey (NHDS), with a probability sample of approximately 200,000 patients discharged annually from approximately 600 hospitals in the United States. The Missouri ratio is only slightly higher, and may be due to differences in the definition of an injury-associated hospitalization. The NHDS estimates exclude traumatic complications, late effects of injury, adverse effects, and complications of surgical and medical care from the possible injury diagnostic codes, whereas these were included in Missouri data. The NHDS estimates were also adjusted downward by approximately 12 percent, based on work of others, to account for rehospitalization for follow-up of an injury that previously resulted in a hospitalization.[8] The Missouri data did not exclude rehospitalizations for follow-up care.

The most common causes of injury were similar when Missouri data and national estimates were compared for hospitalized patients. In Missouri, falls (33.3%) were most common, followed by motor vehicle crashes (12.0%), poisonings (8.7%), firearms (2.4%), burns (2.2%), and drownings (0.1%). Other causes were documented in 35.4 percent of injuries and 15.8 percent had unknown causes.

Comparison of the Missouri ED injury visits to the National Health Interview Survey is difficult. The NHIS includes injuries not resulting in hospitalization that occurred within two weeks of the interview and injuries that required medical attention, or at least one full day of restricted activity. It would be expected that the ratio of nonhospitalized injuries to deaths would be much higher because the NHIS information includes injured patients who may not have gone to the ED for treatment. Despite the different methodology, the distribution of injury causes for nonhospitalized events was generally similar between Missouri data and national estimates. In Missouri, the leading injury causes for ED visits were falls (21.1%), motor vehicle crashes (10.4%), poisonings (3.1%), burns (2.3%), firearms (0.3%), and drownings (0.4%). Other causes were documented in 47.1 percent of injuries, and 15.9 percent had unknown causes. In Missouri, these data suggest that falls, poisonings, and firearms make up a relatively smaller component of the cause of nonhospitalized injuries compared to those who were hospitalized. These differences point out the importance of comprehensive data describing ED injuries and their causes in developing the most appropriate injury control strategies.

The statewide data can also provide useful information regarding differences in injury causes for individual areas of the state. The Springfield MSA had higher rates for five of the six specific categories of injury cause than statewide data, even after adjustment for the differences in E-code reporting rates. The increased rate of firearm-caused injury in older patients and decreased rate of firearm-caused injury in younger patients described in the Springfield MSA data suggest that different injury control strategies should be used to decrease firearm-caused injuries in the Springfield area. The ability of the data to allow local customization of injury control programs further strengthens the value of the Missouri injury data. The importance of local action on future progress in injury control has recently been stressed.[9] Focusing cause of injury data to individual hospitals would also be useful in focusing institutional resources and educational programs.[10]

While evaluation of the 1993 injury data reported to the Missouri Center for Health Statistics demonstrates the feasibility and potential value of this information, there are a number of additional issues that should be addressed in the interpretation of these data. As presented in this evaluation, the frequency of injuries, outcomes, and injury causes is based on the frequency of reports in medical records and death reports. The number of actual injury events and the number of different individuals involved in the injuries were not evaluated. Since one person may be injured multiple times and a single event may injure more than one person, hospital and ED records may not correctly reflect the impact of injury on all aspects of public health. The quantity of information obtained and documented necessary to assign E-codes and the accuracy of E-code assignment have recently been discussed, and methods to improve documentation and accuracy suggested.[11,12]

Linking the death, hospital, and ED injury data to law enforcement and emergency medical services records would enhance understanding of the causes of injury and their impact on public health. The availability of E-coded records in Missouri has facilitated the development of a firearms surveillance system. This information will also be used to improve the linkage with police report data in the Missouri Crash Outcome Data Evaluation System.

• • •

The Missouri experience with required reporting of hospitalized and ED records demonstrates that a comprehensive, centralized system to capture information regarding injuries is feasible. The reported data provide, for the first time, a quantified determination of the extent and cost of nonfatal injuries in Missouri. The database also allows individual communities in the state to assess the problem of injury specific to their region so that customized injury control programs can be established and unique injury cause problems can be identified.

REFERENCES

1. Committee on Trauma Research. *Injury in America*. Washington, D.C.: National Academy Press, 1988.
2. Committee To Review the Status and Progress of the Injury Control Program at the CDC. *Injury Control: A Review of the Status and Progress of the Injury Control Program at the CDC*. Washington, D.C.: National Academy Press, 1988.
3. U.S. National Center for Health Statistics. *Persons Injured and Disability Days by Detailed Type and Class of Accident, United States—1971–72*. Vital and Health Statistics, Series 10, No. 105. DHEW Pub. No. (HRA) 76-1532. Washington, D.C.: U.S. Department of Health, Education and Welfare, 1976.
4. R.L. Muelleman et al. "Decoding the E-Code," *Nebraska Medical Journal* 78 (1993): 184–185.
5. U.S. Department of Health and Human Services. *Healthy People 2000: National Health Promotion and Disease Prevention Objectives*. DHHS Pub. No. (PHS) 91-50212. Washington, D.C.: Government Printing Office, 1990.
6. U.S. Department of Health and Human Services. *International Classification of Diseases*, Ninth Revision. DHHS Pub. No. (PHS) 91-1260. Washington, D.C.: Government Printing Office, 1989.
7. U.S. Department of Health and Human Services. *Report on the Need To Collect External Cause of Injury Codes in Hospital Discharge Data*. NCHS Working Paper, Series No. 38. Hyattsville, Md.: Government Printing Office, 1991.
8. D.P. Rice and E.J. Mackenzie and Associates. *Cost of Injury in the United States: A Report to Congress*. San Francisco, Calif.: Institute for Health and Aging, University of California and Injury Prevention Center, The Johns Hopkins University, 1989.
9. *Injury Control in the 1990s. A National Plan for Action*. A Report to the Second World Conference on Injury Control. Atlanta, Ga.: Centers for Disease Control and Prevention, 1993.
10. W.A. Watson et al. "E-Codes from Emergency Department Records," *Academic Emergency Medicine* 2 (1995): 569–570.
11. R.J. Schwartz et al. "The Quantity of Cause of Injury Information Documented on the Medical Record: An Appeal for Injury Prevention," *Academic Emergency Medicine* 2 (1995): 98–103.
12. R.J. Schwartz et al. "Accuracy of E-Codes Assigned to Emergency Department Records," *Academic Emergency Medicine* 2 (1995): 615–620.

6

Cardiovascular Disease Control Efforts among Local Health Departments

Nilsa E. Mack, Ross C. Brownson, Michael Pratt,
Carol A. Brownson, Cynthia Dean, and Sue Dabney

Cardiovascular diseases (CVDs) are the leading cause of illness, disability, death, and escalating medical costs in the United States.[1] Systematic prevention and control of modifiable CVD risk factors (e.g., smoking, high blood pressure, high blood cholesterol, physical inactivity, and obesity) are important public health priorities, as reflected in Healthy People 2000 objectives and model standards for state and local action.[2,3] Attainment of these objectives will depend substantially on community-based programs to promote health and prevent disease.[4]

Among community-based programs designed to decrease CVD risk factors, favorable results have been reported for health knowledge, smoking, blood pressure, and physical activity.[5-9] However, recently in the Minnesota Heart Health Program, significant progress was not observed for most risk factors against the background of strong favorable secular trends.[9]

State and local health departments are vital resources that can enable communities to achieve the Healthy People 2000 objectives for prevention and control of CVD and associated risk factors; however, coordinated leadership, support, and resources for these efforts are lacking.[10] For example, a 1989 nationwide survey disclosed that almost a third of the local health departments did not undertake any chronic disease control measures and that activity at the local level was often limited to only a few interventions, such as hypertension screening.[11] A more recent national survey of local health department services conducted during 1992–1993

This project was funded in part by Centers for Disease Control and Prevention cooperative agreement U58/CCU700950, awarded to the Missouri Department of Health. The authors are grateful for the technical assistance of Theophili Murayi and Eduardo Simoes, Division of Chronic Disease Prevention and Health Promotion, Missouri Department of Health, and Russell Roegner, Division of Chronic Disease Control and Community Intervention, Centers for Disease Control and Prevention.

J Public Health Management Practice, 1997, 3(2), 71–77

by the National Association of County and City Health Officials and the Centers for Disease Control and Prevention (CDC) supports the finding that hypertension screening (85%) is the most frequently performed chronic disease control activity at the local level, followed by diabetes (60%) and cancer screenings (54%).[12] Further, preliminary data from a 1993 nationwide survey of local health department activities and expenditures in chronic disease control revealed that only 5.9 percent of financial resources and 13.5 percent of staff time were dedicated to chronic disease activities.[13]

Despite recent national surveys, few state-based surveys of local health department risk-reduction activities have been conducted or published. In 1989, the Missouri Department of Health, in a cooperative agreement with CDC, began a community-based CVD risk-reduction project (The Bootheel Heart Health Project) in a six-county rural area of the state known as the Bootheel. Project objectives focused on reducing the major modifiable CVD risk factors through community-based interventions. A key component in achieving these objectives was the involvement of local health departments in local coalition building, program planning, program implementation, and evaluation of CVD prevention and control interventions.[14]

To evaluate risk reduction activities at the local level, and to better understand how local health departments might participate more effectively in the development of CVD control coalitions, the Missouri Department of Health conducted baseline and follow-up surveys in 1990 and 1994. In this report, we compare changes in knowledge, attitudes, and activities related to CVD prevention and control among local health departments.

METHODS

Background

The Bootheel is located in the southeastern corner of the state and includes the counties of Dunklin, Mississippi, New Madrid, Pemiscot, Scott, and Stoddard. These counties were chosen for intervention because of their high coronary heart disease mortality and an absence of CVD risk-reduction programs in the area.[4,14] Also, this region of the state has relatively large economically disadvantaged and minority populations.[4,14]

Project activities at the state and local level, including the process of coalition development, have been described previously and are discussed only briefly here.[15] Among activities at the state level were the establishment of a Cardiovascular Health Task Force and the development of the Missouri Cardiovascular Health Plan and the CVD Control Resource Directory, both of which were widely disseminated to health organizations across the state, including all local health departments.[14]

At the local level, coalitions coordinated by the local health departments were developed in each of the six Bootheel counties. The development of these coalitions was guided by the principles of the Planned Approach to Community Health (PATCH).[16] By the end of the study period, community members in the area had organized 17 sub-coalitions within the six-county region. These local coalitions allowed for tailored interventions and helped minimize members' travel. From 1991 to 1994, each of the six-county coalitions received about $5,000 per year to implement community-based interventions. Examples of coalitions' activities included: walking clubs, aerobic classes, heart healthy cooking demonstrations, community blood pressure and cholesterol screenings, and CVD education programs.[17] Local health agencies were a key component in the coalition development process as they provided assistance in many areas including blood pressure and cholesterol screenings, training, and distribution of local funds for coalition activities. These coalitions are being run by local citizens and volunteers and are addressing the major modifiable CVD risk factors.

Local health department surveys

Baseline and follow-up surveys were mailed to all health departments in Missouri (city, county, and district). The baseline survey was conducted from June through August 1990 (n = 119) and the follow-up survey from July through August 1994 (n = 120). Response rates were similar for the baseline and the follow-up surveys (95 percent vs. 92 percent). Major areas covered on both surveys were the relative importance of various diseases in terms of morbidity and mortality, knowledge of CVD risk factors, and health department activity levels in various health care services.[4] Most of the questions were closed-ended and standardized from other surveys.[18,19] The majority of the questions on both surveys were identical, with the exception of statements about attitudes toward CVD control. At baseline, respondents were asked about possible barriers to CVD control, whereas at follow-up, those questions were eliminated and respondents were asked if there had been increased CVD risk-reduction counseling, visits, and awareness of services among minority groups during the project period. In addition, at follow-up, local health departments in the Bootheel area were asked if they were more active in CVD prevention and control as a result of the county heart health coalition and if the county heart health coalition had a beneficial effect.

Answers to questions pertaining to CVD risk factor knowledge and activity levels in various health care services were ranked on three- and five-point scales, respectively. Numerical values of 0, 1, 2, 3, and 4 were assigned to the different response options (Tables 1 and 2). Mean scores were then calculated by summing the values and dividing by the total number of respondents for each item. For statewide local health departments, differences in mean scores were obtained by

Table 1 Comparison of local health departments' activity scores of health care services

Health care services	Statewide (n = 103)			Bootheel (n = 7)		
	1990 Activity score*	1994 Activity score*	p-value	1990 Activity score*	1994 Activity score*	p-value
Immunizations	3.7	3.6	0.03	3.5	3.6	> 0.10
Child health care	3.3	3.0	< 0.001	3.7	3.2	0.06
Blood pressure screening	3.1	3.0	0.08	2.8	3.4	0.06
Nutrition education & counseling	2.7	2.7	> 0.10	3.2	3.2	> 0.10
Maternal health care	2.6	2.5	> 0.10	2.0	2.8	> 0.10
Home health visits	2.5	2.2	0.03	1.3	0.4	0.06
General health education	2.4	2.6	> 0.10	2.0	2.8	> 0.10
Diabetes screening	2.2	2.3	> 0.10	1.7	2.4	> 0.10
Family planning	2.0	2.3	0.07	2.7	3.6	> 0.10
Cholesterol screening	1.6	1.1	< 0.001	1.0	0.4	> 0.10
AIDS education & counseling	1.5	1.9	0.02	1.0	2.6	> 0.10
Smoking cessation education & counseling	1.4	1.4	> 0.10	0.5	1.8	> 0.10
Physical exams	1.4	1.3	> 0.10	2.5	1.6	> 0.10
Cancer screening	1.2	1.5	0.04	0.7	2.0	> 0.10

*The activity score is a mean value based on the following levels of assessment of health care services: no activity = 0; low activity = 1; medium activity = 2; high activity = 3; very high activity = 4.

comparing mean activity scores at baseline for each local health department with mean activity scores for that local health department at follow-up. The difference between the two sets of scores was analyzed by paired-comparison t test.[20] For Bootheel local health departments, the difference between baseline and follow-up scores was analyzed using the Wilcoxon matched-pairs signed-rank test.[21]

RESULTS

More than 50 percent of the surveys were completed by a health department administrator/non-nurse (Table 3). From a list of 10 health issues, CVD was identified as the most important in terms of morbidity and mortality at both baseline (98 percent) and follow-up (96 percent). Other chronic diseases, such as cancer, diabetes, and chronic lung disease, also were viewed as having major health impacts in the population. Table 1 shows state and Bootheel local health departments' assessment of health care services that their units provided at baseline and follow-up. Among non-CVD–related activities, immunization and child health care received a high activity score. Nutrition education and counseling was also ranked relatively high. For activities related to CVD control, only hypertension screening was rated high at both baseline and follow-up for the state and the Bootheel area.

Among non-CVD–related activities statewide, significantly lower activity scores were found at follow-up for immunization ($p = 0.03$), child health care ($p = <0.001$), and home health visits ($p = 0.03$); whereas significantly higher activity scores were found for acquired immune deficiency syndrome education ($p = 0.02$) and cancer early detection screening ($p = 0.04$) (Table 1). For activities related to CVD prevention and control (e.g., blood pressure screening, diabetes screening, cholesterol screening, and smoking cessation education and counseling), no significant differences were found at follow-up except for cholesterol screening, which showed a lower activity score ($p = <0.001$) (Table 1). Among Bootheel local health departments, no significant difference was found between baseline and follow-up surveys for CVD- and non-CVD–related activities.

Table 2 presents local health departments' assessment of the importance of major CVD risk factors at baseline and at follow-up. Mean scores on CVD risk factors were similar for both surveys. Hypertension, cigarette smoking, obesity, and a high-fat diet were rated as the most important risk factors for CVD.

At baseline, 95 percent of local health departments acknowledged the need for increased CVD prevention and screening efforts in their areas, and 60 percent selected patient education as the most effective method for increasing CVD control efforts. Results were similar at follow-up. Several important barriers to CVD risk-reduction activities in the local health department setting were identified at baseline. These were lack of time for counseling, deficiencies in reimbursement,

Table 2 Local health departments' assessment of the effects of CVD risk factors in reducing the risk of a person developing CVD

Risk factor	1990		1994	
	Number	Knowledge score*	Number	Knowledge score*
Hypertension	113	1.9	109	1.8
Cigarette smoking	113	1.8	109	1.8
Overweight	113	1.8	109	1.7
High-fat diet	113	1.8	109	1.8
Elevated blood cholesterol	111	1.6	109	1.6
Diabetes	113	1.5	108	1.5
Sedentary lifestyle	113	1.5	109	1.6
Type A behavior/stress	113	1.4	108	1.4

*The knowledge score is a mean value based on the following levels of assessment of the effects of various risk factors: little or no effect = 0; moderate effect = 1; large effect = 2.

and lack of technical training. At follow-up, attitudes on the Bootheel Heart Health coalitions were measured by means of a series of statements about the impact and perceived benefit of the Bootheel Heart Health coalitions on the county health departments. Six out of seven (86%) of the Bootheel local health departments agreed with the statement that their participation in CVD control activities and awareness of services among minority groups had increased during the project period. Four out of seven (57%) of the Bootheel local health departments agreed with the statement that visits of minority groups had increased. However, there was considerable variation in the way the health departments responded to statements regarding Bootheel Heart Health coalition benefit and impact. Three out of seven (43%) agreed with the statement that their local health department was more active in CVD prevention and control as a result of the county coalition, whereas the same number of respondents (three of seven) disagreed with this statement. Also, three (43%) of the Bootheel local health departments neither agreed nor disagreed with the statement regarding the beneficial effect of coalitions. Among the other four respondents, two (29%) agreed and two (29%) disagreed strongly with this statement.

DISCUSSION

The present study is the first one to assess changes in local health departments' CVD prevention and control activities throughout a longitudinal period. Our sur-

Table 3 Summary characteristics of local health departments

	1990		*1994*	
Characteristics	*No.*	*(%)*	*No.*	*(%)*
Type of health unit				
District	7	(6.2)	7	(6.4)
County	101	(89.4)	100	(90.9)
City	5	(4.4)	3	(2.7)
Position classification of respondents				
Administrator/non-nurse	63	(55.8)	55	(50.0)
Administrator/community health nurse	21	(18.6)	16	(14.5)
Community health nurse	22	(19.5)	30	(27.3)
Other	7	(6.3)	9	(8.1)
Range and median of full-time equivalents				
District	7	(11.0–48.0) median = 23.0	7	(6.0–62.0) median = 54.0
County	101	(2.6–522.0) median = 7.0	97	(2.0–500.0) median = 10.0
City	5	(13.0–300.0) median = 42.0	3	(27.0–120.0) median = 29.0

vey findings are similar to recent national survey results in that they demonstrated the following: (a) local health department activity in CVD health-related services is relatively low and what services do exist are usually limited to hypertension screening; (b) the most common non-CVD–related prevention services identified were immunization, and maternal and infant health; and (c) major barriers reported were inadequate funding, staff, and training.[11-13]

On the basis of comparisons of survey responses from 1990 and 1994, local health departments in Missouri (statewide and Bootheel) revealed no significant changes in CVD knowledge, attitudes, and activities, except for cholesterol screening. Cholesterol screening declined at follow-up among Missouri's local health departments ($p = <0.001$). This decline could be attributed to the lack of financial resources and difficulties in obtaining qualified personnel, which may have prevented some of the local health departments from meeting cholesterol testing requirements (operational and quality control) established under the Clinical Laboratory Improvement Amendment (CLIA '88).[22] Among non-CVD activities, the increase in cancer screening at the local health departments could be due to the implementation in 1992 of the Missouri Breast and Cervical Cancer Control Project, which provides free breast and cervical cancer screening to economically disadvantaged women. Currently, more than one-third of local health departments throughout the state participate in the project. Nutrition education was ranked relatively high, although much of this activity is probably focused on maternal/ child health issues and is not targeted directly toward CVD control.

Among Bootheel local health departments, there was considerable variation in most of the mean score ratings between baseline and follow-up surveys for CVD- and non-CVD–related activities; however, no significant differences were found. The small sample size along with a highly variable distribution of responses from Bootheel surveys may partially explain the nonsignificant differences. Bootheel local health department differences in responses to attitude questions regarding county coalitions' beneficial effect were marked. Precise reasons for the differences in experience among Bootheel local health departments cannot be ascertained from these data. Despite uncertainty in the Bootheel local health departments' perceived success of the Bootheel Heart Health Project, empirical data showed a decrease in the prevalence of physical inactivity and an increase in having had cholesterol screening within the past two years in communities where coalitions were developed.[23]

The survey results also suggested that respondents typically preferred more traditional one-to-one CVD education methods and considered other proven strategies (e.g., communitywide efforts) to be less effective.[5–8] This finding emphasizes that local health departments need further information and training about the benefits of coalition building and community-based programs for preventing and controlling CVD.

Our study is limited by the self-reported nature of the data and by the fact that the selection of the local health departments was nonrandom. Another limitation is that the validity and reliability of the survey were not fully evaluated.

Prevention and control of CVD is a key objective at national, state, and local levels. This is an opportune time for evaluating the role of public health in CVD control. There is a move away from patient care/clinical services to assessment, policy development, and assurance. Efforts to improve cardiovascular health and achieve the Healthy People 2000 objectives must rely on a combination of national, state, and local programs.[10] To accomplish this goal, local health departments should expand their priorities to assure positive outcomes in CVD control activities, obtain additional resources, provide personnel adequately trained in risk-reduction methodologies, and move from clinical-based programs to participation and leadership in community-based initiatives.

•   •   •

The Missouri experience demonstrates that CVD prevention and control activities at the local level are lower than other health-related services. Surveys such as ours are inexpensive and can become a routine surveillance mechanism and be used for planning, implementing, and evaluating public health programs. Such surveillance systems are currently lacking for many areas of chronic disease prevention.[24]

REFERENCES

1. American Heart Association. *American Heart Association: 1991 Heart Facts*. Dallas, Tex: AHA, 1991.

2. U.S. Department of Health and Human Services. *Healthy People 2000: National Health Promotion and Disease Prevention Objectives*. DHHS, Pub. No. (PHS) 91-50212. Washington, D.C.: Government Printing Press, 1990.

3. American Public Health Association. *Healthy Communities 2000: Model Standards*. Guidelines for Community Attainment of the Year 2000 National Health Objectives. Washington, D.C.: APHA, 1991.

4. Brownson, R., et al. "Controlling Cardiovascular Disease: The Role of the Local Health Department." *American Journal of Public Health* 82 (1992): 1414–1416.

5. Farquhar, J.W., et al. "Effects of Communitywide Education on Cardiovascular Disease Risk Factors: The Stanford Five-City Project." *Journal of the American Medical Association* 264 (1990): 359–365.

6. Fortmann, S.P., et al. "Changes in Adult Cigarette Smoking Prevalence after 5 Years of Community Health Education: The Stanford Five-City Project." *American Journal of Epidemiology* 137 (1993): 82–96.

7. Lando, H.A., et al. "Changes in Adult Cigarette Smoking in the Minnesota Heart Health Program." *American Journal of Public Health* 85 (1995): 201–208.

8. Fortmann, S.P., et al. "Effect of Long-Term Community Health Education on Blood Pressure and Hypertension Control: The Stanford Five-City Project." *American Journal of Epidemiology* 132 (1990): 629–646.

9. Luepker, R.V., et al. "Community Education for Cardiovascular Disease Prevention: Risk Factors Changes in the Minnesota Heart Health Program." *American Journal of Public Health* 84 (1994): 1383–1393.

10. Association of State and Territorial Chronic Disease Program Directors. *Preventing Death and Disability from Cardiovascular Diseases: A State-Based Plan for Action*. Washington, D.C.: 1994.

11. National Association of County Health Officials. *National Profile of Local Health Departments*. Washington, D.C.: NACHO, 1990.

12. Centers for Disease Control and Prevention. "Selected Characteristics of Local Health Departments—United States, 1992–1993," *Morbidity and Mortality Weekly Report* 43: 839–843.

13. Madden, S., et al. *Chronic Disease Prevention and Control: The Extent of Local Health Department Activity*. (Preliminary Results). Presentation made at the Ninth National Conference on Chronic Disease Control, Washington, D.C., 1994.

14. Missouri Department of Health. *Missouri Chronic Disease Risk Reduction Project* [grant application submitted to CDC]. Columbia, Mo.: Division of Chronic Disease Prevention and Health Promotion, 1989.

15. Brownson, C.A., et al. "Cardiovascular Risk Reduction in Rural Minority Communities: The Bootheel Heart Health Project." *Health Education.* In press.

16. *Journal of Health Education* 23:3 (1992). Entire issue was dedicated to descriptions and accounts of PATCH Program.

17. Dabney, S., et al. "Missouri Builds Heart Health Coalitions in the Bootheel." *Chronic Disease Notes Report* 6 (1993): 11–13.

18. Schucker, B., et al. "Change in Physician Perspective on Cholesterol and Heart Disease." *Journal of the American Medical Association* 258 (1987): 3521–3526.

19. Davis, J.R., et al. "Cancer Control and Public Health in Missouri: A Time for Action." *Missouri Medicine* 87 (1990): 82–85.

20. Statistical Analysis System Institute. *SAS User's Guide: Statistics,* Version 5 Edition. Cary, N.C.: SAS Institute, 1985.

21. Siegel, S. "The Wilcoxon Matched-Pairs Signed-Ranks Test." In *Nonparametric Statistics For The Behavioral Sciences*. New York: McGraw-Hill, 1956.

22. *Clinical Laboratory Improvement Amendment CLIA 88*. Federal Register/Vol. 57, No. 40. Friday, February 28, 1992 /Rules and Regulations: 7163–7172.

23. Brownson, R.C., et al. "Preventing Cardiovascular Disease Through Community-Based Risk Reduction: Five-Year Results of the Bootheel Heart Health Project." *American Journal of Public Health* 86 (1996): 206–213.

24. Thacker, S.B., et al. "Public Health Surveillance for Chronic Conditions: A Scientific Basis for Decisions." *Statistics In Medicine* 13 (1994): 1–12.

7

A Cooperative Effort To Pass Tobacco Control Ordinances

Karen Pippert, Larry Jecha, Steven Coen, Patricia MacDonald, Julia Francisco, and Stephen Pickard

In the United States, the first local ordinances that attempted to limit the exposure of nonsmokers to environmental tobacco smoke (ETS) were passed in the 1970s, several years before the first studies appeared in literature, which reported associations between ETS and chronic disease among nonsmoking adults.[1,2] By the middle of 1992, 542 local governments in 33 states had passed ordinances that restricted indoor smoking in various public or commercial buildings.[1] Initial ordinances tended to restrict smoking to designated areas and applied to few buildings.[1] However, during the 1980s and 1990s, local ordinances increasingly restricted smoking within a broad range of buildings used by the public, and increasingly banned indoor smoking rather than designating indoor smoking areas.[1,2]

During this same period, many municipalities passed ordinances that attempted to restrict minors' access to tobacco.[1,3,4] The passage of local youth access ordinances was likely motivated by the perceived ineffectiveness of state youth access laws.[1,3,4] In 1992, all but three states had a law prohibiting the sale of tobacco to children under 18 years old[1,5]; nonetheless, sale of tobacco to minors and access to tobacco through vending machines was common.[1,3,4] By mid-1992, 181 communities in 21 states had passed ordinances restricting minors' access to tobacco products.[1] Typical local ordinances imposed a civil penalty on merchants who sold to minors and attempted to make vending machines less accessible to minors.[1,3,4] Enforcement was placed in the hands of a local agency.[1,3]

Tobacco control ordinances met with strong resistance in many communities.[6] Tobacco companies played an active role in opposing local ordinances by organizing and financing smokers' rights organizations or business coalitions.[6] In some

This chapter is based on a paper presented at the Annual Meeting and Exhibition of the American Public Health Association (APHA): "Public Health and Diversity," October 30–November 3, 1994, Washington, D.C.

J Public Health Management Practice, 1995, 1(2), 18–22
© 1995 Aspen Publishers, Inc.

communities, this resulted in the repeal of ordinances already passed.[6] In the face of organized opposition, tobacco ordinances were unlikely to pass unless supported by active coalitions of tobacco control proponents.[6] This chapter will: (1) describe how a combination of local public health leadership, community advocacy, media coverage, private financial support, and state technical assistance collaborated to strengthen tobacco control ordinances in Wichita, Kansas, and (2) present results from a population-based community survey of public opinions about tobacco and tobacco control conducted in Sedgwick County, Kansas (population = 435,000).

INTERVENTION METHODS

In the spring of 1993, the Wichita–Sedgwick County Health Department (WSCHD) enlisted the support of Tobacco-Free Wichita (TFW) to pass city ordinances that would substantially strengthen tobacco control in Wichita. Passage of ordinances required approval of the board of health and the city council. TFW contacted Americans for Non-Smokers Rights, a California-based nonprofit organization, from whom they obtained model ordinances and outlines of successful strategies. The two ordinances subsequently presented to the board of health prohibited smoking in all places used by the public, and required merchants to obtain a local license to sell tobacco. Local licensure was contingent on a merchant's refusal to sell tobacco to minors and placement of tobacco vending machines in locations inaccessible to minors.

The media, especially the local newspaper, became the primary forum of public debate for the proposed ordinances several months before they were presented to the board of health. Editorial media coverage was predominantly negative and seemed to suggest a lack of public support for the ordinances. Opposition developed quickly from the local restaurant association, vending machine owners, and smokers' rights groups.

Given the negative reception, TFW concluded that the measures would fail unless evidence of strong public support for the ordinances could be demonstrated to the city council. Strategies included obtaining letters of support from local physicians, small business owners, and corporate interests, staging public events to increase media attention, and surveying the population to determine the level of popular support for the ordinances.

In July 1993, TFW contacted the Behavioral Risk Factor Surveillance Unit (BRFSU) in the Kansas Department of Health and Environment (KDHE) to request assistance in obtaining survey data. The BRFSU, which had routinely collected health risk behavior data for Kansas since 1990 as part of the Behavioral Risk Factor Surveillance System (BRFSS) coordinated by the Centers for Disease Control and Prevention, agreed to conduct a community survey.

In order to sustain continuous media attention and editorial comment between the meeting of the board of health and the meeting of the city council, TFW waited to release survey methodology and results to the press until one week prior to the meeting of the board of health, and embargoed the information until the board meeting. This one-week period gave the press time to research the methodology and confirm the validity of the data. Approval of the ordinances by the board of health was followed by a well-publicized rally that successfully drew a small number of picketers from smokers' rights groups. By the time the ordinances were initially presented to the city council, public interest was high, so the council deferred discussion to a formal public hearing. The release of the data to the media, and approval of the ordinances by the board of health, marked the beginning of a transition in media coverage from negative to guardedly positive.

The presentation at the public hearing was planned. TFW identified each communication point that needed to be presented at the public hearing and a prominent member of the professional or business community to present it. A survey specialist from the BRFSU presented survey results. In addition, 13- and 14-year-old teenagers who had participated in a tobacco sting operation presented data that demonstrated the ability of minors to purchase tobacco from Wichita merchants. The teenagers also used the opportunity to present testimonials before the council about the devastating health impact of tobacco on their families.

TFW was able to control the council meeting; proponents of the ordinances appeared to be sensible and mainstream while opponents appeared to be radical. Subsequent follow-up with council members suggested that the votes of several council members who opposed the ordinances before the meeting were reversed by the presentation.

SURVEY METHODS

The survey instrument was developed by the BRFSU; whenever possible, questions for the survey were borrowed from other surveys. Survey methodology used for this survey was similar to that used to collect BRFSS data. From a list of all prefixes in use in Sedgwick County, the BRFSU generated a simple random sample of telephone numbers to be called. Any household in Sedgwick County with one or more persons 18 years or older was eligible to participate in the survey. Using a random selection procedure, the interviewer selected a single household member to be interviewed from among those eligible. If that person was unavailable, an appointment was made to contact the person at a later date. Refusals were recontacted three times to reattempt the interview before the refusal was accepted. From July 18 to July 30, 1993, interviewers contacted 806 eligible persons, of which 703 persons completed the interview, 72 persons refused to be interviewed, and 31 did not or could not complete the interview.

The BRFSU weighted the data by the age and sex distribution of Sedgwick County, and by number of persons in the household. Ninety-five percent confidence intervals were calculated from the standard error of a proportion.

SURVEY RESULTS

Age, sex, and race distributions for the survey population were similar to the age, sex, and race distribution of Sedgwick County. Twenty-two percent of those surveyed were smokers, compared to 21 percent smoking prevalence among Kansans (1990 Kansas BRFSS data). Seventy-eight percent of respondents were registered to vote; however, for most questions, responses obtained from registered voters were not statistically different from those obtained from the entire survey population.

The survey found that 83% (95% CI = 79% to 85%) of Sedgwick County adults believed that breathing another person's tobacco smoke is harmful to a nonsmoker's health; 90 percent of nonsmokers and 59 percent of smokers believed that breathing another person's tobacco smoke is harmful to a nonsmoker's health (Table 1). Among Sedgwick County adults, 54 percent (95% CI = 50% to 58%) supported a ban on smoking in all places used by the general public; however, support for a smoking ban varied by public site. While support for banning smoking in day care centers, museums/libraries, schools, day care homes, and hospitals was greater than 70 percent, support for banning smoking in government buildings, restaurants, shopping malls, universities, private workplaces, and bars/clubs was below 50 percent. Combined support for either restricting smoking to designated areas or banning smoking was greater than 90 percent for all sites except bars/clubs.

Among Sedgwick County adults, 9 percent (95% CI = 7% to 11%) believed that minors should be allowed to purchase tobacco, 73% (95% CI = 70% to 76%) believed that possession of tobacco by minors should be illegal, and 62 percent (95% CI = 58% to 66%) believed that cigarette vending machines should be banned. Eighty-four percent (95% CI = 81% to 87%) believed that merchants who sell tobacco to minors should be penalized; 44 percent (95% CI = 40% to 48%) believed that the penalty should include loss of license to sell tobacco products, and 40% (95% CI = 36% to 44%) believed that a fine alone was indicated.

RESULTS OF THE INTERVENTION

Ordinances restricting minors' access to tobacco passed the council easily. The council empowered the WSCHD to license merchants who sell tobacco and fine or suspend the local license of merchants caught selling tobacco to minors. Al-

Table 1 Weighted percent of responses among adult Sedgwick County residents, 1993

Question	Yes or Favor (%)	95% CI (%)
Do you believe that exposure to another person's tobacco smoke is harmful to a nonsmoker's health?	83	79–85
Nonsmokers	90	88–92
Smokers	59	55–63
Would you favor or oppose a complete ban on smoking in all areas used by the general public?	54	50–58
Do you think people under the age of 18 should be able to buy tobacco products?	9	7–11
Do you think it should be illegal for people under the age of 18 to have cigarettes in their possession?	72	69–75
Do you think all cigarette vending machines should be banned from all areas used by the general public?	62	58–66
Do you think merchants who sell tobacco products to people under the age of 18 should:		
Be fined?	40	36–44
Lose their privilege to sell tobacco?	7	5–9
Be both fined and lose their privilege to sell tobacco products?	37	33–41
Not be penalized?	11	9–13

though the original ordinance restricting the placement of vending machines did not pass, a compromise ordinance that required vending machines placed in areas accessible to minors be fitted with locking devices and required vending machines be licensed by the city did pass. A complete ban on smoking in all public places was not passed, but a compromise ordinance that exempts bars from the ordinance is under discussion. Follow-up efforts will focus on passing similar ordinances in other smaller municipalities within Sedgwick County.

DISCUSSION

The success of tobacco control efforts in Wichita appeared to depend on several factors, which were orchestrated by a strong local coalition. First, TFW developed a strategic plan based on demonstrating professional and communitywide support and effectively using the media. The rationale for this approach was that (1) obtaining the support of the medical community would increase the legitimacy of tobacco as a community health concern, (2) obtaining the support of businesses would help assuage fears that strict tobacco control ordinances would create an unacceptable business climate, (3) obtaining survey data would demonstrate to the city council the willingness of the public to control the sale and use of tobacco, and (4) obtaining high media visibility would involve the public in the debate, making the issue difficult for the city council to ignore, as well as providing an opportunity for TFW to educate persons about tobacco.

Second, the effort was local. TFW and KDHE communicated early in the planning process and agreed to limit KDHE involvement to providing a contract service for which the agency would be reimbursed.

Third, conducting the campaign and collecting survey data required financial resources. Tobacco companies provide financial support to organizations that oppose tobacco control ordinances; however, organizations attempting to pass tobacco control ordinances do not have similar corporate sponsorship.[6] In Wichita, the money to finance the campaign came from within TFW; the strength of the coalition made this possible.

Fourth, the survey data were scientifically sound. Organized opposition was expected from representatives of the tobacco companies; consequently, the survey data collection and analysis needed to use techniques of proven validity, and sample a population of sufficiently large size to obtain narrow confidence limits.

Fifth, defense of the ordinances before the city council was carefully planned. Prior to the council meeting, council opinion appeared to be strongly against the ordinances. Following the council meeting, vocal opposition within the council was muted, and compromise ordinances were passable. This positive outcome appeared to be a consequence of both the strength of TFW and unexpected weakness from the opposition.

●   ●   ●

Interpretation of the survey findings is subject to some limitations. First, the survey was conducted in Sedgwick County only and results may not be generalizable to the rest of the state, other urban areas of the state, or the nation. Even if data are representative of a geographic area broader than Sedgwick County, actions taken by local governments may be strongly influenced by the availability of local data. Second, only persons with telephones could be reached for the survey. Since low telephone ownership is strongly correlated with low income and education, the survey results may underrepresent persons of low socioeconomic status.[7] The nonresponse rate was low, so bias introduced by nonresponse was likely to be small.

In conclusion, community ordinances strictly controlling tobacco have become increasingly common. A strong local community coalition and data that demonstrate community support for tobacco control can be effective tools for passing tobacco control ordinances.

REFERENCES

1. U.S. Department of Health and Human Services, Public Health Service. *Major Local Tobacco Control Ordinances in the United States.* NIH Pub. No. 93–3532. Washington, D.C.: National Institutes of Health, 1993.

2. Rigotti, N.A., and Pashos, C.L. "No-Smoking Laws in the United States." *Journal of the American Medical Association* 266 (1991): 3162–3167.

3. Jason, L.A., et al. "Active Enforcement of Cigarette Control Law in the Prevention of Cigarette Sales to Minors." *Journal of the American Medical Association* 266 (1991): 3159–3161.

4. Altman, D.G., et al. "Reducing the Illegal Sale of Cigarettes to Minors." *Journal of the American Medical Association* 261 (1989): 80–83.

5. O'Connor, C., ed. *State Legislated Actions on Tobacco Issues.* Washington, D.C.: Coalition on Smoking OR Health, 1992.

6. Samuels, B., and Glantz, S.A. "The Politics of Local Tobacco Control." *Journal of the American Medical Association* 266 (1991): 2110–2117.

7. Thornberry, O.T., Jr., and Massey, J.T. "Trends in Telephone Coverage Across Time and Subgroups." In *Telephone Survey Methodology*, edited by R.M. Groves, et al. New York: John Wiley, 1988.

8

Conducting a Participatory Community-Based Survey

Amy J. Schulz, Edith A. Parker, Barbara A. Israel,
Adam B. Becker, Barbara J. Maciak, and Rose Hollis

In the past decade there has been a resurgence of interest in community-based initiatives to address differentials in health status associated with social inequalities.[1-5] Among the many questions that face practitioners, researchers, and policy makers who seek to enhance health in community settings are: (1) Whom to work with; (2) How to work together most effectively; and (3) How to understand and address both global and local social, economic, and political processes that affect the health of particular communities.[3,6-9]

In this chapter we describe a participatory action research process that brought together community members, representatives from community-based organizations (CBOs) and service providers, and academic researchers to collect, interpret, and apply community information to address issues related to the health of women and children in a geographically defined urban area. Specifically, we describe the development and administration of a community-based survey designed to inform the work of the East Side Village Health Worker Partnership in Detroit, Michigan. We discuss issues that arose in the ongoing process of engaging representatives from CBOs, health care institutions, key informants, and other community members in the development of the community-based survey. Finally, we examine the

The East Side Village Health Worker Partnership was developed in conjunction with the Detroit Community-Academic Prevention Research Center, funded through a cooperative agreement with the Centers for Disease Control and Prevention. We are indebted to the members of the East Side Village Health Worker Partnership (Butzel Family Center, Detroit Health Department, Friends of Parkside, Henry Ford Health Systems, Kettering Butzel Health Initiative, Mack Alive, Warren Conner Development Coalition), the Survey Committee, and the residents of Detroit's East Side who helped bring this project to fruition. In addition, we thank Sue Andersen for her invaluable assistance in the preparation of this manuscript.

J Public Health Management Practice, 1998, 4(2), 10–24

diverse contributions of the participants, the negotiation of priorities, and implications for research and collective action in community settings.

COMMUNITY-BASED AND PARTICIPATORY ACTION RESEARCH

There are nearly as many definitions of "community-based" research and interventions as there are definitions of "community."[10–13] Community may refer to geographically defined areas, groups that share a common history or interest, a sense of collective identity, shared values and norms, mutual influence among members, common symbols, or some combination of these dimensions.[3,14] In the research described here, we began with a geographically defined area, a neighborhood whose residents share some common history and social ties. Other more relational dimensions of community, such as the extent to which residents share values and norms, interact with each other, and exert mutual influence, are among the variables of interest in the survey.

Like community, the term community-based requires a more explicit definition. We use "community-based research" to refer to research that engages members of a community—in this case, a geographic area—in all phases of the research process, including the application of results to guide planned community change.[13,15–20] This definition draws upon principles of participatory action research to integrate community participation and influence in each stage of the research process: setting the direction for the research; defining the study problem; constructing the research design; collecting, analyzing, and interpreting the data; and applying the data to inform subsequent action. This model of research brings together participants who represent a variety of perspectives and experiences to contribute to and learn from each other's theories and experiences.[21–23] The knowledge-building process is connected to planned community change as participants work together to define and critically analyze neighborhood concerns, and to plan, implement, and evaluate actions to address those concerns.[16,23] Thus, community-based research does not refer to research that is simply conducted in community settings. We use this term to refer to research that centers on community strengths and issues and that explicitly engages those who live in the community in the research process. The insights and perspectives of community participants enhance the knowledge and understanding of researchers about community dynamics and conditions. This research seeks to strengthen the skills of community members in gathering and using data to facilitate planned community change.[20]

THE EAST SIDE VILLAGE HEALTH WORKER PARTNERSHIP

The East Side Village Health Worker (VHW) Partnership is one project developed as part of the Detroit Community-Academic Prevention Research Center (hereafter the Detroit PRC), funded in October 1995 through a cooperative agreement with the Centers for Disease Control and Prevention (CDC) as part of its Urban Research Centers initiative. The VHW Partnership includes representatives from the local health department, hospitals, CBOs (e.g., community development organizations, citizen action groups, community centers), and academic institutions. The overall goal of the Detroit PRC is to promote and conduct collaborative, community-based prevention research that strengthens the ability of communities to address and expand the knowledgebase of public health regarding the health of women and children. In early 1996, the Detroit PRC adapted research principles initially developed by the Detroit Genesee-County Community-Based Public Health Consortium.[15] These principles encourage participatory research processes that engage a variety of community groups in all phases of research conducted under the rubric of the Detroit PRC, with the broad aim that the research benefit the community.[24]

The academic and health department partners developed the conceptual framework for the Detroit PRC and the VHW Partnership, drawing upon their past history of collaboration, expertise, and interests, and using census and vital statistics data to define priority areas. Key informants, individuals who were knowledgeable about and respected in the community, helped to identify four CBOs located on Detroit's East Side with a history of effective community-level collaboration. These organizations were invited to work with the academic and health department partners and funding was included to support their participation. Representatives from each of these organizations comprised the Steering Committee for the East Side Village Health Worker Partnership. The first six months of the project were dedicated to establishing working relationships and specific objectives that drew on the local knowledge of committee members and key informants. Within the first year, based on recommendations from the Steering Committee, three additional CBOs joined the committee.

The Steering Committee agreed upon three specific aims for the Partnership: (1) to design, implement, and evaluate a collaborative VHW intervention[2,25–27] to address the factors associated with women's and children's health on Detroit's East Side; (2) to identify personal, interpersonal, organizational, community, and policy factors associated with poor health outcomes for women and children on Detroit's East Side; (3) to increase knowledge among participants in the VHW Project and among community members about these risk factors and protective factors, and to increase participation in strategies to modify these factors to improve the health of women and children. The VHW Partnership intervention and evaluation plans are discussed in more detail elsewhere.[24]

DEVELOPING THE SURVEY

This chapter focuses on a description and analysis of the process of designing and administering a community survey to inform and assess the VHW intervention. The tasks and timeline for the survey are shown in Table 1, and described below. The chapter draws on field notes and in-depth interviews collected as part

Table 1 Tasks and timeline to conduct a participatory community survey

Task	Timeline
Develop and maintain working relationships with members of the Steering Committee	January 1996–ongoing
Define specific aims for the Partnership	January–March 1996
Define the purpose of the survey	March–April 1996
Develop conceptual model	March–April 1996
Define the survey population	March–May 1996
Define the survey items	March–May 1996
Develop and pretest the questionnaire	March–June 1996
Blocklisting	May 1996
Draw the sample	May 1996
Send letters to selected households and area police departments to inform them of the survey	May 1996
Recruit and train community members as interviewers	May–July 1996
Establish field office and procedures	June 1996
Administer survey	June–December 1996
Monitor survey administration	June–December 1996
Feedback from interviewers	November–December 1996
Enter survey data into database	November 1996–January 1997
Data management/scale construction	January–March 1997
Begin analysis of data	February 1997
Preliminary feedback of survey results to Steering Committee and other community members	March–June 1997
Discuss implications of survey results with community members	April 1997–ongoing
Analyze data for basic research purposes	April 1997–ongoing
Prepare manuscripts for publication/ presentation	April 1997–ongoing

of the overall evaluation plan, which also includes pre- and post-training assessments, documentation of activities, and focus group interviews.[24,28]

Developing structures and setting the course

One of the first Steering Committee tasks was to develop and administer a survey of the community in which the intervention would be implemented. In doing so, they worked with a university-based Survey Committee, made up of individuals with expertise in survey design and methods, community organizing, women's and children's health, health behavior and health education, epidemiology, health services management, biostatistics, sociology, nutrition, and environmental health. The Survey Committee was to ensure that the survey would be constructed and conducted in a manner that would produce reliable and valid information that could be used to inform and evaluate the intervention and contribute to the body of knowledge in public health. The Steering Committee was responsible for: determining the boundaries of the community or neighborhoods that would be part of the survey; operationalizing the conceptual framework underlying the project and the intervention in these neighborhoods; helping to define the study population; and deciding upon the most effective strategies for administering the survey. A core support team of faculty and staff were members of both the Survey and Steering Committees, and conducted support work between meetings (e.g., minutes, background research). The two committees worked intensively, meeting every other week for a period of several months to define the study population and discuss survey design issues, content of the questionnaire, and the process for administering the questionnaire.

Conceptualizing the survey

Broadly, the purposes of the survey were defined as: (1) to assess community concerns and resources to guide the intervention; (2) to gather baseline data in order to evaluate the effects of the intervention on community-level change; and (3) to test the stress process model (described below) as a conceptual framework linking stressors to enduring health outcomes for women and children living in an urban community. The survey questionnaire was developed by bringing together information from the literature on women's and children's health with the particular local knowledge of community members.

Building on the work of Israel and colleagues,[14,29] House,[30] and Katz and Kahn,[31] we developed an initial conceptual framework that postulated that stressors (psychosocial and environmental conditions conducive to stress) in women's environments contribute to increases in perceived stress, and that this may in turn be linked to short-term responses and enduring health outcomes for women and their children. Conditioning variables such as knowledge, skills, social support, community problem-solving abilities, and accessible health and social services could reduce the potential for negative short-term or enduring health outcomes associated with exposure to stressors (see Figure 1). The stress model[24] provided an initial conceptual framework that linked social, structural, and physical factors in the environment with enduring health outcomes for women and children, consistent with the literature in this area.[5,11,32–40] This framework provided the broad outline for the survey questionnaire. The next steps were to define the study population and operationalize the model for women living in this particular urban area.

Defining the survey items

The Steering Committee participated in a series of discussions to translate the conceptual framework of the stress model to the specific experience of women living on Detroit's East Side. They first identified sources of stress for women caring for children living on the East Side, and how people feel and respond to these sources of stress. Next, they talked about the health and social effects of these stressors over long periods of time, and finally what might keep these stressors from having a negative effect on people's health in the long run. In a group session, Steering Committee members drew upon personal experiences and the experiences of friends, relatives, and, in some cases, clients to generate a list of 49 stressors experienced by women who live on the East Side and who care for children. They discussed conditions that created or supported these stressors in this community, and followed a similar process of identifying and discussing each of the other components of the stress model.

Through this process, the Steering Committee began to define the particular stressors experienced by women living on the East Side of Detroit, and pathways through which they might translate into enduring health outcomes. These stressors and conditioning variables were used to define broad sections of the questionnaire and to develop specific items within each section. For example, a section of the questionnaire on "problems and worries" included items developed from those identified by the Steering Committee (e.g., how often do you worry about your children's safety when they play outside in your neighborhood). In other instances, standardized items from other questionnaires were used that tapped into the dimensions identified by Steering Committee members (e.g., access to health services), allowing us to compare our results with those from national surveys. Table 2 shows selected results from the Steering Committee discussions and corresponding items developed for the questionnaire.

Pretesting the questionnaire

An early version of the questionnaire was reviewed by Steering Committee members and revised substantially based on their comments. Community mem-

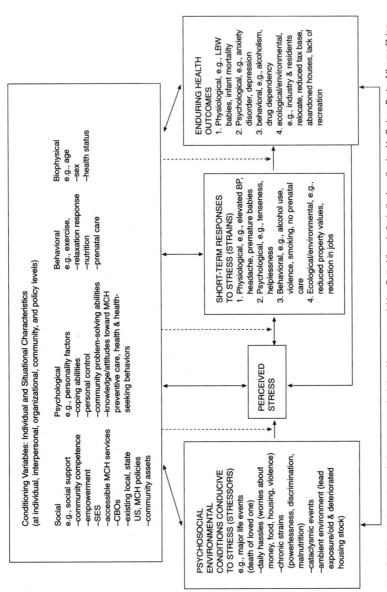

Conditioning Variables: Individual and Situational Characteristics
(at individual, interpersonal, organizational, community, and policy levels)

Social
e.g., social support
  -community competence
  -empowerment
  -SES
  -accessible MCH services
  -CBOs
  -existing local, state
    US, MCH policies
  -community assets

Psychological
e.g., personality factors
  -coping abilities
  -personal control
  -community problem-solving abilities
  -knowledge/attitudes toward MCH
    preventive care, health & health-
    seeking behaviors

Behavioral
e.g., exercise,
  -relaxation response
  -nutrition
  -prenatal care

Biophysical
e.g., age
  -sex
  -health status

ENDURING HEALTH
OUTCOMES
1. Physiological, e.g., LBW
   babies, infant mortality
2. Psychological, e.g., anxiety
   disorder, depression
3. behavioral, e.g., alcoholism,
   drug dependency
4. ecological/environmental,
   e.g., industry & residents
   relocate, reduced tax base,
   abandoned houses, lack of
   recreation

SHORT-TERM RESPONSES
TO STRESS (STRAINS)
1. Physiological, e.g., elevated BP,
   headache, premature babies
2. Psychological, e.g., tenseness,
   helplessness
3. Behavioral, e.g., alcohol use,
   violence, smoking, no prenatal
   care
4. Ecological/environmental, e.g.,
   reduced property values,
   reduction in jobs

PERCEIVED
STRESS

PSYCHOSOCIAL
ENVIRONMENTAL
CONDITIONS CONDUCIVE
TO STRESS (STRESSORS)
e.g., major life events
  (death of loved one)
  -daily hassles (worries about
    money, food, housing, violence)
  -chronic strains
    (powerlessness, discrimination,
    malnutrition)
  -cataclysmic events
  -ambient environment (lead
    exposure/old & deteriorated
    housing stock)

Note: Solid lines between boxes indicate presumed relationships among variables. Dotted lines indicate the hypothesized buffering effects of the modifying variables on the relationship between stressors and perceived stress, between perceived stress and short-term responses, and between short-term responses and enduring health outcomes.

Figure 1. Stress model as it relates to maternal-child health.

Table 2 Selected results from steering committee group discussions and examples of corresponding survey items

	Results from steering committee discussions	Example survey items
Stressors	Long waiting times for scheduled medical care appointments	The last time you went to see your usual health care provider, how well would you say they did in terms of seeing you close to the time you arrived? (excellent, good, fair, poor)
	Poor neighborhood environment (abandoned cars and lots, weeds, vacant homes, illegal dumping, not safe)	How often are the following a problem (in your neighborhood): • Not safe being on the street during the day? • Gangs in your neighborhood? • Litter, garbage, or dumping in vacant lots?
	Poor housing, lack of good housing	How often are the following a problem for you: • Poor housing? • Vacant housing?
	Worries about children	How often do you worry about: • Your child getting involved in gangs? • Your children's safety when they play outside in your neighborhood?
Conditioning variables	Social support	If you needed someone to watch your children for a few hours, how often could you get somebody to help without paying them?
	Religion/spirituality	In general, how important is your faith or spiritual beliefs as a source of strength in your day-to-day life?
	Perceived influence	By working together with others in this neighborhood, I can influence decisions that affect the neighborhood
	Neighborhood ties	Thinking about the last twelve months, how often have you asked one of your neighbors over to your house or gone over to their house for a meal, to play cards, to watch TV, or just to socialize?

bers in training as field interviewers (described in a later section) also pretested the questionnaire, and their comments were used to make further revisions. The process of developing and pretesting the questionnaire occurred over several months: the feedback from Steering Committee and other community members was essential to the development of the final questionnaire.

Negotiating the survey-intervention balance

The initial grant application proposed that the community survey would be conducted within the first year of the project. This meant that the multiple partners involved needed to develop working relationships, decide on the intervention area, agree upon specific intervention aims, establish a locally determined conceptual model, and develop and conduct the survey within the first twelve months. This timeline was set to ensure that baseline data collection would be completed before the first Village Health Workers were trained and began their work, and to maximize the intervention period before final evaluation data were collected.

This timeline was renegotiated through a series of discussions during the first year, with some Steering Committee members arguing strongly for the intervention to begin sooner, while academic and some community partners argued for a slower time line to conduct the survey and to implement the "reputational" method to recruit lay health advisors, as described in the literature.[41] Ultimately the Steering Committee agreed to begin the survey in mid-May and complete it July 30, with recruitment of Village Health Workers to begin in August and the first Village Health Worker training to occur in October 1996.

DECIDING WHO TO INTERVIEW

Defining the study population

Determining who would be included in the survey involved a series of decisions: defining the geographic community and the population of interest within that community, developing the sampling frame, and deciding on a sampling strategy. In agreement with the initial grant proposal, both committees believed that the effectiveness of the Village Health Workers would be strengthened if the intervention and documentation efforts were concentrated in an area smaller than the overall area involved in the Detroit PRC (1990 population of 82,182).

Over a period of several months, the Steering Committee examined information related to Detroit's East Side and discussed how to use this information to define the geographic area for the intervention. Resources and infrastructure in the sub-communities were examined, and knowledgeable residents were interviewed to learn about the community, including the history of collective action and perceived problems, as well as resources in the area. Census data describing household income, proportion of households headed by women, proportion of households with children under the age of 18, and vital statistics data such as infant morbidity and mortality rates were also considered in this process. Using criteria that included available resources (e.g., churches, block clubs), history of collaboration or community organizing, interest of community members, the potential for ongoing institutional support for the Village Health Workers, the size and shape of local networks and catchment areas, available data about social and health indicators, and ongoing initiatives or activities within the area, the Steering Committee defined an area within the East Side within which they would focus the efforts of VHW Partnership. This area, bounded by four major East Side streets, contained approximately 6,000 households.

At the same time, the Survey Committee discussed sample size, sampling frame, and the definition of the study population (e.g., whether survey respondents would include both men and women, women of childbearing age, all women over the age of 18). Ultimately, based on estimated eligibility and response rates, and projected attrition between the two waves of the survey (the second wave to be conducted three years later) the Survey Committee recommended that the study area include approximately 5,000 households (roughly 20,000 people), and set a goal of 1,000 completed interviews. The Steering and Survey Committees together defined eligibility for the study as women 18 years and older with responsibility for the care of children under the age of 18 for five hours a week or more.

PREPARING TO CONDUCT THE SURVEY

Blocklisting

Once the geographic area for the survey and intervention had been defined, a process called "blocklisting" was carried out to develop a sampling frame of individual housing units within that area. Blocklisting involves listing each individual housing unit on a given block.[42] Steering Committee members identified individuals who lived in the area, who were paired with university students, faculty, and staff researchers. Folders were prepared for each census block within the survey area, and each team was given a set of folders containing a detailed map of the area and forms for listing the addresses of individual housing units. A formal half-day training on blocklisting procedures was held to explain the process, and blocklisting was conducted over a series of several weekends. Community residents who participated in the blocklisting process contributed invaluable knowledge of the community by locating hard-to-find units, identifying vacant units, accessing apartment buildings, explaining the presence of university participants to community members, and offering practical guidance on safety-related concerns.

Sampling

A two-stage simple random sampling process was used to generate the sample for this survey. As a first step, 2,800 households were randomly selected from the sampling frame of 6,124 households blocklisted. These represented the estimated number of households needed to achieve the desired 1,000 completed interviews based on one interview per household and an estimated 60 percent eligibility rate, 85 percent occupancy rate, and 70 percent response rate.[43,44] Within households with more than one eligible member, a Kish selection table was used to randomly select one respondent.[45]

Letters of introduction were developed by the core support team, signed by locally recognized Steering Committee members, and sent to the selected addresses. The letters explained the purpose of the survey and indicated that an interviewer would soon be visiting. For units with an illegible address, and for unnumbered units within large apartment buildings, letters were hand-delivered using directions and maps produced by the blocklisting teams. In addition, letters were sent to police precincts in the survey areas, alerting them that interviewers affiliated with the VHW Partnership would be in the area during the survey time period.

A unique address/sample identification label was prepared for each address to be visited, and a cover sheet was designed to introduce the survey; establish eligibility; and, as needed, randomly select one eligible respondent by applying a Kish selection table to the household listing.[45] The cover sheet also documented informed consent, collected recontact information, provided a "call record" of attempted contacts with that household, and recorded the final outcome (i.e., completed interview, noneligible, vacant unit, refusal, other).

Recruitment and training of interviewers

The Steering Committee decided to hire and train residents of the neighborhood to administer the survey for several reasons, including:

- The interviews would be conducted by individuals who were familiar with the neighborhood and its concerns;
- The potential respondents would be more likely to participate in an interview conducted by someone from the area;
- The quality of the data would be enhanced due to greater trust between the interviewer and interviewee;
- Local interviewers would set the tone for the community-based nature of the research and the intervention that would follow;
- This would provide employment, although temporary and part time, in an area with an unemployment rate of 19 percent.[44]

The Steering Committee contributed to the development of a job description that specified interviewer qualifications, and helped to determine reasonable compensation for the interviewers.

Steering Committee members were actively involved in recruiting interviewers, distributing fliers, and contacting individuals they felt might be interested in the positions. Applicants were screened to determine eligibility, with questions that included past experience with survey interviewing, residence, community involvement, availability for the training and the survey field period, and their perceived strengths and challenges in conducting survey interviews. Those who were invited to attend the training were paid for the training time, and informed that the final decision about who would be hired as interviewers would be made at the end of the training period. Because all respondents would be assured of the confidential and anonymous nature of the interview, professionals (such as social workers and educators) whose state licenses required them to report certain activities (e.g., suspected child abuse) were considered ineligible.

The training, which included lecture, group discussion, role plays, and group and individual practice and feedback, was based on curricula developed by the Detroit Area Study and the Institute for Social Research at the University of Michigan, supplemented by materials developed by the University of North Carolina at Chapel Hill Breast Cancer Screening Program. (In addition, the Collaborative Initial Glaucoma Study-Interviewing Center and the Women Take Pride Project, both based at the University of Michigan School of Public Health, shared strategies for training interviewers.) Trainees received 17 hours of formal training that included basic information about survey research, descriptions of random sampling techniques, information on obtaining respondent participation, instruction on use of the survey instrument, confidentiality, use of standardized probes and responses to questions from respondents, and verification of interviews. Of 62 individuals who were screened for the training, 50 attended at least one training session, 23 completed the training sequence and were selected to work as interviewers, and 19 worked for one week or more.

Final preparations and getting into the field

As the date initially set for beginning the survey approached, many details remained to be addressed. Faculty and staff involved in the survey administration spent weeks preparing and conducting the interviewer training, blocklisting, sampling, mailing letters to residents and area police precincts, and preparing cover sheets and folders for the interviewers. The folders, bearing the same address/sample ID label, contained the cover sheet and all supplies needed to conduct the interview: questionnaire, respondent booklet, incentive coupon, and neighborhood resource directory (to be distributed to those who completed interviews), VHW Partnership brochure; appointment cards, interviewer labels, and copies of introductory letters sent to households and local police precincts.

Further, as pretesting of the questionnaire progressed, revisions of the survey instrument were required, which in turn led to changes in the interviewer training and field office procedures. In the press to begin the survey on time, it was a challenge to involve all members of the Steering Committee in making decisions about the questionnaire content and its administration. For example, in the hurry to mail letters to selected households in time for the initial interviews to start according to the set timeline, the letters were mailed without the approval of the Steering Committee members. They were subsequently revised and approved by the Steering Committee, but this could have become a serious division within the Committee had there not been a prior history of working relationships and trust developed over the preceding months. The time and energy involved in this process, and the importance of the contributions of all participants, should not be underestimated. Even with the hard work of Steering Committee members and the students, staff, and faculty who supported the survey process, the field period began in the second week of June, two weeks later than scheduled.

CONDUCTING THE SURVEY

Survey administration

The survey field office was established at Butzel Family Center, a member of the VHW Partnership. A team of field supervisors consisting of researchers and students was recruited and at least one supervisor was available in the field office at all times that interviewers were in the field. Field supervisors were responsible for checking out survey folders to interviewers at the beginning of their shift, and for debriefing with interviewers at shift's end. This involved reviewing all cover sheets, call records, and completed interviews with the interviewer; noting any discrepancies; providing inservice training where needed; and discussing any interviewer problems or concerns. Completed interviews were logged on a standard tracking form (adapted from those used by the Detroit Area Study in the University of Michigan's Sociology Department), and follow-up appointments were noted in an appointment log book. The first six interviews completed by each interviewer were verified by phone or in person, followed by verification of every sixth interview thereafter. Verifications were completed by field supervisors and a community member who was hired to assist with this task.

Nine interviewers began interviewing in mid-June. A second training was conducted in July and 12 additional interviewers joined the team. At the suggestion of Steering Committee members, respondents were given a copy of the "Kettering-

Butzel Community Resource Directory," a listing of community programs and service providers developed by the Kettering Butzel Health Initiative (a Steering Committee member), along with a small gift certificate to a local retail center. The community interviewers were clearly an asset; their knowledge of the community, long hours, and ability to encourage community members to be interviewed contributed to the success of the survey. In the few instances when problems arose (e.g., interviewers not returning on schedule; interviews conducted at the wrong address; improper procedures followed), the Steering Committee was invaluable in finding ways to address them, and in supporting decisions made by the office staff. It was particularly important that decisions made by those who managed the survey office be informed and supported by members of the Steering Committee, since the survey would be followed by the community intervention and was the first introduction of the VHW Partnership to the community. For the same reason, it was important to maintain positive working relationships among university staff and community interviewers. Toward this end, periodic group meetings were held with the interviewers to inform them of progress, changes in procedures, and elicit feedback and discussion of concerns and challenges they faced in the field.

Despite the long hours worked and the commitment of the field office staff and the interviewers, the field period continued two months longer than initially anticipated as we sought to reach the goal of 1,000 completed interviews. At the end of August, with about 660 interviews completed, several hundred cover sheets remained to be closed out and the graduate students and faculty who had staffed the field office needed to return to their other academic responsibilities. At this point, the Steering Committee established the procedures under which a transition would be made from the community interviewers to professional interviewers. To ensure that the professional interviewers who completed the survey were familiar with community norms and that they were as similar to the community interviewers as possible, the Steering Committee requested that the professional interviewers hired be African-American, live in Detroit, and modify their interviewing techniques somewhat (e.g., be less assertive about following up with soft refusals than they might have been if the survey were not linked to a subsequent intervention in the community). Eight interviewers were hired and worked for four months to follow up on the remaining cover sheets.

Response rates

Altogether, 700 interviews were completed and verified as usable interviews. In 1,075 of the households selected to be part of the sample, no resident met the eligibility criteria. There were 307 vacant houses, 43 at which no interviewer was ever able to establish contact with a resident, and 104 selected households were classified as "other." In 84 households an eligible respondent was identified but refused to participate, and 40 additional interviews were completed but were not usable for a variety of reasons (e.g., incomplete, conducted at the wrong address). Thus, the completed interview rate (the number of completed interviews divided by the number of eligible households in the sample) was 81 percent.

Feedback from the interviewers

Debriefing sessions were conducted with community interviewers after the end of the interview period, providing information about which neighborhoods had strong networks and which were more fragmented, stressors discussed by women in the community that were not included in the survey (e.g., lack of safe recreation for children), and additional resources (e.g., strong family networks). Interviewers described strategies that they had used to obtain interviews and minimize risks (e.g., how to conduct interviews in distracting situations, how to identify potentially unsafe houses, safety precautions). These insights are helpful to inform the intervention and future interviewer training sessions. In addition, interviewers were encouraged to reflect on aspects of the interviewer/supervisor relationship that could be improved in the second wave of the survey.

NEXT STEPS

Dissemination of results

We are beginning to disseminate preliminary survey results to community members. The Steering Committee is developing processes that will allow community members and researchers to examine the stressors and conditioning variables identified, and discuss ways to reduce the stressors or strengthen the protective factors (e.g., enhance control, social support). Initially envisioned as a single large community forum, other options now being considered for disseminating the survey results include: printed summaries made available to neighborhood residents, presentations at block club meetings and other small groups working to address local concerns, presentations at local police precinct meetings, and a half-day "retreat" with Village Health Workers and Steering Committee members.

Determine priorities and change strategies

We anticipate that community members will want more than information about the problems in their communities. As one Steering Committee member noted, "This community has been researched to death—they're going to want to hear solutions, not just the survey results." Recognizing this, one goal of this project is to work together to prioritize community concerns and develop solutions.

A part of this process will involve disentangling concerns that are amenable to change at the community level from those more effectively addressed through state and federal policies. For example, the social, political, and economic processes that reduce access to resources within Detroit and that contribute to the health problems of residents are connected to patterns of production and processes of racial and class segregation that may not be within the range of influence of members of those communities.[46–49] These processes may not be immediately responsive to local influence. On the other hand, as residents of marginalized communities mobilize to address social, economic, and political patterns within their communities that are linked with differentials in health status, they may also address some of these broader political and economic processes. Further, the development of coalitions and alliances within and beyond the boundaries of the immediate community can expand the resources available to leverage change at the policy level. Determining priorities and building skills, organizations, and other resources necessary to promote change is essential to the development of influence at the local level and beyond.

Implications for linking research with health promotion at the community level

Our experience highlights some of the dynamics that may shape participatory research that is linked to community interventions. As we indicated at the beginning of this chapter, one of the challenges is that of defining community, what dimensions of community are important, and how to tap into them. These may emerge and evolve over time, as new information is gathered and as participants develop new understandings of community dynamics and their relation to particular health issues.

Steering Committee members familiar with the community were essential to begin to understand the social and economic worlds of women living in this neighborhood. They helped to identify a smaller geographic area and determine the extent to which it was a community, shape the research questions, define the survey population, develop questionnaire items, select interviewers, and make other day-to-day decisions about the administration of the survey. The expertise, credibility, and support of members of the Steering Committee will be critical throughout the upcoming community dialogues about the survey results and their implications for action. This is particularly relevant considering the differences of ethnicity and class that continue to separate many academic practitioners from communities of color, and the mistrust associated with those differences and with the history of health-related research within disenfranchised communities.[20,50]

While practitioners engaged in community research are strongly encouraged to create a community advisory board, they should be aware of the time commitment, vigilance, and energy required to effectively maintain open lines of communication and trust. Among members of the VHW Steering Committee, there were different perspectives, priorities, and resources, and these translated at times into differences of opinion. Some of these differences arose from the pressures and politics that shape the lives of researchers based in academic settings and those who work in larger service organizations such as health departments. These pressures are not always visible or acceptable to those who are working in small CBOs, who face their own sets of pressures and politics that may be equally invisible to those based in larger institutions or outside of the community. Other differences arise between representatives from CBOs based on their distinct experiences within and views about the communities in which they live and work. Thus, the ability of the Steering Committee to work together to come to consensus despite these differences depends on members' ability to educate each other about the pressures and politics of their organizations, and establish a level of trust that allows open dialogue. It demands a willingness to discuss problems, listen, forge solutions to which all members can agree, challenge each other, address conflicts, and, when necessary, apologize and move beyond mistakes made by one or more of the partners. Effective community-based research hinges on the ability of Steering Committee members to engage in honest and productive dialogue that examines pressures and conflicts and the way that they shape the research process, the information that is gathered, and the way that it is interpreted and used.

LIMITATIONS

The use of the survey as one aspect of a community-based intervention is a time and resource intensive process for gathering information about the community itself. The decision to use a participatory research approach increased the number of persons involved in the decision-making process, and thus increased the time spent in negotiation and discussion. At the same time, we believe that this approach increased the number of different perspectives that informed the survey and enhanced its relevance to community members.

The Survey and Steering Committees decided not to conduct a parallel survey in a comparison community. The decision was based on the desire to maximize the use of available resources, ethical considerations in not providing an intervention subsequently in the comparison community, and concerns articulated in the literature and expressed by some members of our research team about the ability to adequately match and the usefulness and interpretability of data from a "control" community.[20,28,51,52] Without power to control, or resources to monitor in enough detail, changes that might occur in a "control" community, real questions arose about the extent to which such a study design would contribute to an understanding of the process or effects of the intervention. Instead resources were focused on documenting change within the intervention community.

Interpretations and generalizations made on the basis of the results of this survey will be applicable to women 18 years and older living in this community who are responsible for the care of children under the age of 18 for five hours a week or more; that is, the study population. Care must be taken in generalizing to other populations—including other communities—on the basis of these results. Further, we are limited in making some kinds of comparisons. For example, because of the small number of Caucasian respondents included in this survey (1%), we cannot test for differential neighborhood effects by race of respondent. In addition, we cannot use these data to make comparisons between African-American women living in this community and other, perhaps less economically marginalized, communities. This survey, because of the purposes for which it was conducted and the decisions made about sampling and eligibility, provides a rich description of the experiences of women living in the community. These decisions were based on the goals and objectives for the survey data and the intervention. They are not limitations of the use of a participatory process per se, but are limitations (and strengths) of the data, based on decisions that were made through a participatory process.

●   ●   ●

This chapter describes a participatory action research process that brought together community members with health service providers and academic researchers. As practitioners and researchers work together with community members to understand and to intervene in social conditions associated with health and illness, the processes that are used to collect and interpret information about the community may reflect or challenge the very social inequalities that shape differentials in health status. Processes that involve community members in framing the research questions, collecting and interpreting data, and determining the uses of the information in community change efforts, can both contribute to the scientific literature and to the social resources available to residents of disenfranchised communities.

Explicit attention to power relationships between researchers and community members is linked to theories of the social construction of knowledge as well as to a history of activist research in the social sciences.[53,54] Questions of who participates in the process of creating knowledge, what kind of influence they have, and implications for those who are not represented or who have less influence become particularly salient.[20] These questions of representation and participation are directly linked to the history of local political and social processes, and have important implications for research and interventions developed at the local level.[8,46,55] Specifically, we suggest that community research and interventions that seek to address the social inequalities that are fundamental to differentials in health should explicitly work to establish more equitable power relationships among participants, and between those who participate and other subgroups within geographically defined communities.[10,20,56] Community-based research that is grounded in community concerns and linked with reflection and action can begin to address underlying social and political inequalities that contribute to differentials in health status.

REFERENCES

1. W.K. Kellogg Foundation. *Community-Based Public Health Initiative*. Battle Creek, Mich.: 1992.
2. U.S. Department of Health and Human Services, Centers for Disease Control and Prevention. *Cooperative Agreement Program for Urban Center(s) in Applied Research in Public Health*. Program Announcement No. 515. Washington, D.C.: Government Printing Office, 1994.
3. M. Schlessinger. "Paradigms Lost: The Persisting Search for Community in American Health Policy." *Journal of Health Politics, Policy and Law* 22, no. 4 (1997): 937–992.
4. Institute of Medicine, Committee for the Study of the Future of Public Health. *The Future of Public Health*. Washington, D.C.: National Academy Press, 1988.
5. U.S. Department of Health and Human Services, Public Health Service. *Healthy People 2000. National Health Promotion and Disease Prevention Objectives*. Boston: Jones & Bartlett Publishers, 1992.
6. D.W. Light. "The Rhetorics and Realities of Community Health Care: The Limits of Countervailing Powers to Meet the Health Care Needs of the 21st Century." *Journal of Health Politics* 22, no. 1 (1997): 105–145.
7. K. Blankenship and A.J. Schulz. Approaches and Dilemmas in Community-Based Research and Action. (Paper presented at the Society for the Study of Social Problems Annual Meeting, New York, August 15–17, 1996.)
8. C. Schneider and N. Freudenberg. "Local Response to HIV and Substance Abuse: An Ethnographic Study of Four Puerto Rican Low Income Neighborhoods in New York City, 1993–94." Unpublished.
9. C. Brown. "Systemic Power in Community Decision Making: A Restatement of Stratification Theory." *The American Political Science Review* 74 (1980): 978–990.
10. R. Labonte. "The View from Here: Community Development and Partnerships." *Canadian Journal of Public Health* 84, no. 4 (1993): 237–238.
11. E.R. Brown. "Community Action for Health Promotion: A Strategy to Empower Individuals and Communities." *International Journal of Health Services* 21, no. 3 (1991): 441–456.
12. L.W. Green and M.W. Kreuter. "CDC's Planned Approach to Community Health as an Application of PRECEDE and an Inspiration for PROCEED." *Journal of Health Education* 23, no. 3 (1992): 140–147.
13. J. Hatch et al. "Community Research: Partnership in Black Communities." *American Journal of Preventive Medicine* 9, suppl., no. 6 (1993): 27–31.
14. B.A. Israel et al. "Health Education and Community Empowerment: Conceptualizing and Measuring Perceptions of Individual, Organizational and Community Control." *Health Education Quarterly* 21, no. 2 (1994): 149–170.

15. A.J. Schulz et al. "Development and Implementation of Principles for Community-Based Research in Public Health." *Journal of Community Practice*, in press.

16. R. Stoeker and E. Bonacich. "Why Participatory Research? Guest Editors' Introduction." *The American Sociologist* 23, no. 4 (1992): 5–14.

17. R. Stoeker and D. Beckwith. "Advancing Toledo's Neighborhood Movement through Participatory Action Research: Integrating Activist and Academic Approaches." *Clinical Sociology Review* 10 (1992): 198–213.

18. M. Elden. "Sharing the Research Work: Participative Research and Its Role Demands." In *Human Inquiry: A Sourcebook of New Paradigm Research*, eds. P. Reason and J. Rowan. New York: John Wiley and Sons, 1987, 253–266.

19. C.A. Heaney et al. "Industrial Relations, Worksite Stress Reduction, and Employee Well-Being: A Participatory Action Research Investigation." *Journal of Organizational Behavior* 14 (1993): 495–510.

20. B.A. Israel et al. "Community-Based Research: A Partnership Approach to Improve Public Health." *Annual Review of Public Health*, in press.

21. M. Singer. "Knowledge for Use: Anthropology and Community-Centered Substance Abuse Research." *Social Science and Medicine* 37, no. 1 (1993): 15–25.

22. B. Hall. "From Margins to Center? The Development and Purpose of Participatory Research." *The American Sociologist* 23, no. 4 (1992): 15–28.

23. B.A. Israel et al. "Action Research on Occupational Stress: Involving Workers as Researchers." *International Journal of Health Services* 19 (1989): 135–155.

24. E.A. Parker et al. "East Side Village Health Worker Partnership: Community-Based Health Advisor Intervention in an Urban Area." *Health Education & Behavior,* in press.

25. E. Eng and J. Hatch. "Networking Between Agencies and Black Churches: The Lay Health Advisor Model." *Journal of Prevention in Human Services* 10, no. 1 (1991): 123–146.

26. E. Eng and R. Young. "Lay Health Advisors as Community Change Agents." *Family and Community Health* 15, no. 1 (1992): 24–40.

27. A.H. Collins and D.L. Pancoast. *Natural Helping Networks: A Strategy for Prevention.* Washington, D.C.: The National Association of Social Workers, Inc., 1981.

28. B.A. Israel et al. "Evaluation of Health Education Programs: Current Assessment and Future Directions." *Health Education Quarterly*, 22, no. 3 (1995): 364–389.

29. B.A. Israel. "Social Networks and Social Support: Linking Theory, Research and Practice." *Patient Counseling and Health Education* 4 (1982): 65–79.

30. J.S. House. *Work, Stress and Social Support.* Reading, Mass.: Addison-Wesley Publishing Co., 1981.

31. D. Katz and R.L. Kahn. *The Social Psychology of Organizations*, 2nd ed. New York: John Wiley & Sons, 1978.

32. A.T. Geronimus. "The Effects of Race, Residence and Prenatal Care on the Relationship of Maternal Age to Neonatal Mortality." *American Journal of Public Health* 76 (1986): 1416–1421.

33. A.T. Geronimus. "The Weathering Hypothesis and the Health of African-American Women and Infants: Evidence and Speculations." *Ethnicity and Disease* 2 (1992): 207–221.

34. T.A. LaViest. "The Political Empowerment and Health Status of African-Americans: Mapping a New Territory." *American Journal of Sociology* 97, no. 4 (1992): 1080–1095.

35. N. Krieger et al. "Racism, Sexism and Social Class: Implications for Studies of Health, Disease and Well-Being." *American Journal of Preventive Medicine* 9, suppl., no. 6 (1993): 82–122.

36. A.T. Geronimus et al. "Excess Mortality among Blacks and Whites in the United States." *New England Journal of Medicine* 335 (November 21, 1996): 1552–1558.

37. K.G. Reeb et al. "Predicting Low Birthweight and Complicated Labor in Urban Black Women: A Biopsychosocial Perspective." *Social Science and Medicine* 25, no. 12 (1987): 1321.

38. J.S. Norbeck et al. "Life Stress, Social Support and Emotional Disequilibrium in Complications of Pregnancy: A Prospective, Multivariate Study." *Journal of Health and Social Behavior* 24 (1983): 30–46.

39. S.A. James. "Foreword: Racial Differences in Preterm Delivery." *American Journal of Preventive Medicine* 9, suppl., no. 6 (1993): v–vi.

40. K.R. McLeroy et al. "An Ecological Perspective on Health Promotion Programs." *Health Education Quarterly* 15 (1988): 351–377.

41. C. Service et al. "Identification and Recruitment of Facilitators." *Community Health Education: The Lay Health Advisor Approach*, eds. C. Service and E.J. Salber. Durham, N.C.: Duke University Health Care Systems, 1979.

42. Survey Research Center. "Detroit Area Study Blocklisting Manual" (modified from *Survey Research Center Sampling Manual*). Ann Arbor, Mich.: Institute for Social Research, University of Michigan.

43. Survey Research Center. *Survey Research Center Sampling Manual*. Institute for Social Research, University of Michigan, Ann Arbor, Mich.

44. Southeast Michigan Census Council, Inc. *1990 Census Subcommunity Profiles for the City of Detroit, Michigan*. Detroit, Mich.: Metropolitan Information Center, Center for Urban Studies, Wayne State University, United Community Services of Metropolitan Detroit, October 1993.

45. G. Kalton. *Introduction to Survey Sampling*. Sage University Series "Quantitative Applications in the Social Sciences," no. 35. Beverly Hills, Calif.: Sage Publications, 1983.

46. T.J. Sugrue. *The Origins of the Urban Crisis: Race and Inequality in Postwar Detroit*. Princeton, N.J.: University Press, 1996.

47. L.J.D. Wacquant and W.J. Wilson. "The Cost of Racial and Class Exclusion in the Inner City." *Annals of the American Academy of Political and Social Science* 501 (1989): 8–25.

48. J.D Kasarda. "Urban Industrial Transition and the Underclass." *The Annals of the American Academy of Political and Social Science* 501 (1989): 26–47.

49. D.S. Massey and N.A. Denton. *American Apartheid: Segregation and the Making of the Underclass*. Cambridge, Mass.: Harvard University Press, 1993.

50. J.H. Jones. *Bad Blood: The Tuskegee Syphilis Experiment*. New York: The Free Press, 1993.

51. M. Susser. "The Tribulations of Trials-Intervention in Communities." *American Journal of Public Health* 85 (1995): 156–158.

52. M.B. Mittlemark et al. "Realistic Outcomes: Lessons from Community-Based Research and Demonstration Programs for the Prevention of Cardiovascular Diseases." *Journal of Public Health Policy* 14 (1993): 437–462.

53. K. Lewin. "Action Research and Minority Problems." *Journal of Social Issues* 2, no. 4 (1946): 34–46.

54. D. Bailey. "Using Participatory Research in Community Consortia Development and Evaluation: Lessons from the Beginning of a Story." *The American Sociologist* 23, no. 4 (1992): 71–82.

55. G.W. Steuart. "Social and Behavioral Change Strategies." In *Aging and Public Health*, eds. H.T. Phillips and S.A. Gaylord. New York: Springer, 1985.

56. P. Maguire. *Doing Participatory Research: A Feminist Approach*. Amherst, Mass.: The Center for International Education, School of Education, 1990.

PART III

Intervention Development and Implementation

This section provides examples of community-based intervention projects. Several of the chapters describe national initiatives that are implemented at the local level, whereas others describe national efforts to develop local initiatives. These projects highlight some of the components that are common in community-based interventions including: the use of coalitions, program implementation at multiple sites, the use of both secondary and primary data for program planning, and the importance of media involvement.

The first chapter describes the National 5 A Day for Better Health Program. Although this is a national initiative, local community organizations, governmental officials, and local businesses tailor the program to meet local needs. The chapter provides a good example of a program that intervenes at multiple levels of the ecological framework (e.g., individual behavior change and policy change), uses coalitions for planning and implementing activities, and is implemented at multiple sites (e.g., workplaces, schools, and supermarkets). The chapter also raises the issue of sustainability of community-based initiatives.

The second and third chapters in this section describe the Breast and Cervical Cancer Early Detection Program (BCCDP). As with the National 5 A Day for Better Health Program, the BCCDP is a national initiative that is developed and implemented at a local level. Henson et al. present the national picture of this program. One of the critical issues that is raised in this chapter is the importance of understanding local needs and issues prior to the development of local program activities. The authors note that program success requires working with already existing organizations. The third chapter, "Progress in Breast Cancer Screening," describes how the state of Vermont has modified the national initiative to meet the local needs. The authors make the point that successful modification requires the collection of primary data, both qualitative and quantitative. Moreover, the chapter provides an example of a coalition that is addressing multiple issues, rather than a single issue, in the community. The authors also mention the role of managed care in providing screening opportunities.

The last chapter in this section, "Demonstration Projects in Community-Based Prevention," describes the CDC-funded Prevention Research Centers (PRCs) and the W.K. Kellogg Foundation-funded Community-Based Public Health (CBPH) Initiative. The PRCs are an example of a national effort to develop local initiatives to change risky health behaviors, whereas the CBPH projects focus on building academic-community-practice partnerships to address locally defined needs. Multiple strategies are used in each of these efforts, and both attend to multiple levels of the ecological framework, use a multidisciplinary approach, and incorporate coalitions or consortia to assist in program planning and implementation. The chapter highlights some of the lessons learned including the importance of: community member participation, using existing data, using appropriate methods for evaluating community-based interventions, and acknowledging the amount of time these projects take for completion.

As you read these chapters, consider the following set of questions:

Objectives and Data Sources

1. Are the objectives of each of the interventions clearly described? Why is this important?
2. One of the intentions of the BCCDP is to enhance utilization of breast and cervical cancer screening among traditionally underserved populations. What are some ways in which a local project can do this? What type of data would be important to gather to ensure that the program meets the specific needs of these women?
3. What sources of already existing data would be helpful to a local community that is developing a 5 a day or BCCDP program?

Methods and Strategies

4. How were coalitions used in each of the interventions described? To what extent were community members, as opposed to community organizations, incorporated into program activities? How might this affect program effectiveness?
5. How was the media used to enhance community-based initiatives?
6. What policy changes were enacted in each of the programs described? What other types of policy changes might be appropriate for the future?
7. What are the advantages of using multiple sites for program implementation?

8. When state health departments initiate multiple site interventions in cooperation with local health agencies, should they fund all local health agencies or issue requests for proposals (competitive funding)?
9. What efforts are being pursued to conduct long-term evaluations of these intervention programs?

Dissemination and Implications for Public Health Practice

10. What are the advantages and disadvantages of national initiatives with local implementation? What are the advantages and disadvantages of national efforts to develop local initiatives? In what instances might one be preferable to another?
11. Should public health efforts focus on changing behaviors that negatively affect health outcomes, or on enhancing relationships between the different partners that work in the public health arena?

9

The National 5 A Day for Better Health Program: A Large-Scale Nutrition Intervention

Jerianne Heimendinger, Mary Ann Van Duyn, Daria Chapelsky, Susan Foerster, and Gloria Stables

Over the past decade, consensus about the science base for dietary change has grown steadily. Seminal publications include Doll and Peto's Causes of Cancer; the NCI's Cancer Control Objectives, 1985–2000; the Surgeon General's Report on Nutrition and Health (USDHHS, Surgeon General, 1988); Diet and Health: Implications for Reducing Chronic Disease Risk; Healthy People 2000 National Health Promotion and Disease Prevention Objectives; and the Dietary Guidelines for Americans.[1-6] These reports provide a basis for consistent policy making in diet and health issues and enable national, state, and local governments to move ahead with nutrition programs that address national goals.

In a parallel development, the National Cancer Institute (NCI) awarded grants in 1986 to build technical capacity in state health departments for implementing cancer prevention and control programs in screening, tobacco control, and diet. Of the nine funded grants, only the California Department of Health assumed the challenge of implementing a statewide dietary intervention, which became the California 5 A Day for Better Health campaign.

Based on the strength of the science base linking fruit and vegetable consumption and cancer prevention and the tested state-based prototype, the NCI launched the 5 A Day Program as a national public health initiative for nutrition and cancer in 1991.[7-14]

DESCRIPTION OF THE NATIONAL 5 A DAY PROGRAM

The 5 A Day Program is a national partnership between the fruit and vegetable industry, represented by the Produce for Better Health Foundation (PBH) and the NCI. This partnership has a vision for modifying national dietary behaviors, using

J Public Health Management Practice, 1996, 2(2), 27–35

as tools the scientific credibility of the NCI and the ability of the industry to reach the entire U.S. population.

The 5 A Day Program endeavors to transmit its message through the mass media, government, industry, community channels, and research efforts.[15] Using social marketing techniques and theory driven strategies, the NCI and PBH work together to develop, implement, and evaluate a variety of interventions. The major program components are mass media, point of sale, community, and research. The national media campaign is designed to increase public awareness of the 5 A Day message and communicate the skills-building information needed to encourage Americans to eat more fruits and vegetables.

The national program facilitates partnering and assures consistent execution of the 5 A Day message in all channels by setting standards and establishing agreements with all partners participating in the program. The NCI has currently licensed 55 of the 56 state and territorial health departments as health authorities to organize state-level 5 A Day programs, and it has delegated to PBH the authority to license industry partners. National program guidelines have been developed for a variety of partners such as the health departments, supermarkets, restaurants and food service, merchandisers and suppliers.[16]

At present, approximately 1,200 industry partners, including retailers (with chains representing more than 30,000 supermarkets nationwide), state and federal agricultural commodity boards, branded companies, wholesalers, merchandisers, suppliers, and food services, are licensed to participate. The purpose of the retail component of the program is to reach consumers with informational and motivational messages at the point of purchase. The retailers and their suppliers participate in 5 A Day by displaying promotional materials and the logo on eligible products, incorporating the 5 A Day message in print and broadcast advertisements, developing interactive events in the supermarket such as taste tests and supermarket tours, and in resource-sharing with the community component through the state 5 A Day coalitions. Restaurants and food service operators are recent additions to the point of sale component.

Finally, both intervention research and nationwide evaluation are well underway. The research component consists of nine community-based research studies, funded by NCI in 1993 for four years.[17] These grants represent a second generation of community-based research, using community channels as the unit of randomization, a strategy that provides more power than the larger community-wide nonrandomized designs. The purpose of these grants is to implement and evaluate interventions aimed at increasing fruit and vegetable consumption among specific population segments in specific community channels, including worksites, schools, churches, and the Supplemental Food Program for Women, Infants, and Children.[17] The NCI will conduct a national survey to measure consumption in 1996 and a process evaluation of intervention activities by states and the industry.

In addition, the NCI funded in 1994 and 1995, in coordination with the Centers for Disease Control and Prevention (CDC), eight grants to evaluate 5 A Day activities implemented at the state level within specific community channels. In 1994 and 1995, CDC funded more than 30 intervention grants for one year addressing 5 A Day project areas.

PROGENITORS TO 5 A DAY

The origins of the 5 A Day Program are found in the previous community heart disease prevention trials and behavioral change research. The California Campaign adapted for its own use the elements of mass media information, education, community organization, and food system change from the North Karelia, Stanford, Minnesota Heart Health, and Pawtucket trials.[18–25] Execution of the campaign focused on channels with the greatest reach to the public, namely mass media, supermarkets, and government programs. A public-initiated partnership was developed between the produce industry and state health and agriculture departments. As the prototype was adapted for national use, strategies were modified to meet national needs.

PUBLIC/PRIVATE PARTNERSHIPS

Use of a public/private partnership as the mechanism to formulate and disseminate the 5 A Day message is one of the essential features of the National 5 A Day Program. Previous community trials and the Project LEAN initiative laid the groundwork for this approach (Table 1).[18–19,24,26] In North Karelia, partnerships were formed with the food industry.[18] Minnesota Heart Health, California, and Project LEAN built on and expanded this concept.[14,24,26] In addition, public confidence in messages from a credible health agency such as the NCI and promoted by industry had been shown to be a key factor in affecting consumer buying patterns.[27] Sales of high-fiber cereals rose dramatically after a national advertising campaign by the cereal industry that utilized government-approved health information.[28]

Development of a national partnership between the NCI and the fruit and vegetable industry was made possible by the formation of the PBH, a nonprofit consumer education organization representing the highly diverse fruit and vegetable industry. PBH represents the first time that the fruit and vegetable industry has collaborated on such a large scale with a health partner toward a common objective that embraced fresh, frozen, canned, and dried products. The prototype California 5 A Day Campaign had demonstrated the feasibility of a state health agency working in partnership with agriculture boards and commissions, branded fruit and vegetable companies, and supermarkets to deliver large-scale interventions with modest government resources. It also demonstrated the existence of substan-

Table 1 Key components of the 5 A Day program by community nutrition interventions

Key Components in 5 A Day	North Karelia Project	Stanford 3-Community	Stanford 5-City	Minnesota Heart Health Program	Minnesota Heart Health Program	Project LEAN
Nutrition	+	+	+	+	+	+
Simple specific message	–	–	–	–	–	+
Public/private partnership	+	–	–	+	–	+
Community involvement	+	+	+	+	+	+
Mass media	+	+	+	+	+	+
Theory based	+	+	+	+	+	+

tial interest in participation by states and industry groups outside California.[14] With the formation of PBH, it became feasible to elevate the partnership to a national level. The agreement between the NCI and PBH calls for the NCI to serve as the program's scientific voice to the public, secure health and government partners, conduct evaluation, and advance intervention research. PBH's role is to facilitate implementation in the food industry, work with the NCI to develop guidelines and program direction, assure that program standards are maintained by industry partners, and assist with evaluation.

Together, the NCI and PBH provide nationwide leadership, an infrastructure, and a template for action that transfers to the state and local levels. Nationally, the NCI and PBH conduct market research, develop promotional themes and materials, and generate publicity to support all partner activities. At the state and local levels, partners can build on these to organize and run complementary interventions with regional or locally relevant "hooks." As the program matures, additional collaborations with other national organizations, such as the American Dietetic Association (ADA), are being developed. The ADA will use its consumer hotline to reach consumers and urge its 65,000 members to participate in 5 A Day activities. This three-tiered approach of complementary national, state, and local roles represents a potentially powerful way to modify American eating habits.

MASS MEDIA

Mass media plays an essential role in the national 5 A Day Program. The Stanford trials of the '70s and the North Karelia Project showed that media are highly effective in increasing awareness and knowledge and can produce behavior change, but are more effective in achieving behavior change when combined with interactive components.[18,20] Results from the Pawtucket studies demonstrated the power of simple targeted messages delivered through the mass media channel in increasing awareness among a blue-collar population.[29]

Building upon these lessons and using a theory-driven, social marketing approach, the mass media component of the 5 A Day Program is implemented in a complementary fashion at the national level by NCI's Office of Cancer Communications and by PBH.[30] Focus group research was used to design targeted messages to the program's primary audience, identified currently as healthy members of the general public who are eating two to three servings of fruits and vegetables daily. Routine feedback from consumers, a central concept in the social marketing approach, helps ensure that the 5 A Day messages maintain their freshness and relevance.

Events held throughout the year promote the 5 A Day message in the media and to the public. These initiatives involve broadcast media, use of national spokespersons, print materials, and paid media events. Special 5 A Day events, such as the World's Largest Fruit Basket, involve the local community and create media interest. National 5 A Day Week, held each September, allows all partners to join forces for a period of high visibility, theme-related promotion. In 1995, the 5 A Day Week theme of "Take the 5 A Day Challenge" aimed to move consumers beyond awareness toward behavior change.

STATE AND COMMUNITY INVOLVEMENT

State and community involvement are key components of the 5 A Day Program. The program relies heavily on its state and community leaders to operationalize the 5 A Day Program. The importance of community involvement is drawn from the experiences in the North Karelia and Minnesota Heart Health studies, in particular. Both these projects successfully used a community organization approach to involve a network of leaders and organizations, led by advisory boards, to plan and deliver the interventions.[18,19,24]

Within the 5 A Day Program, state health agencies are licensed by the NCI to coordinate statewide 5 A Day activities at the state level. States are encouraged to develop coalitions as a forum for collaboration between the public and private sectors. State 5 A Day coalitions include representatives from state and local government, the fruit and vegetable industry, commodity boards/commissions, farmers' markets, food assistance programs, professional and voluntary organizations, community groups, medical centers, schools, universities, print and broadcast media, and business. The actual structure and composition of these coalitions is left to the discretion of the state program coordinators, in order to tailor program design to meet the needs of each state. The program guidelines provide a national template for state and local activities.[16]

By using the same standards, all recipes, photography, advertising, publicity, and other intervention materials have the potential for being used by partners throughout the country. Similarly, because all partners agree to participate in at least one promotion a year, a standard is set for a minimum level of promotional activity.

THEORETICAL UNDERPINNINGS

Theoretical models play an important role in developing the interventions, strategies, and media messages used at the national and state levels and in designing an outcome evaluation. Most of these same theoretical models have also been applied in varying degrees in the cardiovascular disease community trials and programs. North Karelia, the Stanford Trials, Minnesota Heart Health, Pawtucket, and Project LEAN used awareness, knowledge, motivation, skills development, and environmental constructs in their interventions.[18,21–26]

The specific objectives of the 5 A Day Program are to enhance public awareness of the need to eat five or more servings of fruits and vegetables daily and to create positive dietary behavior change. The latter is accomplished by employing strategies that build consumer skills, provide social support, and make the structural changes necessary to create positive dietary behavior.

Program communications are designed to recognize that people will be at different points in their readiness to act upon the 5 A Day message. Some people will be unaware of the message or aware of it but not yet ready to take action, others will be at the point of planning or acting upon the message, and still others will be looking for ways to maintain the behavior of eating five servings of fruits and vegetables or more daily. To reach these multiple segments that are at different points in the behavior change process, the program encourages partners to use a mix of both awareness and skills-building activities. This concept of behavior change as a stage-based process is drawn from the stages of change or transtheoretical model, and provides an overarching framework for guiding the translation of 5 A Day programming through the end of the decade.[31,32]

Stimulating awareness among Americans of the need to increase fruit and vegetable intake is a first step in promoting the 5 A Day message. The awareness construct, a cornerstone of the communication-persuasion approaches, is recognized as an important mediating variable between the acquisition of new knowledge and behavior change.[33,34] Motivation is also an important prerequisite to stimulating healthy behavior change. Drawing upon theories of persuasion such as Consumer Information Processing proposed by McGuire, many of the messages developed within the 5 A Day Program are framed to motivate, in addition to creating awareness and enhancing knowledge.[33] Understanding the consumer's perceived benefits of and barriers to eating more fruits and vegetables, constructs drawn from the Health Belief Model, has helped the 5 A Day Program develop convincing and timely messages and strategies.[35,36]

Once people are aware, interested in, and motivated to change their eating behaviors, they are ready to participate in the more action-oriented or interactive components of behavioral change. To assist them in this process, the 5 A Day Program has incorporated concepts from the social learning (or cognitive) theory.[37,38] These include efforts to increase self-efficacy through skills building and modeling activities; providing cues to reinforce the message at point of sale; and encouraging more supportive normative behavior within media, peer, family, community, and food purchasing environments.

Within the 5 A Day Program, the theoretical framework—or template—for dietary behavior change is established at the national level; it is operationalized at the state level. Working closely with the state licensees, the program encourages them to apply these theoretical approaches in the design and evaluation of their intervention efforts. The goal is to achieve longer-range, theory-driven strategies at national and state levels to affect and maintain positive dietary behavior change. The most important theoretical constructs by channels have been placed in a matrix that is valuable for program planning (Table 2). The matrix helps ensure that all of the elements thought to be necessary for behavior change are considered in design.

CHANNELS

Channels are a valuable organizing tool for community interventions and they provide for consistency in the delivery of 5 A Day messages and activities to millions of consumers.[14] Channels, like schools, supermarkets, worksites, churches,

Table 2 Matrix of theoretical constructs by channel

Channels	Awareness/ Knowledge	Motivation	Social Support	Skills Building	Environment	Policy
Media						
Supermarkets						
Schools						
Worksites						
Food assistance programs						
Churches						
Food service/ restaurants						
Health care settings						

food assistance programs, restaurants, and civic and service organizations can provide both educational opportunities and increased access to healthy foods. Channels are also open systems, interfacing with the larger community at a number of points, and thus, provide opportunities for changing social norms. Three commonly used channels are supermarkets, schools, and worksites.

Nutrition interventions in supermarkets have the potential of reaching consumers in all demographic strata. In the 5 A Day Program, the supermarket channel was initiated first and has received the most attention, including the use of the 5 A Day theme and logo in print and broadcast ads. The program encourages the inclusion of interactive events, such as supermarket tours and taste tests, within this channel to attract the attention of consumers and actively engage them in the program. For example, the Dole Food Company Supermarket Tours Initiative, which provides store tours for schoolchildren and features the 5 A Day message, is currently in use among a large number of schools across the nation. In this manner, supermarkets can also serve as a medium for cross-channel activity.

Periodic promotional campaigns that focus on specific themes, such as salads, fitness, entertaining, or microwaving, keep the program fresh and visible in grocery stores. Licensed states are encouraged to adapt these themes to their own state-based interventions.

Next to the supermarket channel, schools are one of the channels most frequently used as a setting for 5 A Day interventions. Expanding upon the experiences in the North Karelia Project, Minnesota Heart Health Program, Pawtucket Study, and Project LEAN, 5 A Day school-based interventions frequently consist of, classroom (e.g., curricula) and cafeteria activities.[18,19,24,26] By encouraging a combination of both types of activities, the program aims both to enhance knowledge and awareness of the 5 A Day message within the classroom and increase the visibility and availability of fruits and vegetables in the cafeteria. Four of the nine NCI 5 A Day grants include school-based interventions that incorporate classroom and cafeteria components, as well as parental involvement.[17] Several state agencies and industry partners have developed curricula for use in schools, such as the Indiana State Health Department and the Washington Apple Commission. Others have designed and implemented various school activities that complement other curricula, such as the California Department of Health Services, the Montana Department of Health and Environmental Sciences, and the Dole Food Company.

A third channel that is frequently used in the 5 A Day Program is worksites. The setting offers access to a substantial proportion of the adult population and includes social support systems to assist individuals in changing their behaviors. Worksites were used in the North Karelia, Pawtucket Study, and Project LEAN.[18,26,40] In addition, recent findings from the Working Well Trial, a randomized trial of 114 worksites that had core interventions aimed at individual and environmental change, demonstrated positive changes in fruit and vegetable, fat and fiber dietary behaviors among treatment compared with control worksites. Working Well strategies included campaigns, group activities, self-help materials, and environmental activities such as labeling of foods in cafeterias and vending machines and use of catering policies.[41,42]

In 5 A Day, states are spreading the 5 A Day message in worksites through employee paycheck stuffers and worksite wellness programs. Three of the nine NCI 5 A Day research grants are also conducting worksite specific interventions involving interpersonal networks of peer educational programs and family support in changing eating habits at the worksite.[17]

SUMMARY AND CONCLUSION

Distinguishing features of the national 5 A Day Program are activation of government and food industry systems at the national, state, and local levels, the creation of public/private and national/state/local partnerships, the development of periodic and theme-related mass media, the generation of activity in organized channels that reaches the public directly, and the use of constructs from a variety of behavior change theories. Drawn from past community-based intervention trials, these elements form the framework for the program. Although the overall results of the community intervention trials have been disappointing, the components of the interventions, upon which the 5 A Day Program was modeled, were deemed to be effective.[43]

The 5 A Day Program has expanded on the common program elements that link these trials, but differs from them in scope and design. All the programs mentioned, with the exception of Project LEAN, were research endeavors. Nutrition was a part of the mix of factors addressed. They were communitywide in scope with small sample sizes (two to six communities) and nonrandomized quasi-experimental designs. Project LEAN was a national nutrition campaign to reduce dietary fat consumption, generated by the Kaiser Family Foundation, with the support of a broad partnership of organizations and community-based projects.[26] The 5 A Day program is a national public/private partnership that combines research with a national health promotion program. Its research strategy differs from the first generation of community trials in the following ways: (1) the intervention addresses a single, simple nutrition message; and (2) the research is focused in specific community channels to allow for random assignment of large sample sizes (n = 12 to 24), a design that provides more power than the communitywide trials. This design will also produce tested interventions for a variety of settings that can be combined into a communitywide or national effort.

In looking to the future, the 5 A Day Program envisions a need for more channel-specific, theory-driven interventions that are proven effective in changing eating behavior. Some channels that provide a challenge for research are restaurants, food assistance programs, child care programs, community organizations, and physicians' offices. Not only 5 A Day but the field of nutrition would profit from more research on environmental supports for sustaining dietary behavior changes. This would include an exploration of the impact of changes in eating environments (restaurants, airlines, airports, school lunch), the food system (food producers and manufacturers), legislation and policies (catering policies), and on eating behavior.

For 5 A Day to succeed in changing national dietary behaviors, it must reach broader audiences more frequently than its current penetration. In order to do this, it must have more of a media presence and more action through the industry and community components. Both industry and government need to make a renewed commitment to support the program with staff and financial resources if this is to happen. The future of the 5 A Day for Better Health Program lies in capitalizing on the partnerships and the extensive diffusion infrastructure of licensed state health agency and industry partners, working through state and local coalitions. Providing the states with the capacity to implement tested channel-specific, theory driven interventions will be key in building on the current momentum of the 5 A Day Program. Unfortunately, resources for states are extremely limited. Although each state has a designated 5 A Day Program coordinator, no funds were available for implementation until 1994, when the CDC, working with NCI, provided funds for half the states for one year. To mount a sustained effort in which local retailers, restaurateurs, and other coalition members are consistently active requires staffing time dedicated to the program. The activation of this program network is a rare opportunity for both research and potential national impact on dietary behavior change. A national partnership of this nature is difficult to initiate and maintain. It would be a sadly missed opportunity if adequate resources were not made available to sustain such a good beginning.

Important new directions for the program include cross promotion with foods outside the fruit and vegetable category to increase the reach of 5 A Day. The 5 A Day model could also be used by other food groups such as grains. Other nations have already requested program information in order to develop their own programs. Results of the 1996 survey on consumption and results from the nine grants expected in 1997 will provide more data for future program directions.

•   •   •

As the entire field of community interventions reexamines its future directions based on the recent results of communitywide interventions, the 5 A Day Program has the capacity to test new approaches using its existing infrastructure.[44] A new series of grants should be funded, allowing researchers to test new ideas using a simple, targeted message. The strategy of focusing research in specific channels enables better control of the environmental component of change, and could provide progress in this arena. With continued funding made available through the program, research can be done on improved methods of dietary assessment, biomarkers for consumption, tested behavioral theories, the testing of environmental and policy initiatives, and other issues of concern to the larger field of community nutrition. The 5 A Day Program has the potential to serve as a national laboratory for research in testing new strategies and diffusing successful innovations.

REFERENCES

1. Doll, R., and Peto, R. "The Causes of Cancer: Quantitative Estimates of Avoidable Risk of Cancer in the United States Today." *Journal of the National Cancer Institute* 66 (1981): 1191–1308.

2. U.S. Department of Health and Human Services. *Cancer Control Objectives for the Nation: 1985–2000,* edited by P. Greenwald and E. Sondik. National Cancer Institute Monographs (2). Rockville, Md.: DHHS, 1986.

3. U.S. Department of Health and Human Services, Public Health Service. *The Surgeon General's Report on Nutrition and Health.* Washington, D.C.: Government Printing Office, 1988.

4. National Academy of Sciences. *Diet and Health: Implications for Reducing Chronic Disease Risk.* Washington, D.C.: National Academy Press, 1989.

5. U.S. Department of Health and Human Services. *Healthy People 2000: National Health Promotion and Disease Prevention Objectives.* DHHS Pub. No. (PHS) 91-50212. Washington, D.C.: Government Printing Office, 1990.

6. U.S. Departments of Agriculture and Health and Human Services. *Nutrition and Your Health: Dietary Guidelines for Americans.* Home and Garden Bull. No. 232. Washington, D.C.: 1995.

7. Steinmetz, K.A., and Potter, J.D. "Vegetables, Fruit and Cancer. I. Epidemiology." *Cancer Causes and Control* 2 (1991): 325–357.

8. Block, G., Patterson, B., and Subar, A. "Fruit, Vegetables, and Cancer Prevention: A Review of the Epidemiological Evidence." *Nutrition and Cancer* 18 (1992): 1–29.

9. Ziegler, R.G. "Vegetables, Fruits, and Carotenoids and the Risk of Cancer." *American Journal of Clinical Nutrition* 53 (1991): 251S–259S.

10. Ziegler, R.G., et al. "Does Beta Carotene Explain Why Reduced Cancer Risk Is Associated with Vegetable and Fruit intake." *Cancer Research* (1992): 2060S–2066S.

11. Negri, E., et al. "Vegetable and Fruit Consumption and Cancer Risk." *International Journal of Cancer* 48 (1991): 350–354.

12. Willett, W.C. "Vitamin A and Lung Cancer." *Nutrition Review* 48, no. 5 (1990): 201–211.

13. Steinmetz, K.A., and Potter, J.D. Vegetables, Fruit, and Cancer. II. Mechanisms." *Cancer Causes and Control* 2 (1991): 427–441.

14. Foerster, S.B., et al. "California's 'Five a Day—for Better Health!' Campaign: An Innovative Population-Based Effort to Effect Large-Scale Dietary Change." *American Journal of Preventive Medicine* 11, no. 2 (1995): 124–131.

15. Heimendinger, J., and Van Duyn, M.A. "Dietary Behavior Change: The Challenge of Recasting the Role of Fruit and Vegetables in the American Diet." *American Journal of Clinical Nutrition* 61, suppl. (1995): 1397S–1401S.

16. National Cancer Institute. *5 A Day for Better Health Program. Program Guidebook.* Bethesda, Md.: National Cancer Institute, 1994.

17. Havas, S., et al. "5 A Day for Better Health: A New Research Initiative." *Journal of the American Dietetic Association* 94 (1994): 32–36.

18. Puska, P., et al. "The Community-Based Strategy to Prevent Coronary Heart Disease: Conclusions from the Ten Years of the North Karelia Project." *Annual Review of Public Health* 6 (1985): 147–193.

19. Nissinen, A., Tuomilehto, J., and Puska, P. "From Pilot Project to National Implementation: Experiences from the North Karelia Project." *Scandinavian Journal of Primary Health Care,* suppl. 1 (1988): 49–56.

20. Farquhar, J., et al. "Community Education for Cardiovascular Disease." *Lancet* 1 (1977): 1192–1195.

21. Stern, M., et al. "Results of a Two-Year Health Education Campaign on Dietary Behavior." *Circulation* 54 (1976): 826–833.

22. Fortmann, S.P. "Effect of Health Education on Dietary Behavior: The Stanford 3 Community Study." *American Journal of Clinical Nutrition* 34 (1981): 2030–2038.

23. Farquhar, J.W. "The Stanford Five-City Project: Design and Methods." *American Journal of Epidemiology* 122, no. 2 (1985): 323–334.

24. Mittelmark, M., et al. "Community-wide Prevention and Cardiovascular Disease: Education Strategies of the Minnesota Heart Health Program." *Preventive Medicine* 15 (1986): 1–17.

25. Lefebvre, R.C., et al. "Theory and Delivery of Health Programming in the Community: The Pawtucket Heart Health Program." *Preventive Medicine* 16 (1987): 80–95.

26. Samuels, S.E. "Project LEAN—Lessons Learned from a National Social Marketing Campaign." *Public Health Reports* 108, no. 1 (1933): 45–53.

27. Hammond, S. *Health Advertising: The Credibility of Organizational Sources.* Paper presented to International Communication Association's annual meeting, Health Communication Division, Chicago, Ill., 1986.

28. Levy, A., and Stokes, R. "Effect of a Health Promotion Advertising Campaign on Sales of Ready-to-Eat Cereal." *Public Health Report* 102 (1987): 398–403.

29. Wallack, L. "Mass Media Campaigns: The Odds Against Finding Behavior Change." *Health Education Quarterly* 8 (1981): 209–260.

30. Kotler, P., and Roberto, E.L. *Social Marketing: Strategies for Changing Public Behavior.* New York: Free Press, 1989.

31. Prochaska, J.O., and DiClemente, C.C. "Transtheoretical Therapy: Toward a More Integrative Model of Change." *Psychotherapy: Theory, Research, and Practice* 20 (1982): 161–173.

32. Prochaska, J.O., and DiClemente, C.C. "Stages of Change in the Modification of Problem Behaviors." In *Progress in Behavior Modification,* edited by M. Hersen, R.M. Eisler, and P.M. Millers. New York: Academic Press, 1992.

33. McGuire, W.J. "Attitudes and Attitudes Change." In *Handbook of Social Psychology,* Vol. 2, 3rd ed., edited by G. Lindzey and E. Aronsen. New York: Random House, 1985.

34. Cialdini, R.B., Petty, R.E., and Cacioppo, J.T. "Attitude and Attitude Change." *Annual Reviews in Psychology* 32 (1981): 357–404.

35. Janz, N.K., and Becker, M.H. "The Health Belief Model: A Decade Later." *Health Education Monographs* 11 (1984): 1–47.

36. Rosenstock, I.M. "The Health Belief Model: Explaining Health Behavior Through Expectancies." In *Health Behavior and Health Education: Theory, Research and Practice,* edited by K. Glanz, F.M. Lewis, and B.K. Rimer. San Francisco: Jossey-Bass Publishers, 1990.

37. Bandura, A. *Social Learning Theory.* Englewood Cliffs, N.J.: Prentice-Hall, 1977.

38. Glanz, Z., Lewis, F.M., and Rimer, B.K. *Health Behavior and Health Education: Theory, Research and Practice.* San Francisco: Jossey-Bass Publishers, 1990.

39. Carleton, R.A., et al. "The Pawtucket Heart Health Program: Community Changes in Cardiovascular Risk Factors and Projected Disease Risk." *American Journal of Public Health* 85 (1995): 777–785.

40. Linnan, L.A., et al. "Marketing Cardiovascular Disease Risk Reduction Programs at the Workplace: The Pawtucket Heart Health Program Experience." *American Association of Occupational Health Nurses* 38, no. 9 (1990): 409–418.

41. Heimendinger, J., et al. "The Working Well Trial: Baseline Dietary and Smoking Behaviors of Employees and Other Worksite Characteristics." *Preventive Medicine* 24 (1995): 180–193.

42. Sorensen, G., et al. "Working Well: Results from a Worksite-Based Cancer Prevention Trial." *American Journal of Public Health.*

43. Fortmann, S.P., et al. "Community Intervention Trials: Reflections on the Stanford Five-City Project Experience." *American Journal of Epidemiology* 142, no. 6 (1995): 576–586.

44. Luepker, R.V., et al. "Community Education for Cardiovascular Disease Prevention: Risk Factor Changes in the Minnesota Heart Health Program." *American Journal of Public Health* 84 (1994): 1383–1393.

10

The National Breast and Cervical Cancer Early Detection Program

Rosemarie M. Henson, Stephen W. Wyatt, and Nancy C. Lee

Breast cancer is the most commonly diagnosed cancer and the second leading cause of cancer death among women in the United States. For 1995, the American Cancer Society estimates that breast cancer will be diagnosed in 180,000 women, and 46,000 women will die from the disease.[1] We currently do not know how to prevent breast cancer from occurring. Thus, detecting carcinoma of the breast at an early stage is the key to more treatment options, improved survival, and decreased mortality.[2] Research has shown that the use of mammography can reduce the mortality due to breast cancer among women 50 years and older by 30 percent.[3,4]

The overall incidence of invasive cervical cancer has decreased steadily over the past several decades, but in recent years this rate has increased among women who are less than 50 years old. In 1995, invasive cervical cancer will be diagnosed in approximately 15,800 women, and carcinoma in situ will be diagnosed in about 65,000 women. In this same year, about 4,800 women will die of cervical cancer.[1] The primary goal of cervical cancer screening is to increase detection and treatment of precancerous cervical lesions and thus prevent the occurrence of cervical cancer. Although no clinical trials have studied the efficacy of the Papanicolaou (Pap) test in reducing cervical cancer mortality, experts agree that it is an effective technology.[5] Since the introduction of the Pap test in the 1940s, cervical cancer mortality rates have decreased by 75 percent.[5]

Although mammograms and Pap tests are crucial components of a cancer prevention and control strategy, they are routinely underused. In *Healthy People 2000,* the Public Health Service (PHS) established that by the year 2000, 60 percent of women aged 50 years and older should receive a mammogram every two

The authors acknowledge the assistance of Janet Abrams, Kate Egan, and Sara Craig who obtained the legislative information that documents the history of the Breast and Cervical Cancer Mortality Prevention Act of 1990.

J Public Health Management Practice, 1996, 2(2), 36–47

years.[6] However, the baseline data on mammography use from the 1987 National Health Interview Survey (NHIS) showed that only 23 percent of women 50 years and older reported having received a mammogram within the past three years. This proportion was lower for racial and ethnic minority women, for women who had less than a high school education, for women who were over age 75 years, and for women who were living below the poverty level.[7]

In 1991, the PHS established that, by the year 2000, 85 percent of women should be receiving a Pap test within the preceding one to three years.[6] Baseline data on the use of the Pap test from the 1987 NHIS indicated that only 65 percent of women aged 18 years and older reported having received a Pap test within the past three years.[7] As with the use of mammography screening, this proportion was lower for racial and ethnic minority women, for women who had less than a high school education, for women who were over age 75 years, and for women who had low incomes.

Studies have consistently shown multiple barriers to the routine use of breast and cervical cancer screening services. These barriers have included the costs associated with the screening tests, lack of physician recommendation for screening, lack of knowledge about the importance of early detection, and fear of learning of a diagnosis of cancer.[8] Studies have also shown that women without health insurance are less likely than those with insurance to seek and obtain clinical preventive services. Kaluzny et al. report that low income and old age translate into low use of cancer screening services.[8] Studies show that these barriers remain consistent, but the extent to which they play a role in the underutilization of these screening tools tends to vary between individuals and communities.

The complex problem of increasing access to cancer-screening services cannot be adequately addressed by interventions that target only one barrier at a time. Rather, the design and implementation of carefully coordinated comprehensive programs that use innovative strategies to address multiple barriers are essential if the use of screening services is to be increased. In response to this need, the Centers for Disease Control and Prevention (CDC) established the National Breast and Cervical Cancer Early Detection Program (NBCCEDP) in 1990. This Program forms the foundation for a comprehensive, national effort for the control of breast and cervical cancer.

ORGANIZATIONAL SETTING

Founded in 1946, the CDC is an agency within the PHS. It is internationally renowned for its critical work in controlling infectious illnesses, such as malaria, smallpox, polio, and Legionnaires' disease. In the mid-1980s, CDC expanded its activities in chronic disease control and made a strong commitment to reducing morbidity and mortality from chronic illnesses. A review of CDC's chronic disease control functions revealed that many of the activities were located in different organizational settings throughout the agency and lacked a concentrated focus. In 1985, a limited budget of approximately $3 million was provided to teams within CDC to award competitive grants for chronic disease projects. In 1988, the chronic disease functions and activities within the agency were reorganized into the National Center for Chronic Disease Prevention and Health Promotion (NCCDPHP).

The mission of NCCDPHP is to prevent premature death and disability from chronic diseases and to promote healthy personal behaviors. Breast and cervical cancer control was identified as a top priority for the new center. It was the vision of CDC that the same public health strategies used to manage infectious diseases should be used to successfully combat breast and cervical cancer. The control of these cancers should be incorporated into the public health system in much the same way as programs that promote the control of tuberculosis, sexually transmitted diseases, and the acquired immunodeficiency syndrome epidemic.

As the nation's prevention agency, CDC enjoys a strong working relationship with state and local health agencies across the country. Placing state health agencies in a leadership role for the development of intervention programs for cancer control was viewed as a natural progression from their efforts in implementing infectious disease program. The presence of such programs would recognize the critical role health agencies need to play in the prevention and control of breast and cervical cancer.[9] In 1990, the passage of the Breast and Cervical Cancer Mortality Prevention Act created the first opportunity for state health agencies to build a state and local public health infrastructure for cancer control and broadly for chronic disease prevention and control.[10]

CONGRESS RESPONDS

The passage of the Breast and Cervical Cancer Mortality Prevention Act of 1990 was a product of rapid bipartisan action by the Congress and the Executive Branch.[10] This act, which was authored and introduced by Congressman Henry Waxman in the House of Representatives, established a nationwide, comprehensive public health program to increase access to breast and cervical screening services for women who are medically underserved.

The health care climate at the time was one of increasing public and congressional concern about women's health issues. Through the 1970s and 1980s, many prominent women became active in the fight against breast cancer. In 1989, the Executive and Legislative branches of the federal government became increasingly concerned about the disease burden from breast cancer and missed opportunities to detect and treat premalignant and preinvasive cervical neoplasia. Many policy makers recognized the importance of establishing a nationwide infrastructure to increase the use of mammography and Pap test screenings among all women by implementing early detection programs designed to address multiple barriers to screening. Of special concern to congressional and government leaders was the poor use of these screening tests among women who were uninsured and underinsured and among racial and ethnic minority women.

As the Congress moved forward to draft the legislation, the PHS began to lay the foundation for a national early detection effort. In fiscal year (FY) 1990, CDC received appropriations of $5 million to establish partnerships with several state health agencies to design early detection programs for medically underserved women. The CDC awarded grants of approximately $400,000 to $555,000 to four states: Colorado, Minnesota, South Carolina, and West Virginia. These resources were used to establish state breast and cervical cancer activities that would start to build the infrastructure for early detection efforts.

In early 1990, Henry Waxman, Chairman of the Subcommittee on Health and Environment of the House Energy and Commerce Committee, introduced a bill to establish a state-based initiative offering free breast and cervical cancer screening services to women with low incomes. The program, which was to be administered by CDC, also provided for public and professional education, quality assurance, and surveillance and evaluation systems to monitor program activities. Waxman's initiative received bipartisan support and was passed in June of 1990. Senator Barbara Mikulski championed the bill in the Senate and secured passage with a wide majority in August 1990. Marilyn Quayle provided strong support for the program. Once the legislation was passed by Congress, it was signed into law by President George Bush on August 10, 1990. The landmark legislation marked important progress in the fight to prevent and control chronic diseases and contributed momentum to the wave of national interest in women's health issues.

The legislation, Public Law (PL) 101-354, established a program of grants to states to carry out activities in six key areas:

1. to screen medically underserved women for breast and cervical cancer,
2. to provide appropriate and timely referrals for medical treatment for women with abnormal screening tests and ensure the provision of follow-up services,
3. to develop and disseminate public information and education related to the detection and control of breast and cervical cancer,
4. to improve training of health professionals in the detection and control of breast and cervical cancer,
5. to establish mechanisms for monitoring the quality of screening procedures and the quality of interpretation of such procedures, and
6. to evaluate program activities through the establishment of surveillance systems.[10]

The act specifies that at least 60 percent of funds received by a state should be expended on screening and referral services.[10] The other 40 percent of funds can be used to support public and provider education, quality assurance, and surveillance and evaluation activities. Only 10 percent of the state funds can be used for administrative expenses. The NBCCEDP is the payer of last resort for screening services. Grant monies cannot be used to pay for services if other coverage is available through any state fund, private health insurance, or other government health benefits program, such as Medicaid and Medicare. States are also required to contribute $1 for every $3 of federal funds. States are allowed to donate personnel and other services as part of their match to the CDC grant.

The issue that has caused the greatest controversy concerns the availability of funds to pay for the treatment of women diagnosed with cancerous or precancerous lesions. Congressman Waxman was concerned that uninsured women who were diagnosed with breast and cervical cancers would be stranded in the health care system with no ability to pay for treatment. Because the use of federal monies to pay for treatment services might rapidly deplete the funds available for screening services, Congress decided that the states would be required to ensure that women with cancerous and precancerous lesions receive timely and appropriate treatment services. However, these services could not be reimbursed through the NBCCEDP funds.

THE NATIONAL STRATEGIC PLAN

The enactment of legislation in 1990 coincided with a charge to CDC from the Department of Health and Human Services to lead a planning effort that would result in the development of a National Strategic Plan for the early detection and control of breast and cervical cancers.[9] This charge was issued by the Assistant Secretary for Health of PHS after members of the Association of State and Territorial Health Officials, the National Association of County Health Officials, and the United States Conference of Local Health Officials called on PHS to strengthen the federal emphasis on those cancers that primarily affect women. The process of developing the national plan was coordinated by three PHS agencies: the CDC, the Food and Drug Administration (FDA), and the National Institutes of Health. A series of interactive meetings were initiated by these three agencies to obtain input from the public, private, and voluntary sectors. More than 75 national organizations provided guidance during the process. This guidance resulted in the development and publication of the National Strategic Plan in 1993. The plan addressed cancer control issues in five critical areas: (1) the integration and coordination of screening services, (2) public education, (3) professional education and practice, (4) quality assurance, and (5) surveillance and evaluation. During implementation of the NBCCEDP, the plan was a valuable guide to CDC. Many of the priority issues identified in the plan are now addressed by CDC, state and local health agencies and their partners as they implement breast and cervical cancer early detection programs.

BUILDING STATE AND TRIBAL INFRASTRUCTURE

The Congress appropriated $30 million in FY 1991 for the first year of this program. In the summer of 1991, CDC used a competitive application process to fund the first eight states. State health agencies were given grants averaging $3 million to fund comprehensive screening programs in California, Colorado, Michigan, Minnesota, New Mexico, South Carolina, Texas, and West Virginia. In FY 1992, appropriations increased to $50 million, and CDC was able to expand the number of states receiving support for comprehensive screening program from 8 to 12. In January 1992, CDC added four new states—Maryland, Missouri, Nebraska, and North Carolina.

During the first two years of implementation, CDC recognized that the initial 12 states would have benefited from resources for planning and for developing an infrastructure before the infusion of funds for screening services. In these states, start-up time averaged 15 months before screening actually began. Start-up activities included: (1) recruiting and hiring a cancer control staff; (2) identifying and contracting with provider organizations to deliver screening services; (3) building partnerships with hospitals and community-based organizations to obtain support for diagnostic, treatment, and support services; (4) developing billing and reimbursement systems that are coordinated with other third party payers, such as Medicare and Medicaid; (5) designing public education and outreach strategies; and (6) establishing a surveillance system to track and follow women.

To allow time for infrastructure development, CDC established the Capacity Building Program in October 1992. A competitive application process was used to award grants that ranged from $225,000 to $280,000 to 18 additional states to help them prepare for the delivery of screening programs. These capacity building resources enabled states to hire staff, develop cancer plans and coalitions, carry out public and professional education efforts, improve and monitor quality assurance systems, and design and enhance surveillance activities.

The program continued to expand in FY 1993 with appropriations of $72 million. Using a competitive application process, CDC added six more comprehensive states—Massachusetts, New York, Ohio, Pennsylvania, Washington, and Wisconsin. These six states had all been awarded capacity building grants the previous year. In this same year, an additional nine states joined the Capacity Building Program, and by October 1993, the NBCCEDP was active in 45 states.

Congressional hearings were also held in 1993 on the activities and accomplishments of the NBCCEDP. Following these hearings, Congress reauthorized PL

101-354, the Breast and Cervical Cancer Mortality Prevention Act, and added several key amendments to the legislation. The new legislation, PL 103-183, required CDC to give funding priority to those states with a high disease burden from breast or cervical cancer.[11] Grant funds could only be made available to states that provided coverage for mammograms and Pap tests through their state Medicaid programs. States could pay no more than the Medicare rate for screening and diagnostic procedures.

Congress also directed CDC to establish a grant program with American Indian tribes and tribal organizations to increase screening services among American Indian women. CDC launched this major initiative in 1993 and began to build important relationships with tribal leaders and American Indian organizations across the country. In October 1994, nine tribes and tribal organizations were funded through a competitive application process to establish comprehensive screening programs.

In FY 1994, with an appropriation of $78 million, CDC provided support to 26 states and 9 tribes and tribal organizations for comprehensive screening programs. Twenty-four states, three territories, and the District of Columbia were funded as Capacity Building Programs. The NBCCEDP was truly nationwide.

In FY 1995, CDC entered its fifth year of this program with an appropriation of $100 million. CDC provided funding to 35 states and 9 tribes and tribal organizations for comprehensive screening programs. Fifteen states, three territories, and the District of Columbia received planning and infrastructure grants as part of the Capacity Building Program (Figure 1).

PROGRAM DESIGN AND IMPLEMENTATION

Removing financial barriers to screening is only the first step toward reducing mortality from breast and cervical cancers, particularly among women who are medically underserved. If the health service delivery system is to reach these women, a comprehensive approach is needed that integrates and coordinates the following critical elements: screening, referral, and follow-up services, public education and outreach, professional education, quality assurance, surveillance, and partnership development.

SCREENING, REFERRAL, AND FOLLOW-UP SYSTEM

The NBCCEDP reimburses states for clinical breast exams, screening mammograms, pelvic exams, Pap tests, and some diagnostic procedures. State health agencies contract with a broad range of provider agencies to deliver screening services. Each state has developed its own delivery system based upon available resources.

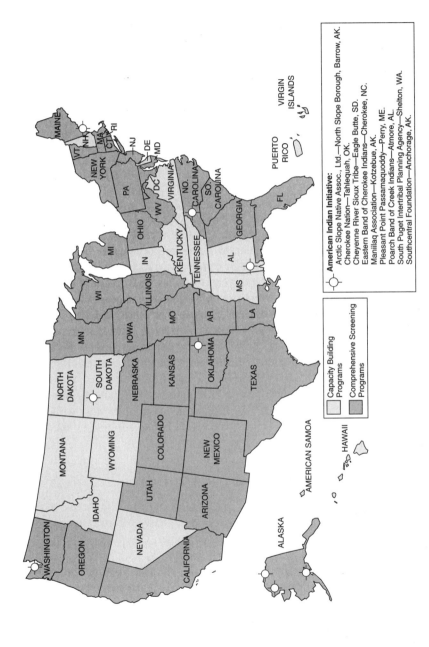

Figure 1. National Breast and Cervical Cancer Early Detection Program—1995.

In Texas, for example, the state health department contracts with community and migrant health centers, Young Women's Christian Associations (YWCA) of the USA, family planning organizations, community-based organizations, and county health departments. In Nebraska, where a county health department system does not exist and where few community-based organizations are established, the state contracts directly with private physicians. Maryland and Michigan contract primarily with local and county health departments. Contracts with these agencies can include support for screening and diagnostic procedures; public education; coalition activities; and clinical, outreach, and administrative support staff.

When PL 101-354 was passed by Congress, states were concerned about the burden that treatment would place on their health care system given that no federal funds were available to pay for treatment and limited resources were available for diagnostic services. Establishing a network of medical providers who are willing to donate these services is a challenge for many states. States have shown creativity and determination in identifying and securing financial resources for diagnostic and treatment services for women who are served by the NBCCEDP. Resources for these services vary across states and are a reflection of state and local government support, medical provider generosity, and community commitment. Examples include county programs for the underserved, state-funded cancer clinics, and legislative mandates to use cigarette tax revenues for diagnostic or treatment services. In some states, community commitment ranges from local efforts to raise funds for diagnostic and treatment services to the willingness of a national or local foundation to pay for these services for women who lack resources for care. For example, the Susan G. Komen Breast Cancer Foundation has donated resources from its annual Race for the Cure for diagnostic and treatment services in several states. Medical providers and hospitals in communities have been critical partners by donating diagnostic and treatment services. Many states have hired case managers to work with provider organizations to ensure that each woman who requires follow-up receives appropriate and timely diagnostic and treatment services.

Public Education and Outreach

Public education and outreach has played an important role in the success of the NBCCEDP. Using a variety of intensive community-based efforts, the program has successfully screened medically underserved women. One of the early important lessons learned was that the NBCCEDP could not expect to reach women in need of screening without developing partnerships with those organizations that have for many years served the priority populations CDC wanted to reach. Public education materials and outreach strategies needed to be sensitive to the groups targeted by the state program with regard to culture, language, and literacy.[12] Examples of innovative community-based strategies have included the following interventions and activities:

- The Texas Department of Health funds the YWCA in Abilene to provide screening services. The YWCA recruits women in this predominantly rural area through churches, clinics, senior centers, and programs affiliated with the YWCA. To facilitate access to screening services, the YWCA provides transportation to the clinic sites. The YWCA also ensures that women with abnormal tests receive appropriate and timely follow-up and identifies financial resources for diagnostic and treatment services.
- In Maryland, the state health department has placed state funded outreach workers at each of the county health departments throughout the state to enhance the program's intervention efforts. The women hired for these positions come from the community and are primarily older minority women. The outreach workers recruit women who are in need of screening services from various sites including senior citizen centers, low-income housing, factories, homemaker clubs, thrift shops, churches, influenza vaccination clinics, and nursing homes.
- In Massachusetts, the program has developed printed materials for women whose primary language is not English or whose reading ability is limited. Focus groups were held with women who were 60 years and older to test concepts and educational materials. Public education materials are provided to program participants in Haitian-Creole, English, French, and Spanish.
- In New York, the state health department established the concept of Breast Health Partnerships as a unique method of delivering screening services throughout the state. The Breast Health Partnerships work to bring the resources of all the partners in a community together to address and overcome barriers to screening. For example, the Batavia community in Genesee County established a Breast Health Partnership with participation from more

---

Professional Organizations

- American Academy of Physician Assistants
- American College of Radiology
- American College of Physicians
- American Medical Women's Association
- American Nurses Association
- Association of Teachers of Preventive Medicine
- National Medical Association

than 30 agencies. The Saint Jerome's Hospital Healthy Living Unit functions as the coordinating agency and the data management center. The YWCA of Genesee County manages the reimbursement of screening services for the partnership. Some of the participating agencies include the ACS, Office for Aging, United Way, the Tonawanda Tribe, Genesee Memorial Hospital, and Planned Parenthood.

Professional Education

Several studies have shown that women are significantly more likely to seek screening if they have a physician's recommendation.[13,14] The National Strategic Plan suggests that each encounter—with an emergency room physician, an obstetrician or gynecologist, an internist, a dentist, or a nurse—is an opportunity for a health care provider to educate women about screening for breast and cervical cancers.

In launching the NBCCEDP, CDC established important relationships with major professional organizations across the country. The CDC has provided resources to these organizations for the development of training materials, physician reminder systems, and educational curricula to improve skills in the areas of screening, quality assurance, communication, and counseling.

State health agencies have targeted many of their professional education efforts to family practitioners, internists, obstetricians and gynecologists, nurses, physicians' assistants, and other allied health professionals. The focus of the training has been on detection and diagnostic procedures, communication skills, guidelines for screening, data collection and reporting requirements, and the strengthening of clinical skills.

QUALITY ASSURANCE

The National Strategic Plan suggests that an effective quality assurance system for a breast cancer screening program provides confidence that a technically satisfactory mammogram was performed, that the results were interpreted properly, and that the results were reported to the referring clinician and the woman in a timely manner.[9]

Quality assurance strategies for cervical cancer screening have focused on both improved specimen collection by the primary care practitioner and on interpretation by the laboratory.[9] The Clinical Laboratory Improvements Act of 1988 (CLIA 88) has increased the federal role in evaluation and oversight of laboratory performance.[15] Quality control measures and proficiency testing are being developed and implemented to improve diagnostic accuracy.

With the passage of PL 101-354 in 1990, Congress recognized the importance of improving the quality of mammography and cytological services nationwide.[10] CDC developed technical guidelines for mammography and cytology services for facilities participating in the NBCCEDP. To ensure high-quality screening tests, all mammography facilities are required to meet standards of the American College of Radiology and all cytology laboratories are required to meet CLIA 88 standards. In 1993, the reauthorization required the state programs to adhere to the new standards for mammography quality assurance developed by FDA.

State health agencies have taken several important steps to develop and improve quality assurance programs for mammography and cytological services. Medical advisory committees have been organized in states to provide technical guidance, assist with training activities, review and develop clinical protocols, and develop guidelines and systems to ensure that the breast and cervical cancer screening process is carried out in a safe and effective manner. Training and education activities have been provided to radiologists, radiologic technologists, and cytotechnologists. Additional staff have been hired in some states to monitor the compliance of mammography facilities and cytopathology laboratories with state and federal quality assurance standards and requirements.

Surveillance

Surveillance activities are necessary to effectively evaluate the program's progress in meeting established goals and objectives. When the NBCCEDP was implemented in 1991, CDC, in collaboration with its state partners, developed a set of minimum data elements to monitor the program's screening, diagnostic, and treatment activities.

For each woman receiving screening services, the states collect and report to CDC information on screening location, demographic characteristics, screening results, diagnostic procedures and outcomes, and initial treatment. The tracking and follow-up of women with abnormal test results has been a labor intensive activity for states. Tracking and reminder systems have been implemented in clinics to ensure timely follow-up of all women with abnormal findings and treatment of all women with cancer or precancerous conditions. Reminder systems have also been implemented to encourage all women with normal screening exams to return for rescreening at the appropriate interval. Many states have a surveillance team that consists of epidemiologic and data management staff to manage the surveillance component of the program.

These data are used to help state health agencies implement, monitor, and evaluate their screening programs; provide Congress and CDC partners with data on the progress and accomplishments of the NBCCEDP; and direct and evaluate CDC's breast and cervical cancer control efforts.

National Partnerships

The ability to implement a national strategic effort to control breast and cervical cancers depends largely on the assistance provided by partners in both the public and private sectors. CDC relies heavily on its partnerships with national, voluntary, and private organizations to build the necessary infrastructure at the community level to provide screening services for all women who need them. These partners have played a critical role in assisting state health agencies in reaching priority populations, such as women with low incomes, racial and ethnic minorities, women with low literacy skills, older women, and lesbians.

At the national and state level, the CDC and its state partners have established a strong working relationship with the ACS. Through its national office and local divisions, ACS assists in the development and delivery of CDC-directed programs. Local ACS divisions serve as active partners with state health agencies to increase access to screening services among women who are medically underserved. CDC collaborates with ACS staff in all programmatic areas, including the implementation of early detection programs, public and provider education, and cosponsorship of conferences.

In 1993, CDC entered into a unique partnership with Avon Products, Inc., YWCA of the USA, The National Alliance of Breast Cancer Organizations (NABCO), and the National Cancer Institute (NCI) to improve access to early detection services. Avon created the Avon Breast Access Fund and raised $10 million to support community-based efforts through the sale of its Breast Cancer Awareness pin and key ring. Avon has funded more than 125 programs through the YWCA of the USA and NABCO. These organizations work closely with state health agencies to provide breast health education, recruitment and outreach, and support services for women.

In 1994, CDC expanded its collaborative network by funding 12 organizations to develop educational strategies and interventions to improve its capacity to reach racial and ethnic minorities, older women, lesbians, and women with low literacy skills (see box entitled National Organizations).

PROGRAM IMPACT

At the state and local level, the NBCCEDP has made remarkable progress in establishing breast and cervical cancer early detection programs. The NBCCEDP surveillance data through January 31, 1995, shows that 556,003 screening tests have been provided to women who are medically underserved. As of this date, the

---

National Organizations

- American Association of Retired Persons
- American Federation of Teachers
- American Indian Health Care Association
- National Caucus and Center for Black Aged, Inc.
- National Coalition of Hispanic Health and Human Services Organizations
- National Education Association
- National Hispanic Council on Aging
- National Migrant Resource Program
- Mayo Foundation
- Susan G. Komen Breast Cancer Foundation
- World Education, Inc.
- Young Women's Christian Association of the USA

---

program had provided 220,592 mammograms in 18 states. Of the women who received mammograms, 1,005 were diagnosed with breast cancer. During the same period, 335,411 Pap tests were performed and a total of 14,605 women were diagnosed with cervical intraepithelial neoplasia, a precursor of cervical cancer that can be successfully treated. Invasive cervical cancer was diagnosed in 120 women.

The most important risk factors for breast cancer are being female and older age.[1] The NBCCEDP's guidelines place a high priority on screening women 50 years and older. As of January 31, 1995, 59 percent of the mammograms were provided to women 50 years and older (Figure 2).

Although the incidence of cervical cancer does not rise appreciably with age, mortality from this disease is higher among older women.[16] Further, older women are less likely to receive Pap tests on a regular basis.[5] As of January 31, 1995, 57 percent of the Pap tests were provided to women 40 years and older (Figure 2).

Reaching racial and ethnic minority women with screening services is a high priority for the program. A review of the NBCCEDP's racial and ethnic breakdown reveals that 49 percent of the mammograms were provided to minority women and that 48 percent of all Pap tests were provided to minority women (Figure 3).

The NBCCEDP was established early on in states that had a high proportion of Hispanic women. Thus, 22 percent of the mammograms and 21 percent of Pap tests were provided to Hispanic women. With the implementation of the American Indian Initiative in 1994, the NBCCEDP has improved its capacity to reach American Indian women. The NBCCEDP will enhance its capacity to screen

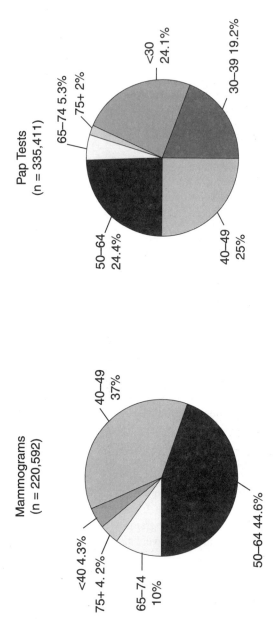

Figure 2. Percent distribution of mammograms and Pap tests, by age group, National Breast and Cervical Cancer Early Detection Program, 1991–1995. Includes mammograms performed for screening or following an abnormal breast examination. *Source:* Minimum Data Elements through 01/31/95.

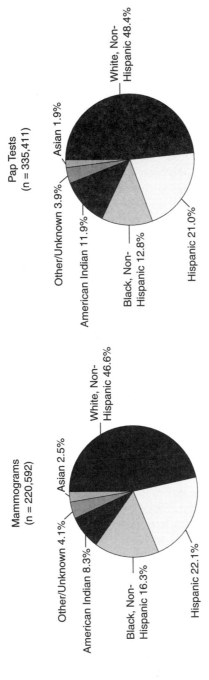

Figure 3. Percent distribution of mammograms and Pap tests, by race and ethnicity, National Breast and Cervical Cancer Early Detection Program, 1991–1995. Includes mammograms performed for screening or following an abnormal breast examination. *Source:* Minimum Data Elements through 01/31/95.

black women with the recent implementation of comprehensive screening programs in states with a high proportion of black women.

DISCUSSION

The Breast and Cervical Cancer Mortality Prevention Act of 1990 laid an important foundation for the development of a public health focus for cancer control in the United States. The CDC's NBCCEDP is one of the largest efforts in chronic disease prevention and control ever undertaken by an agency of the federal government. The legislation provided the first opportunity for the federal and state governments together to address the control of breast and cervical cancer in a concerted and deliberate manner. At the state and community levels, the development of early detection programs has resulted in new organizational capacity and infrastructure for cancer control, increased staff resources and expertise, multiple collaborative partnerships in the private and public sectors, state and community coalitions, and a greater understanding of the challenges in delivering preventive health services to women who are medically underserved. The NBCCEDP's comprehensive approach to breast and cervical cancer control ensures that not only medically underserved women benefit from this early detection effort but that all women gain from the educational activities, public and private partnerships, and quality assurance standards implemented in the states.

The success of NBCCEDP has contributed to the growing pressure on state health agencies to focus more attention and resources on chronic disease prevention and control. This public health foundation for breast and cervical cancer control could significantly benefit efforts of states in developing a comprehensive cancer prevention and control program that would address other cancer sites such as skin, lung, colon, rectum, and prostate.

•   •   •

One of the greatest challenges for the future is to sustain the momentum and commitment of federal and state governments to implement a comprehensive screening program in the remaining 15 states, the District of Columbia, and U.S. territories, and to expand screening coverage in currently funded states and American Indian tribes and tribal organizations. A comprehensive, nationwide program such as the NBCCEDP provides an unique opportunity to improve the use of breast and cervical cancer screening tests among all women. This national effort has allowed the United States to make strides toward the achievement of the Healthy People 2000 objectives for breast and cervical cancer control, particularly among women who are medically underserved.

REFERENCES

1. American Cancer Society. *Cancer Facts and Figures—1995.* Atlanta, Ga.: American Cancer Society, 1995.

2. Shapiro, S. "The Status of Breast Cancer Screening: A Quarter of a Century of Research." *World Journal of Surgery* 13 (1989): 9–18.

3. U.S. Department of Health and Human Services, Public Health Service, National Institutes of Health, National Cancer Institute. *Cancer Statistics Review: 1973–1986.* Bethesda, Md.: Pub. No. 89-2789, May 1989.

4. U.S. Preventive Services Task Force. "Screening for Breast Cancer, 1989." *American Family Physician* 39 (1989): 89–96.

5. Devesa, S.S., et al. "Recent Trends in Cervix Uteri Cancer." *Cancer* 64 (1989): 2184–2190.

6. U.S. Department of Health and Human Services, Public Health Service. *Healthy People 2000: National Health Promotion and Disease Prevention Objectives—Full Report, With Commentary.* DHHS Pub. No. 91-50212. Washington, D.C.: Government Printing Office, 1991.

7. Anderson, L.M., and May, D.S. "Has the Use of Cervical, Breast, and Colorectal Cancer Screening Increased in the United States?" *American Journal of Public Health* 85 (June 1995): 6840–6843.

8. Kaluzny, A.D., Rimer, B., and Harris, R. "The National Cancer Institute and Guideline Development: Lessons from the Breast Cancer Screening Controversy." *Journal of the National Cancer Institute* 86 (1994): 12901–12903.

9. U.S. Department of Health and Human Services, Public Health Service, Centers for Disease Control and Prevention. The National Strategic Plan for the Early Detection and Control of Breast and Cervical Cancers. Atlanta, Ga., 1994.

10. U.S. Congress. "Public Law 101-354: The Breast and Cervical Cancer Mortality Prevention Act of 1990." *Congressional Record* 136, 1990.

11. U.S. Congress. "Public Law 103-183: The Preventive Health Acts of 1993." *Congressional Record,* 1993.

12. Padilla, G.V., and Bulcavage, L.M. "Theories Used in Patient/Health Education." *Seminars in Oncology Nursing* 7 (1991): 2.87–2.96.

13. Mandelblatt, J., and Kanectsky, P.A. "Effectiveness of Interventions to Enhance Physician Screening for Breast Cancer." *Journal of Family Practice* 40 (1995): 2:162–2:171.

14. Dawson, D.A., and Thompson, G.B. "Breast Cancer Risk Factors and Screening: United States, 1987." *Vital and Health Statistics Data from the National Health Survey* 10 (1990): 172,1–60.

15. Helfand, M., et al. "Effect of the Clinical Laboratory Improvement Amendments of 1988 on the Incidence of Invasive Cervical Cancer." *Medical Care* 30 (1992): 12,1067–82.

16. U.S. Department of Health and Human Services, Public Health Service, National Institutes of Health, National Cancer Institute. "Incidence Data from the Surveillance, Epidemiology, and End Results Program, 1973–1990." *Cancer Statistics Review, 1973–1990.* Pub. No. 93-2789, Bethesda, Md.: NCI, 1993.

11

Progress in Breast Cancer Screening

Jan K. Carney, Jean F. Ewing, and Christine A. Finley

Breast cancer is an enormous public health problem in Vermont. Vermont's breast cancer mortality rate from 1960 to 1991 consistently ranked in the highest quartile for age-adjusted breast cancer mortality rates per 100,000 women compared to the rest of the U.S.[1-3]

It is estimated that breast cancer death rates could be reduced by 30 percent if women followed breast cancer screening recommendations.[4,5] However, nationally as of 1990, while nearly two-thirds of women 40 years and older had had at least one mammogram, less than one-third of women in this age group were following mammography screening guidelines.[6]

Although much has been learned and accomplished in recent years to better understand and improve participation in screening for breast cancer, many challenges remain.[7]

This chapter describes Vermont's efforts to reduce mortality from breast cancer by identifying and removing barriers to early detection among Vermont women.

VERMONT DEMOGRAPHICS

Vermont is the most rural state in the nation with a population of 562,758 in 1990; the largest city, Burlington, has a population of only 39,000. Although the age structure of Vermont is similar to the nation, in 1990 only 1.4 percent of the

Many activities described in this publication were supported by grant number 5-UO1-CA50109 from the National Cancer Institute. The contents of this chapter are solely the responsibility of the authors and do not necessarily represent the official views of the National Cancer Institute. We are indebted to Nancy M. Erickson and Julie Royer Wick for their creative efforts in the development of the public awareness campaign: Progress In Breast Cancer Screening: Vermont's Efforts.

J Public Health Management Practice, 1996, 2(2), 57–63

total population was nonwhite and only 0.4 percent of women aged 50 and older reported their race as other than white.[8]

Many of the challenges of providing access to health care services for Vermonters arise from the rural nature of the state as well as from its geography. Vermont's Green Mountains run through the center of the state; both rural and mountain roads as well as climate may restrict travel, especially in winter and spring months.

HISTORY OF VERMONT'S CANCER PREVENTION AND CONTROL EFFORTS

To encourage the translation of cancer control science into public health practice, the NCI awarded Data-based Intervention Research grants. In 1989, the Vermont Department of Health (DOH) was awarded Data-based Intervention Research grant funding for seven years to analyze state-specific data and implement appropriate cancer control strategies to meet the unique needs of the state. It was recognized that to address problems as large and complex as cancer, a comprehensive multifaceted approach involving multiple disciplines, in addition to public health, was required.

The Vermont Coalition on Cancer Prevention and Control was formed by the Vermont DOH in June 1988 to address this need. Forty organizations with interests in cancer prevention and control participated including public, private, and voluntary agencies. Representatives from breast cancer advocacy, the Vermont legislature, managed care, churches, health centers, and others joined the coalition in subsequent years. The coalition guided the development of the Vermont Plan for Cancer Prevention and Control from 1990–1995.[9] Six priority areas were addressed in the plan: (1) tobacco use reduction, (2) dietary modification, (3) screening and early detection, (4) access to state-of-the-art treatment, (5) reducing exposures to environmental and occupational carcinogens, and (6) program evaluation.

In the area of screening and early detection, the goal was to increase access to and utilization of screening and early detection activities. Five recommendations were developed for the 1990–1995 cancer plan: (1) develop interventions to enable high-risk, economically disadvantaged populations to receive screening services, (2) consider legislation to require health insurance carriers to provide coverage of cancer screening examinations, (3) educate primary care physicians and other health care providers to strengthen their role in the adoption and application of early detection guidelines for breast and cervical cancer, (4) promote patient education related to screening activities during contact with medical providers, and (5) integrate cancer control activities into ongoing worksite health promotion activities.

In this same time period the DOH released Healthy Vermonters 2000, Vermont's efforts, based on the U.S. Public Health Service's Healthy People 2000, to set goals and objectives for Vermont for the year 2000.[10] Cancer was one of eleven priority areas chosen with the specific goal to reduce the incidence of cancer and the number of deaths associated with cancer. Specific objectives included increasing the percentage of women who have clinical breast exams and mammograms.

IDENTIFYING BARRIERS TO EARLY DETECTION

In order to further define risk behaviors, screening practices, and barriers to early detection, the first Vermont cancer control survey was completed in 1990. This survey established baseline levels of knowledge, attitudes, and behavior regarding cancer screening, diet, and smoking, and assisted in the formation of program initiatives. The point-in-time survey was repeated in 1993 to determine changes following the multifaceted interventions. Methodology was similar to that of the Behavior Risk Factor Survey (BRFS) that also began in Vermont in 1990.

The sample selection process in both years was designed to provide a representative sample of Vermonters age 18 or over who live in households with either listed or unlisted telephones. The cancer control survey included the six BRFS mammography and clinical breast exam questions and added five questions on mammography, five on physical breast exam, and three on breast self-exam. Some of the additional questions were: Whose idea was it for you to have your last mammogram/physical breast exam?; What is the most important reason why you have not had a mammogram/physical breast exam in the last two years?; About how often do you think a woman age 50 or over should have a mammogram?; About how often do you examine your breasts for lumps? Female interviewers were employed because of the detailed questions concerning women's health practices.

The sample was stratified so that the number of interviews from each county was proportionate to its population. Survey results were weighted with respect to the age, gender, and number of eligible adults in the household in order to obtain statistics representative of the adult Vermont population as a whole. There were 1,314 completed interviews in 1990 and 1,353 in 1993, with 52 percent female for both years. In both years, the survey took place in late winter and was completed in March. Care was taken to follow the BRFS protocol, which included procedures to reduce other potential biases such as calls limited to one time of day.

The 1990 census reported that 4.5 percent of Vermont households were without telephones.[8] Although this represents a potential weakness, response rates of telephone surveys are superior to mail surveys and in-person interviews are impractical in Vermont, due to its rural nature.

Overall (Table 1, 1990 survey), 46 percent of women age 40–49 and 57 percent of women 50 and older had a mammogram within the past two years. In contrast to anecdotal perceptions that cost or lack of insurance was the major barrier to hav-

Table 1 Survey 1990 vs 1993 of women who have had mammograms

Age	1990 (%)	1993 (%)
Have EVER had mammogram:		
40–49	61	82*
50+	68	82*
Had one less than two years ago:		
40–49	46	60*
50+	57	65

Major reasons given by women 40+ for
NOT having had mammograms:

Reason	1990 (%)	1993 (%)
Not needed (lack of awareness)	30	14*
Procrastination	17	20
Doctor didn't recommend it	15	14
Not having any problem	10	10
Cost	9	9

*Significant change p = <0.05

ing a mammogram, 30 percent of women (40 and older) who had not had a mammogram within the past two years were not aware of the benefits of mammography or felt it was not needed. For 9 percent of those women not having a mammogram within the past two years, cost was the major reason. Fifteen percent of the women who had not had a mammogram noted their doctor didn't recommend it. However, 76 percent of women 40 and older reporting they had not had a mammogram within the past two years had seen their physician within the last year. In addition, for women (40 and older) who *had* a mammogram within the past two years, 70 percent said it had been their physician's idea.

VERMONT'S PUBLIC AWARENESS CAMPAIGN

Based on information from the 1990 survey, a public awareness campaign, designed to remove barriers and promote breast cancer screening, began in 1991 and carried over to 1993. The campaign included television and radio ads, posters and brochures, broadcast and print news coverage, community meetings and action groups, letters to physicians, worksite education sessions, and reduced-cost mammography programs.

To ensure that the television ads would effectively reach the target audience of primarily rural women over age 40, three focus groups were held early in the development of the campaign. Focus groups, a form of qualitative research, are used to obtain opinions about a specific topic in small group settings.[11] Findings from these groups, while not definitive because of their small size and nonrandom selection process, are nonetheless helpful in shaping a message and general approach.[12] In the three focus groups, photo storyboards were used to depict the proposed ad, scene by scene. Written open-ended evaluations were completed by focus group members, and a facilitated discussion followed. Through these groups, it was learned that the portrayal of friends or family members helping each other was well received; perceived "affluence" in the actors or their surroundings, and the use of voice-overs (a narrator rather than a character speaking) were seen as negative influences.

Television and radio ads were produced, and air time was paid for with a combination of public and private funds to ensure the ads would receive prime time placement. Approximately $25,000 was contributed by private sources, and television and radio stations contributed "matching" public service air time.

Based on the focus group suggestions, several themes were employed. Two ads, produced for 1991, carried the message: "a mammogram can save your life, and hers." The first ad, a kitchen conversation between two older women, longtime friends, addressed the misperception that screening is not needed until you have symptoms. The second, a conversation between a grandmother, her daughter, and granddaughter at their Vermont farm, addressed the misperception that older women do not need mammograms. Both ads stressed the control women have over their health by seeking screening and encouraged women to help each other to get mammograms and clinical breast exams.

A third ad, produced for 1992, presented a woman in a dream-like setting, sitting alone at a desk, sorting through old letters, toys, and other objects filled with personal memories. A female voice says: "There are many things a woman wants to remember. But there are three things she can't forget . . . regular mammograms, clinical breast exams, and breast self-exams."

All three ads publicized the toll-free 24-hour hotline 1-800-4-CANCER (operated by the NCI), where callers could get information about breast cancer and mammography facilities in Vermont and discuss the procedure itself with a cancer information specialist. Using an established out-of-state hotline was a feasible alternative to funding and staffing a new in-state service. The hotline provided the Vermont DOH with information about the numbers of calls from Vermont.

To launch the campaign, a press conference was held with the governor of Vermont. Health department officials and state cancer experts provided numerous media interviews. Posters carrying the campaign message were distributed to supermarkets, general stores, libraries, laundromats, malls, and other locations around the state.

In advance of the campaign, community outreach meetings were held in five locations around the state, involving a total of 60 women, over a two-month period. These meetings were designed to motivate community leaders to reinforce the public awareness by initiating or promoting educational and reduced-cost screening efforts locally. Community leaders were identified by health department district managers and recruited by telephone and written invitation. A brochure titled "there is something you can do about breast cancer" was produced for these community action groups.

Physician education initiatives included presentations by local physicians to medical staff meetings in several locations. A letter was sent by the Commissioner of Health to all physicians in the state, reinforcing the importance of their advice in influencing their patients' decision to get mammogram and clinical breast exams. Concurrently, hospitals and other mammography facilities throughout the state offered mammograms at reduced cost.

Through the community outreach meetings, worksites were also identified as an important vehicle for providing health education. One community group organized informational sessions at all of the largest businesses in the area. The success of that effort led the Vermont DOH to develop a worksite awareness campaign in cooperation with the University of Vermont, local hospitals, home health agencies, and worksites around the state. Health department staff trained 43 nurses from hospitals and home health agencies to deliver 45-minute interactive educational sessions to women where they worked.

More than 585 women aged 40 and older attended 74 worksite presentations. All participants completed a questionnaire prior to the session, and participants from Vermont's most populous county received a telephone follow-up and comparison with a control group who did not attend sessions. Both evaluations noted that high proportions of the participants were already following the recommended guidelines for breast and cervical cancer. Further, it was noted that most companies that were willing to schedule health education sessions during work time already provide health insurance for all employees, such that access to preventive care was probably greater than the access of many other women in the state.

IMPACT OF AWARENESS CAMPAIGN ON VERMONT SCREENING RATES

Following extensive public awareness efforts, the cancer control survey was repeated in 1993. A significant increase was seen in the percentages of women 40 and over who had ever had a mammogram (Table 1, 1993 survey). In addition, the percentage of women reporting they had a mammogram less than two years ago increased significantly for women aged 40–49. Although from 1990–1993 there was an increase in women over 50 reporting mammograms less than two years ago (57 percent to 65 percent), the change was not statistically significant.

With regard to questions about barriers to mammography among women who had *not* had a mammogram within the past two years, there was a statistically significant decrease noted in the percent of women who had previously identified lack of awareness as the major barrier (30% to 14%), with procrastination being noted as the greatest barrier in 20 percent of the women *not* having a mammogram. Other previously noted barriers to screening had not changed.

In addition, a very high proportion of Vermont women reported *ever* having a clinical breast exam (96 percent), unchanged from 1990 (95 percent). The proportion of women reporting clinical breast exam in the past year was 78 percent in both 1990 and 1993.

DISCUSSION AND FUTURE DIRECTION

Based on cancer control survey data, Vermont's public awareness campaign targeted and impacted Vermont women's behavior in obtaining mammograms. Although the increase in women over 50 from 1990 (57 percent) to 1993 (65 percent) was encouraging, it was not statistically significant and represents an area where continued efforts are needed.

Although there has been increased national attention about breast cancer screening, it is felt that the increases seen in obtaining mammograms were predominantly due to our educational efforts, due to the intensity, timing, and multifaceted nature of the educational campaign. In addition, questions about why women had not had a mammogram in the past two years showed a significant decline from 30 percent to 14 percent in "not needed" (lack of awareness), the area targeted, following our campaign.

Other studies have given estimates of breast cancer screening utilization and changes over time.[13–14] The NCI Screening Consortium[13] reported 46 to 76 percent of non-Hispanic white respondents (aged 50 to 74 years) had had a clinical breast exam within the previous year and only 25 percent to 41 percent had had a mammogram, noting lower rates among older, less educated, and poorer women.[13] The Mammography Attitudes and Usage Study (MAUS) found nearly two-thirds of women age 40 and over had at least one mammogram, an increase over previous surveys, but noted that still less than one-third of women in this age group were following screening guidelines for mammography.[6] Vermont's 1990 percentage of women ever having a mammogram is similar to that reported in the MAUS, but the percentage of Vermont women following screening guidelines was higher during this same year.

Previous earlier studies identified "never thought about it/no problem" and "doctor never recommended it" as the two predominant barriers for women who never had a mammogram.[13–14] Other studies noted absence of physician recommendation in 45 percent of women never having a mammogram.[6] Although direct comparisons are not possible, Vermont's reasons for not having a mammogram within the past two years (in 1990) focused on lack of awareness as the predominant reason (30 percent), followed by procrastination (17 percent) and physician didn't recommend it (15 percent). These differences may reflect Vermont-specific barriers.

Although we noted a decrease in "lack of awareness," "procrastination" remained the predominant reason Vermont women had not had a mammogram in 1993, and this percentage (20 percent) was essentially unchanged from 1990.

Various models have been used to develop educational strategies and promote behavior change. For example the Precede-Proceed model can help both in identifying factors affecting health behavior and developing educational messages.[15] The Transtheoretical model, which relates changes in behavior to progressive stages of precontemplation, contemplation, acting, and maintenance, may be applicable to women currently procrastinating. Increased encouragement by health care providers to follow screening recommendations may be necessary to see improvement in this area and is a focus of our future efforts.[16,17]

The importance of physician advice in women's decisions to get a mammogram has been well documented.[13] Vermont's findings are similar, and the vast majority of Vermont women who had a mammogram had done so on the advice of their physician. However, the percentage of women who had not had a mammogram within the past two years who noted that their doctor didn't recommend it in 1990 (15 percent) was unchanged in 1993 (14 percent). Although our campaign reinforced physicians' important role, more intense effort is needed in this area.

Other studies have found consistent discrepancy between rates of mammograms and clinical breast exams.[13] Our results showed discrepancies, though less pronounced. Although precise contributing factors cannot yet be identified, additional emphasis about the importance of clinical breast exam reinforced by health care providers is needed.

Assessment, policy development, and assurance are key components of a public health agency's work.[18] These are applicable to the specific area of cancer prevention and control. In addition, in the context of national cancer prevention and control, as defined by the NCI and Healthy People 2000, it is the responsibility of state and local public health agencies to prioritize objectives and identify state-specific needs.[19] In Vermont, there are no autonomous county or local health departments and this role is carried out through the state DOH and its 12 local public health offices throughout the state. Through the Data-based Intervention Grant, the development of Vermont's Cancer Plan (1990–1995), the development of Healthy Vermonters 2000, and Vermont's cancer control survey, Vermont cancer prevention and control priorities have been set, Vermont-specific barriers identified, and interim progress evaluated. This is an example of practical application of data from a variety of sources to plan and evaluate cancer control activities.[19]

Our original perception of cost as the most important barrier to screening was not supported by our surveys. However, despite the fact that only 9 percent of women surveyed stated cost as the reason for not having a mammogram, it may represent an underestimate because of the overwhelming lack of awareness reported by women surveyed. Other authors have documented the association between lower incomes and lower screening rates.[6,13] Our 1993 BRFS showed a reduced level of screening (women 50 and older who had a mammogram and clinical breast exam within two years) for women with annual household incomes less than $10,000 per year (39 percent), increasing to 93 percent for those with incomes of $35,000. Future program emphasis will be placed on reducing these disparities.

Our public health approach is based on the premise that a comprehensive and multifaceted approach is needed to address a problem as large and complex as breast cancer, and that this approach is needed at all stages of planning, policy development, and implementation. This concept is reflected in the formation and ongoing work of the Vermont Coalition for Cancer Prevention and Control, the development of the Vermont Cancer Plan, and Healthy Vermonters 2000. Other authors have noted that multi-strategy interventions are more effective than single-strategy interventions, although it may not be possible to sort out the relative strength of each contribution.[14]

Carrying out our awareness campaign required partnership among many groups and organizations, many of whom were active participants in the Cancer Coalition, and the use of both public and private resources. For example, efforts among hospitals, the health department, and the Cancer Coalition helped in increasing the availability of reduced cost mammography. Vermont businesses and worksites collaborated with hospitals, the health department, University of Vermont, and home health agencies (all members of the Vermont Coalition for Cancer Prevention and Control) in the development of the worksite awareness campaign.

In addition, evidence of the broad involvement and support required to impact breast cancer in Vermont is further demonstrated by the Vermont Legislature's passage of a law requiring health insurers to provide coverage for annual screening mammograms for women 50 and older, and under 50 when recommended by a health care provider, one of the original goals of the Vermont Plan for Cancer Prevention and Control. This reflects a growing national trend.[20]

•   •   •

Although Vermont has met the overall year 2000 objective for clinical breast exam and mammography screening for women over 50, additional work is aimed at further increasing screening rates in women over 50. In addition, efforts are being made to identify and address barriers to women of lower incomes and educational attainment, where screening rates are still much lower than year 2000 goals. Further progress will depend on a continued comprehensive and multifaceted approach, partnerships among public and private entities, and impacting all identified barriers to screening for Vermont women.

REFERENCES

1. Riggan, W.B., et al. National Cancer Institute—Environmental Protection Agency Interagency Agreement on Environmental Carcinogenesis. "U.S. Cancer Mortality Rates and Trends, 1950–1979, Volume II." Pub. No. EPA-600/1-83-015b. Washington, D.C.: Government Printing Office, 1983.

2. Ries, L.A.G., et al. (eds). *SEER Cancer Statistics Review, 1973–1991: Tables and Graphs, National Cancer Institute*. NIH Pub. No. 94-2789, Bethesda, Md.: Government Printing Office, 1994.

3. "Chronic Disease Reports: Deaths from Breast Cancer among Women—United States, 1986." *Morbidity and Mortality Weekly Report* 38, (1989): 566–569.

4. Shapiro, S., et al. *Periodic Screening for Breast Cancer: the Health Insurance Plan Project and its Sequelae, 1963–1986*. Baltimore, Md.: Johns Hopkins University Press, 1988.

5. Eddy, D.M. "Screening for Breast Cancer." *Annals of Internal Medicine* 111 (1989): 389–399.

6. "Use of Mammography—United States, 1990." *Morbidity and Mortality Weekly Report* 39 (1990): 621–629.

7. Zapka, J.G. "Promoting Participation in Breast Cancer Screening." *American Journal of Public Health* 84 (1994): 12–13.

8. U.S. Census of Population and Housing. *1990 U.S. Census of Population and Housing for Vermont*. Summary Tape File 3A: Race, Language, and Ethnicity, Vermont State and County Profiles. Burlington, Vt.: Department of Commerce, 1990.

9. Vermont Department of Health. Vermont Coalition on Cancer Prevention and Control. *Vermont Plan for Cancer Prevention and Control 1990–1995*. Burlington, Vt.: October 1989.

10. U.S. Department of Health and Human Services. *Healthy People 2000: National Health Promotion and Disease Prevention Objectives*. DHHS Pub. No. (PHS) 91-50212. Washington, D.C.: Government Printing Office, 1990.

11. Basch, C.E. "Focus Group Interview: An Underutilized Research Technique for Improving Theory and Practice in Health Education." *Health Education Quarterly* 14 (1987): 411–448.

12. Schechter, C., Vanchieri, C.F., and Crofton, C. "Evaluating Women's Attitudes and Perceptions in Developing Mammography Promotion Messages." *Public Health Reports* 105, no. 3 (1990): 253–257.

13. National Cancer Institute. "Screening Mammography: A Missed Clinical Opportunity? Results of the NCI Breast Cancer Screening Consortium and National Health Interview Survey Studies." *Journal of the American Medical Association* 264, no. 1 (1990): 54–58.

14. Rimer, B.K. "Mammography Use in the U.S.: Trends and the Impact of Interventions." *Annals of Behavioral Medicine* 16, no. 4 (1994): 317–326.

15. Centers for Disease Control and Prevention. "Public Education Intervention Strategies For Breast and Cervical Cancers." *Wellness Perspectives—Research, Theory, and Practice* 11, no. 2 (1995).

16. Prochaska, J., DiClemente, C., and Norcross, J.C. "In Search of How People Change: Applications to Addictive Behaviors." *American Psychologist* 47 (1992): 1102–1107.

17. Prochaska, J., and DiClemente, C. "Common Processes of Self-Change in Smoking, Weight Control, and Psychological Distress." In *Coping and Substance Use,* edited by S. Shiffman and T. Willis. New York: Academic Press, 1985.

18. Institute of Medicine. *The Future of Public Health.* Washington, D.C.: National Academy Press, 1988.

19. Boss, L.P., and Suarez, L. "Uses of Data to Plan Cancer Prevention and Control Programs." *Public Health Reports* 105, no. 4 (1990): 354–360.

20. Thompson, G.B., Kessler, L.G., and Boss, L.P. "Breast Cancer Screening Legislation in the United States: A Commentary." *American Journal of Public Health* 79 (1989): 1541–1543.

12

Demonstration Projects in Community-Based Prevention

Ross C. Brownson, Patricia Riley, and Thomas A. Bruce

Over the past several decades, epidemiologic and laboratory sciences have identified many preventable risk factors for the major causes of morbidity, mortality, and disability in westernized societies. This knowledge base has evolved from population-based studies and controlled studies in laboratory and clinical settings to application of research findings in community-level demonstration projects.[1] The National Cancer Institute has described the progression of research through five phases: (1) hypothesis development, (2) methods development, (3) controlled intervention trials, (4) defined population studies, and (5) demonstration and implementation.[2] Mercy et al.[3] have described a similar public health model that progresses from problem definition and etiologic research to community intervention and demonstration (Figure 1).

Thus, demonstration projects—large-scale interventions designed to improve the health of population at community level—represent a final stage in the progression and application of research. Demonstration projects share several important characteristics. Many seek to improve health through the development and effective use of coalitions or consortia—groups of people or organizations whose collective efforts can improve the health of the public much beyond the influence of any single individual or organization. Demonstration projects usually focus on community development to reduce actual causes of death such as tobacco use, physical inactivity, gunshot wounds, and high-risk sexual behavior.[4] These projects often employ a combination of high-risk and population strategies.[5,6]

This project was funded in part through the Centers for Disease Control and Prevention contract U48/CCU710806 (Centers for Research and Demonstration of Health Promotion and Disease Prevention), including support from the Community Prevention Study of the NIH Women's Health Initiative. The CBPH initiative was funded by the W.K. Kellogg Foundation.

J Public Health Management Practice, 1998, 4(2), 66–77

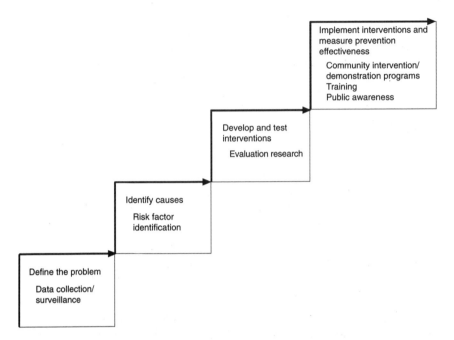

Figure 1. Public health model of a scientific approach to prevention. *Source:* J.A. Mercy et al. "Public Health for Preventing Violence." *Health Affairs* (winter 1993): 7–29. © 1993 The People-to-People Health Foundation, Inc. All rights reserved.

High-risk strategies focus on individuals with the greatest chance of developing adverse health outcomes; population strategies are directed at entire populations, with the goal of altering risk factor prevalence. Finally, demonstration projects often approach health as a complex, multidimensional concept encompassing various physical, mental, behavioral, and social factors.[7,8] These projects take a broad view of prevention that includes attention to individual risk factors (e.g., addiction to nicotine) and personal responsibility for health, environmental factors (e.g., air pollution), and sociocultural factors (e.g., housing, religious faith, employment).[8–13]

Recent multisite demonstration programs for preventing coronary heart disease (CHD) illustrate the evolution of epidemiologic and clinical discoveries into successful community-level interventions. Cardiovascular diseases, among them CHD, have been the leading cause of death in the United States for most of the twentieth century. Large-scale epidemiologic studies such as the Framingham Study have identified[14] modifiable risk factors for CHD (e.g., cigarette smoking, hypertension, physical inactivity, poor nutrition).[13,15] These and other epidemiologic investigations set the stage for demonstration projects such as the National High Blood Pressure Education Program, which began in 1972,[16] and the Stanford Five-City Project,[17] a 14-year trial begun in 1980. Both programs improved awareness and controllability of many CHD risk factors among health professionals and the general public, and may have contributed to a consistent decline in CHD mortality that began in 1968.[18,19]

The literature describes many examples of community-based demonstration projects. We focus on two—the Health Promotion and Disease Prevention Research Center (PRC) Program and the Community-Based Public Health (CBPH) initiative. Each represents a program with the potential to improve health on a large scale and each provides a range of approaches and interventions that include strategies for risk factor reduction, community partnerships, public health education, and attention to other social and environmental needs.

THE PREVENTION RESEARCH CENTERS PROGRAM

Theoretical and programmatic framework

The PRC Program, administered by the Centers for Disease Control and Prevention (CDC), integrates the resources of 14 academic centers committed to research that benefits public health. This national network focuses on health behaviors (e.g., smoking, physical inactivity, unprotected intercourse) that put Americans at risk for health conditions (e.g., heart disease, obesity, HIV infection, teenage pregnancy) that either claim a disproportionate number of lives or have a negative impact on quality of life. The program's goal is to identify effective strategies that promote community health, well-being, and self-sufficiency and thereby to enhance productivity, life span, and quality of life.

Program history

The legal foundation for establishing the PRC program was provided by Public Law 98-551. As originally authorized in 1984, the law specified that PRCs be located within academic centers that: (1) have multidisciplinary expertise relevant to public health, (2) provide graduate training in programs relevant to disease prevention, (3) have a core faculty in specified public health disciplines such as epidemiology, biostatistics, and social and behavioral sciences, (4) conduct residency training in public health or preventive medicine, and (5) demonstrate capacity for curriculum development in disease prevention. With an initial appropriation of $1.5 million in 1986, the PRC Program was housed within the National Center for Chronic Disease Prevention and Health Promotion, the Center within CDC most consistent in theme and mission to the program's conceptual underpinnings.

Since 1986, the Program has grown from three PRCs into a national network of 14. Current core support for the program is about $7.7 million per year. Each PRC dedicates a share of this support to a particular research theme or agenda (Table 1). The PRC program provides a sound basis for promoting health and preventing disease, and works to translate research findings into community-based interventions.

Key contributions

Through high-priority research and demonstration studies and the creation of an environment that enhances such research, the PRC Program contributes essential information about effective strategies for promoting health. Among the program's major accomplishments, four areas are noteworthy. PRCs have (1) improved public health and advanced national health priorities, (2) helped make communities more accessible and amenable to prevention interventions, (3) increased collaboration between health agencies and nontraditional partners, and (4) maximized resources for complex public health research. The following paragraphs discuss examples of successful activities in each area.

Improving public health and advancing national health priorities

In advancing objectives in health promotion and disease prevention as documented in Healthy People 2000,[20] PRCs identify ways to solve many national health concerns such as disability in older adults. For example, studies conducted by the Northwest Prevention Effectiveness Center at the University of Washington have shown that low-cost group exercise programs in community-based senior centers can measurably improve endurance, flexibility, lower-body strength, and self-reported health status among older adults and can reduce the number of falls that result in injury.[21] These improvements have prolonged self-sufficiency and independent living among these people.

Objectives of Healthy People 2000 also address broad themes and identify priority areas related to increasing the span of healthy life of all Americans. One priority is family planning, an important component of which is adolescent sexual development. Three PRCs (at the University of Texas, Johns Hopkins University, and the University of Minnesota) have earmarked adolescent health promotion as a central research theme (Table 1). These three centers are testing various community interventions and strategies among diverse ethnic groups (e.g., American Indians, African-Americans, and Hispanics) that help to increase adolescents' understanding of human sexuality and prevent sexual intercourse and pregnancy. The PRC at the University of Minnesota is exclusively dedicated to the prevention of teenage pregnancy.

Table 1 Prevention Research Center Program: participating institutions and intervention themes

Year established	University	Theme
1986	University of North Carolina at Chapel Hill: Schools of Dentistry, Medicine, Nursing, Pharmacy, Public Health	Workplace health promotion: New approaches to improving worker health
1986	University of Washington, Seattle: School of Public Health and Community Medicine; Group Health Cooperative	Making prevention work with community health partners; health promotion in older adults
1986	The University of Texas School of Public Health	From healthy children to healthy adults
1990	Columbia University School of Public Health	Reduction of excess morbidity and mortality in Harlem
1990	The University of Illinois, Chicago, School of Public Health	Health promotion and disease prevention across the lifespan
1993	The University of California at Berkeley School of Public Health	Families, neighborhoods, and communities: A model for action in chronic disease
1993	The University of South Carolina School of Public Health	Promoting health through physical activity
1993	The Johns Hopkins University School of Public Health	Promoting health and preventing disease among urban and rural adolescents
1993	The University of Alabama, Birmingham, School of Public Health	Risk reduction across the life span in African-American families
1994	Saint Louis University School of Public Health	Chronic disease prevention in low-income, rural communities
1994	The University of Oklahoma College of Public Health	Health behavior promotion and disease prevention in the Native American population
1994	Robert C. Byrd Health Sciences Center of West Virginia University	Risk factors in Appalachia, with emphasis on cardiovascular risk factors
1994	University of New Mexico Medical Center	Promoting healthy lifestyles in American Indian families
1996	University of Minnesota School of Public Health	Preventing teen pregnancy

Making communities accessible and amenable to prevention interventions

The establishment of relationships between PRCs and their surrounding communities bring public health researchers closer to the public. For example, the PRC at Saint Louis University and the Missouri Department of Health have formed coalitions to reach communities in the state's Bootheel and Ozark regions. The coalitions represent a 12-county area that is medically underserved, economically disadvantaged, and burdened with the highest rates of chronic disease in the state. The center, in collaboration with public health agencies and the community members, designs interventions that address the three main risk factors among people of the area: poor diet, smoking, and physical inactivity[22,23]; the coalitions then implement the interventions. Coalitions are comprised of community volunteers and leaders of local public health organizations, and they help teach healthy eating habits to youth, curb tobacco sales to minors, and build walking trails to promote physical activity.

Increase collaboration among agencies and nontraditional partners

Federal agencies must continually find new ways to collaborate with other federal and nonfederal agencies. The PRC Program offers an innovative mechanism for encouraging collaboration. One example is an ongoing collaboration between the PRC Program and the NIH Women's Health Initiative (WHI). Launched in 1991 in response to the critical need to enroll women in medical research, the WHI is a long-term national study focused on strategies to prevent heart disease, breast and colorectal cancer, and osteoporosis in postmenopausal women. As part of the initiative, prevention studies are underway in eight PRCs. The PRCs are conducting 12 community-based studies on physical activity, cardiovascular risk reduction, hysterectomy and hormone replacement therapy, diabetes prevention, and osteoporosis prevention. Each study involves women ages 39–79 years from all races and socioeconomic backgrounds.

One such study, conducted by PRC researchers at the University of South Carolina and the University of New Mexico, is examining physical activity practices among African-American and American Indian women. The researchers have developed innovative survey instruments for identifying the types of physical activity in which these women are most likely to be involved. This information is important because of the well-established link between exercise and health and because other studies of minority women have not addressed physical activity in these specific populations.

All PRCs also conduct at least one demonstration project with a nontraditional partner. One example of this type of collaboration is an ongoing effort by the University of California at Berkeley and Kaiser Permanente to design family-based health maintenance organizations for economically disadvantaged families.

Maximizing resources for complex public health research

The PRC Program not only encourages extramural research in public health but also creates an environment that promotes communication and collaborates among academic centers. For example, a Tobacco Control Network has been established to stimulate interaction and innovative research among multidisciplinary staff at nearly every PRC. The network is coordinated by the University of Illinois and collaborates with CDC's Office on Smoking and Health to select research themes for PRCs. PRCs are researching one such theme—adolescent smoking behaviors.[24] In addition, the network is collaborating with the Robert Wood Johnson Foundation on studies of tobacco advertising and promotion. The Tobacco Control Network has served as a model for others including networks among research institutions that conduct school health initiatives or behavioral risk factor surveillance. Without the structure of the PRC Program, these multifaceted and interinstitutional interactions would be much less likely to occur.

Future directions

As the PRC Program enters its second decade, it has become integral to fulfilling CDC's prevention mandate. A recent Institute of Medicine report on the PRC Program[25] and a 10-year report on the PRCs[25(p.91)] underscored the Program's substantial progress and contributions to health promotion and disease prevention. However, the report also encouraged the program to further expand its vision for the future to encompass:

- a focus on risk conditions and social determinants of health
- an orientation toward the community
- an interdisciplinary approach
- a means for disseminating public health research
- an interactive process for establishing research priorities
- a role in setting national research priorities

Each of these components is fundamental to the program's orientation and overall goal. Together, they offer a framework for future program evaluation and assessment. Ensuring program responsiveness to area defined by these components is essential if the PRC Program is to continue its contributions to public health.

THE KELLOGG COMMUNITY-BASED PUBLIC HEALTH INITIATIVE

Theoretical and programmatic framework

The CBPH initiative was designed to strengthen linkages between public health education and public health practice by forming formal partnerships with people in communities. In part, the initiative reflects recommendations of the Institute of Medicine,[26] the Council on Linkages,[27] and others[28,29] who have called upon schools of public health and other academic health centers to focus educational programs on issues more relevant to public health practice. The initiative acknowledges the large inequalities between the health of "have" and "have not" communities.[30] It reflects the notion that social and behavioral change can best be achieved by working directly with those at greatest risk.[31] And finally, it allows community realities to serve as a powerful stimulus to professional organizational change.[32]

As part of the CBPH initiative, sustainable demonstrations were based in underserved U.S. communities. The intent was to encourage people living in these communities to share responsibility and ownership of public health issues. A professional goal was to shift from a mindset of community "services" to a community "empowerment" perspective—that is, from a professionally administered health delivery system to one with greater reliance on collaboration, community coalitions, and active participation. The vision of the CBPH initiative is that improvements in health and well-being can be achieved by emphasizing the key role of public health engagement in communities and the role of community engagement in public health action.

Program history

The Kellogg Foundation began the CBPH initiative in the early 1990s, following a 1980s focus on health promotion and disease prevention in schools, youth organizations, worksites, senior centers, and college campuses. To be eligible for the program, interested parties had to establish a consortium consisting of (1) a school or an academic program of public health, (2) at least one other health professions school, (3) one or more communities with serious public health problems, and (4) the local public health agencies of these communities. A total of 108 consortia applied to enter the program; from these 15 were selected for one year of leadership training and model development. The models were then implemented by consortia in California, Georgia, Maryland, Massachusetts, Michigan, North Carolina, and Washington (Table 2). These seven consortia were funded in September 1992; awards averaged $2 million each over four years.

Each funded consortium was charged with the following responsibilities:

- Build the capacity of communities to understand and address issues amenable to prevention, including activities that link communities more effectively with health professionals, local resource institutions, and community agencies
- Increase the capacity of academic partners, community partners, and affiliated agencies and organizations to implement culturally relevant, community-based efforts to prevent disease and promote health

Table 2 Community-based public health consortia

State	Public health school	Other health-related schools	Public health agency	Community-based organizations
California	UC Berkeley Sch. of Public Health	UC San Francisco Sch. of Medicine	Alameda County Health Care Services Agency	21 neighborhood groups; 7 youth groups; 16 CBOs in East 14th Crossroads area of City of Oakland
Georgia	Emory Univ. Rollins School of Public Health	Morehouse School of Medicine	Fulton Co. Hlth. Dept.; Cobb Co. Bd. Health	Rose Garden Hills; Kennesaw Village; Fort Hill; and Roosevelt Circle—all in Marietta, GA; initially two public housing units in Atlanta
Maryland	School of Hygiene & Public Health, Johns Hopkins Univ.	Johns Hopkins Univ. Schools of Nursing and Medicine	Baltimore City Health Department	Clergy United for Renewal of East Baltimore (CURE); Heart, Body & Soul, Health Care for the Homeless; Baltimore City Public Schools; The Family Place; The Julie Center
Massachusetts	UMass School of Public Health & Health Sciences	UMass Medical Sch. Dept. of Family Medicine	Mass. Assoc. of Boards of Health; Mass. Dept. of Public Health	Holyoke Latino Community Coalition; Northern Berkshire Community Coalition; Worcester Latino Coalition; North Quabbin Community Coalition
Michigan	Univ. of Michigan Sch. of Public Health	Univ. of Michigan Sch. of Soc. Work; Wayne State Univ. Sch. of Soc. Work; Univ. Detroit-Mercy Sch. Health Sciences; Univ. of Mich-Flint	Detroit Health Dept.; Genesee Co. Health Department	Agape House of Hartford Memorial Baptist Church; Barton McFarlane Neighborhood Assoc.; National Ctr. for Advancement of Blacks in the Health Professions; Flint Odyssey House; Genesee Area Skill Center; Genesee County CAA; Flint Area Cmty. Econ. Dvpt.; Flint Neighborhood Coalition

Table 2 Continued

State	Public health school	Other health-related schools	Public health agency	Community-based organizations
North Carolina	Univ. of NC at Chapel Hill School of Public Health	UNC at Chapel Hill Area Health Educat. Centers	Chatham Co. Hlth. Dpt.; Orange Co. Hlth. Dpt.; Wake Co. Health Dept.; Lee Co. Health Dept.	Joint Orange-Chatham Community Action; Orange-Chatham Comprehensive Health Services; Wake Health Services; Strengthening the Black Family, Inc.
Washington	Univ. of Wash. Sch. of Public Health & Community Medicine	Univ. of Wash. School of Nursing	Seattle-King County Health Dept.; Whatcom Co. Health Dept.	Seattle Urban Health Alliance; Lummi Cedar Project; Group Hlth. Cooperative of Puget Sound

- Carry out essential public health functions; i.e., assessment, policy development, and assurance by community-based approaches[26,31]
- Facilitate the creation of more effective public health policies through the development of integrated action plans at the community level
- Encourage the entry of youth from affected communities into health-related professions through recruitment, education, training, and mentoring

Key contributions

Contributions from the seven consortia were numerous and diverse; brief examples are provided for three of the consortia.

Maryland

Partners of the Maryland consortium can be seen in Table 2. Interventions were focused on an East Baltimore neighborhood surrounding the Johns Hopkins Medical Center. At the time of the intervention, the community's population was approximately 150,000, of which 81 percent was African-American. More than 36 percent of community residents were living in poverty and only 41 percent had completed high school. There were 233 churches in the area—2.1 per city block, and all denominations found there were represented in Clergy United for Renewal of East Baltimore (CURE).

The consortium's overall goal was to create a broad community health program that was church-based and substantially connected to the Johns Hopkins Medical Center. Over a four-year project period, many steps were taken toward fulfilling this goal and improving the health of the community.[33] For example, medical students and residents from the Johns Hopkins School of Medicine began community rotations to provide health care and teach disease prevention. Nursing and public health students were provided in-depth community assignments. Community members were asked to teach community values and perspectives within the university classrooms. The health department provided training for community health workers to enhance their ability to carry out community health interventions—diabetes and tuberculosis control, visual screening, and so forth. Ministers at local churches preached health messages, and congregations expanded societal missions in their neighborhoods. Faculty at Johns Hopkins taught grant-writing skills to community residents, and nearly $2 million in additional funds were obtained from community block grants and other sources. The program became the recipient of a Health Resources and Services Administration "Models of Excellence" award in 1996.

Michigan

The Michigan consortium targeted two communities—one in Northwest Detroit and the other in the Broome section of Flint (60 miles north of Detroit). In both communities a high percentage of the population is below the poverty line, and social problems are prevalent. Most residents in both communities are African-Americans. In Flint, a sizable fraction is retired auto union workers.

Teams were developed in Flint, Detroit, and at the University campus in Ann Arbor. The Genesee County Health Department recruited and trained community residents to serve in public health roles and began a highly visible effort in broad neighborhood development. This later became the model for similar efforts in the public schools and city police departments. In northwest Detroit, health clubs in public schools became more active in encouraging students to pursue careers in the health professions, and summer youth programs addressed critical public health issues such as drugs, violence, and handgun use. Faculty at the University of Michigan were prominently involved in teaching and research using community-based approaches, and they provided leadership in developing community health policy at the state and national levels.

North Carolina

Consortium partners included health and community-based organizations from one urban county (Wake) and three rural counties (Lee, Chatham, and Orange). Interventions were aimed at families residing in the four counties who were identified as at risk for preventable illnesses. Community improvements were made according to local priorities. For example, water and sewer services were extended to isolated homes, a playground was built to enhance friendships between African-American and immigrant Mexican children, and a drug eradication program was launched.

The North Carolina consortium has perhaps the best organizational structure (i.e., constitution and bylaws) of the seven. Its efforts set a standard for effective collaboration among academic, practice, and community partners.

To enhance communication and program development, the University assigned one faculty member and graduate students to each of the four communities. Other program-associated changes included the revision of faculty promotion and tenure guidelines to reflect scholarship in community health. In addition, curricula in CBPH were upgraded, as they were in all seven schools of public health in this initiative, and a new doctoral program in public health practice was initiated.

Future directions

The challenge during the first year of the CBPH initiative was to build the capacity of the community to be a legitimate and valid partner in an ambitious undertaking. At the end of the first year, substantial progress had been made in assembling the staff and personnel to work on the projects in all seven states. Community organizations were better able to understand their unique role in creating more relevant community services. They also had started to encourage some changes in their institutional partners. A great deal of effort was made to develop appropriate governance systems for the consortia.

In the last three years, the institutional partner components have received increasing scrutiny. Public health *agency* policymakers, managers, and staff have considered how their roles and responsibilities should look in a reformed health system. Virtually every aspect of the public health infrastructure has been challenged: administration, funding mechanisms, maintaining quality personnel skills, adapting to a managed care environment, tapping into existing community assets, and responding to dynamic community needs. In the universities, scholarly functions of meticulous research and inspired teaching in community health have been accelerated by all the consortia.

No additional grant funds were provided by Kellogg after the fourth year of funding, and since that time the consortia have been turning to their own resources to sustain their efforts and activities. A CBPH Policy Task Force kept them working together on issues of national public health import, and in late 1997 a new national organization was created, The Center for Advancement of Community-Based Public Health. The mission of this new organization is as follows:

> (The Center) is committed to the advancement of "community-based public health"—the protection and improvement of community health through the full participation of the community. (It) seeks to improve the public's health by 1) building and maintaining local partnerships which include community-based organizations, universities, and public health agencies at the local level, and 2) influencing policy at all levels to promote community-based public health and the partnerships which carry it out.

LESSONS LEARNED

The contributions of large-scale demonstration projects are numerous and diverse. Through project activities, a number of lessons have emerged. We discuss several such lessons; others are described elsewhere.[23,34–37]

Build effective prevention partnerships

Partnerships between public health agencies, community-based organizations, and universities can be ideal vehicles for success in conducting demonstration projects because each entity has a unique set of abilities. In general, public health agencies and community-based organizations have greater access to populations at risk and more experience working at the community level. University researchers can furnish public health agencies with information on relevant theories and promising interventions and can provide expertise for evaluating programs.

Despite the best of intentions, difficulties can arise in building these partnerships. Examples include conflicts over control of funding and confusion over lines of authority. The best mechanisms for overcoming these difficult issues include explicit statement and restatement of project goals, frequent communication, and clear delineation of roles and responsibilities. Obtaining the community's full participation in selecting, designing, and implementing programs is essential. Guidelines for participatory action research (i.e., direct community involvement in the design and conduct of public health research) may enhance methods[38] and are encouraged.

Utilize the potential of community groups to foster change among professional partners

It is unfortunate but commonly true that institutions can develop their own form of bureaucracy and narrow perspective, becoming prone to prescriptive solutions that are irrelevant within the high-risk communities that are the focus of their intervention efforts. Public health agencies and schools can benefit enormously from community partnerships that expose these "blind spots." The resulting methods can lead to more effective and realistic approaches to community health development.

Use and disseminate existing data

Public health agencies collect enormous amounts of health data, as a result of statutory requirements, through ongoing surveillance activities and through prevention programs. In many instances, existing data are underutilized in intervention planning and evaluation.

In our experience, the analysis and dissemination of numerous types of surveillance data is of great value in developing risk reduction programs. Data can be disseminated through various forums including articles in state medical journals, press releases, interviews for radio and television, and fact sheets. In addition, provision of local data (e.g., risk factor surveys) can be beneficial in developing local coalitions and has helped foster early community ownership of intervention projects, which is a key element for program success.

Adopt a causal model in intervention design

Community-based demonstration projects are founded on the notion that action at the level of a social unit can affect health outcomes at the individual level. This notion is embodied in a causal model—one that leads from program inputs (programs and resources) to health outputs (changes in health behaviors or health status) if the program works as intended,[37] and that guides program planners in designing interventions. It is important for evaluation purposes that what has been termed this "small theory" of the intervention be made explicit early in the planning process.[39]

Use appropriate methods for evaluation of community-based interventions

The strongest evaluation designs combine elements of quantitative and qualitative evaluation. In this era of limited public resources, evaluation designs need to be flexible and sensitive enough to assess various community changes, even those that fall short of changes in behavior (e.g., a change in attitudes about physical activity may precede a decline in the behavior of physical activity). Genuine change takes place incrementally over time, in ways that are often not visible to those too close to the intervention.

Risk reduction trials based in communities often involve community-level rather than individual-level units of analysis. Therefore, evaluation methods should include sampling and analytic techniques that account for intraclass correlations.[34,37] Evaluations also may need to assess positive changes that are not directly related to health promotion or disease prevention. For example one measure of success may be the increased participation and influence of coalition members through election to city councils and school boards. Another may be the increasing ability of individual community members to serve as change agents or advocates for health improvement.

Encourage policy change as the intervention

As public health agencies shift their focus away from direct delivery of services[29] and as agencies and research institutions increasingly recognize the importance of policy as a form of intervention,[40] there is a need to emphasize ways to foster positive policy changes at the community level. This emphasis is present not only in the two models profiled in this chapter, but also in the Healthy Cities/ Healthy Communities Movements,[41] and in international movements such as the Victoria Declaration,[42] all of which have adopted a policy-oriented vision to address disease prevention and health promotion. Program success requires the removal of barriers to policy development and the enactment of policies that encourage healthy behavior. The potential for informed and engaged communities to be effective partners in health policy development should not be underestimated.

Allow sufficient time for intervention and evaluation

The process of developing community-based interventions is complex and time consuming. Often, practitioners and researchers may attempt to measure health outcomes before communities have been sufficiently empowered and exposed to interventions. As a result, demonstrating a significant effect may become virtually impossible early in the process. It is critical that funding agencies, public health organizations, and persons working at the community level realize that it may take several years for the necessary local infrastructure to be developed before the intervention can even *begin*. This point is essential for determining which programs are effective and deserving of replication.

•   •   •

A large and continually developing body of evidence supports the usefulness of large-scale community demonstration projects. These projects are logical extensions of decades of research on the etiology of various health conditions. The experience of recent demonstration projects, such as those discussed here, can benefit public health practitioners who are designing, implementing, or evaluating health promotion projects.

REFERENCES

1. R.C. Brownson. "Measuring the Impacts of Prevention Research on Public Health Practice." *American Journal of Public Health*, submitted for publication.

2. P. Greenwald. "Introduction: History of Cancer Prevention and Control." In *Cancer Prevention and Control,* eds. P. Greenwald et al. New York: Marcel Dekker, 1995.

3. J.A. Mercy et al. "Public Health for Preventing Violence." *Health Affairs* Winter 12 (1993): 7–29.

4. J.M. McGinnis et al. "Actual Causes of Death in the United States." *Journal of the American Medical Association* 270 (1993): 2207–2212.

5. G. Rose. "Sick Individuals and Sick Populations." *International Journal of Epidemiology* 14 (1985): 32–38.

6. G. Rose. *The Strategy of Preventive Medicine.* New York: Oxford University Press, 1992.

7. World Health Organization. "Constitution of the World Health Organization." In *Handbook of Basic Documents.* Geneva: WHO, 1948.

8. L.A. Aday. "Health Status of Vulnerable Populations." *Annual Review of Public Health* 15 (1994): 487–509.

9. D.E. Beauchamp. "Public Health as Social Justice." *Inquiry* 13 (1996): 3–14.

10. S. Tesh. "Disease Causality and Politics." *Journal Health Politics, Policy and Law* 6 (1981): 369–380.

11. M. Aguirre-Molina and D.M. Gorman. "Community-Based Approaches for the Prevention of Alcohol, Tobacco, and Other Drug Use." *Annual Review of Public Health* 17 (1996): 337–358.

12. R.G. Evans and G.L. Stoddart. "Producing Health, Consuming Health Care." *Social Science Medicine* 31 (1990): 1347–1363.

13. J.E. Fielding. "Successes of Prevention." *Milbank Memorial Fund Quarterly* 56 (1978): 274–302.

14. T.R. Dawber. *The Framingham Study: The Epidemiology of Coronary Heart Disease.* Cambridge, Mass.: Harvard University Press, 1980.

15. L. Goldman and E.F. Cook. "Reasons for the Decline in Coronary Heart Disease Mortality: Medical Interventions Versus Life-Style Changes." In *Trends in Coronary Heart Disease Mortality: The Influence of Medical Care*, eds. M.W. Higgins and R.V. Luepker. New York: Oxford University Press, 1988.

16. E.J. Roccella and M.J. Horan. "The National High Blood Pressure Education Program: Measuring Progress and Assessing Its Impact." *Health Psychology* 7, suppl. (1988): 297–303.

17. J.W. Farquhar. "Effects of Communitywide Education on Cardiovascular Disease Risk Factors." *Journal of the American Medical Association* 264 (1990): 359–365.

18. W.B. Kannel. "Clinical Misconceptions Dispelled By Epidemiological Research [Review]." *Circulation* 92 (1995): 3350–3360.

19. M.G.M. Hunink et al. "The Recent Decline in Mortality from Coronary Heart Disease, 1980–1990. The Effect of Secular Trends in Risk Factors and Treatment." *Journal of the American Medical Association* 277 (1997): 535–542.

20. U.S. Department of Health and Human Services. *Healthy People 2000: National Health Promotion and Disease Prevention.* Pub. No. 017-001-00473-1. Washington, D.C.: Government Printing Office, 1990.

21. J. Novice et al. "Effects, Safety and Compliance with an Exercise Program in a Senior Center: A Randomized Trial." *Journal of the American Geriatrics Society* (May 20, 1994).

22. R.C. Brownson et al. "Preventing Cardiovascular Disease Through Community-Based Risk Reduction: The Bootheel Heart Health Project." *American Journal Public Health* 86 (1996): 206–213.

23. R.C. Brownson et al. "Developing and Evaluating a Cardiovascular Risk Reduction Project." *American Journal Health Behavior* 21 (1997): 333–344.

24. R. Robinson and R.J. Mermelstein. *Explanations of Race and Gender Differences in Teen Tobacco Use.* Presentation at the 124th Annual Meeting and Exposition of the American Public Health Association, New York, November 19, 1996.

25. Institute of Medicine. *Linking Research and Public Health Practice. A Review of CDC's Program of Centers for Research and Demonstration of Health Promotion and Disease Prevention.* Washington, D.C.: National Academy Press, 1997.

26. Institute of Medicine. *The Future of Public Health.* Washington, D.C.: National Academy Press, 1988.

27. A.A. Sorensen and R.G. Bialek, eds. *The Public Health Faculty/Agency Forum: Linking Graduate Education and Practice, Final Report.* Gainesville, Fla.: University Press of Florida, 1992.

28. J. Showstack et al. "Health of the Public. The Academic Response." *Journal of the American Medical Association* 267 (1992): 2497–2502.

29. R.C. Brownson et al. "Future Trends Affecting Public Health: Challenges and Opportunities." *Journal of Public Health Management and Practice* 3, no. 2 (1997): 49–60.

30. P.R. Lee et al. "Report on NIH Conference Measuring Social Inequalities in Health." *Public Health Reports* 110 (1995): 302–305.

31. Institute of Medicine. Committee on Public Health, M.A. Stoto et al., eds. *Healthy Communities: New Partnerships for the Future of Public Health.* Washington, D.C.: National Academy Press, 1996.

32. R. Bellah et al. *The Good Society.* New York: Alfred A. Knopf, 1991.

33. D.M. Levine et al. "Community-Academic Health Center Partnership for Underserved Minority Populations—One Solution to a National Crisis." *Journal of the American Medical Association* 272 (1994): 309–311.

34. T.D. Koepsell et al. "Selected Methodological Issues in Evaluating Community-Based Health Promotion and Disease Prevention Programs." *Annual Review Public Health* 13 (1992): 31–57.

35. M.B. Mittlemark et al. "Realistic Outcomes: Lessons Learned From Community-Based Research and Demonstration Programs for the Prevention of Cardiovascular Diseases." *Journal of Public Health Policy* (Winter 1993): 437–462.

36. R.C. Brownson et al. "Policy Research for Disease Prevention: Challenges and Practical Recommendations." *American Journal Public Health* 87 (1997): 735–739.

37. T.D. Koepsell. "Epidemiologic Issues in the Design of Community Intervention Trials." In *Applied Epidemiology: Theory to Practice*, eds. R.C. Brownson and D. B. Pettiti. New York: Oxford University Press, 1998: 177–212.

38. Institute of Health Promotion Research, University of British Columbia, and B.C. Consortium for Health Promotion Research. *Study of Participatory Research in Health Promotion. Review and Recommendations for the Development of Participatory Research in Health Promotion in Canada.* Vancouver, British Columbia: The Royal Society of Canada, 1995.

39. M.W. Lipsey. "Theory as Method: Small Theories of Treatment." In *Research Methodology: Strengthening Causal Interpretations of Nonexperimental Data*, ed. L. Sechrest et al. DHHS Pub. No. (PHS) 90-3454. Washington, D.C.: Government Printing Office, 1990.

40. T.L. Schmid et al. "Policy as Intervention: Environmental and Policy Approaches to the Prevention of Cardiovascular Disease." *American Journal Public Health* 85 (1995): 1207–1211.

41. T. Hancock. "The Evolution, Impact and Significance of the Healthy Cities/Healthy Communities Movement." *Journal of Public Health Policy* 14 (1993): 5–18.

42. Advisory Board of the International Heart Health Conference. *The Victoria Declaration on Heart Health.* Victoria, British Columbia: British Columbia Ministry of Health, 1992.

PART IV

Coalition Building

This section discusses the various uses of coalition building in community-based health promotion and prevention programs. Coalitions bring together members of various organizations to work together for a common purpose. These coalitions may include individuals representing various agencies and organizations (e.g., local health departments, American Cancer Society, neighborhood organizations) as well as individuals from the community of interest. Coalitions may be used for various purposes including collecting data, program development and implementation, and policy development and change.

Each of the chapters in this section provide some insight into the common elements of coalitions including the use of coalitions to prioritize health issues and develop strategies to address health issues, and to enhance community capacity to engage in problem solving. These examples also illustrate the capacity of coalitions to bring individuals and organizations who are not typically part of health care decision making into key decision-making positions. These examples also highlight the importance of building trust among coalition members, and sharing power within the coalition. Lastly, each of the coalitions described either implicitly or explicitly used coalitions as a means to enhance the appropriateness of services with the intent of increasing utilization of services and ultimately improving community health.

In the first chapter, True presents a case study of the Breast Health Partnerships. These coalitions were "categorical" coalitions (i.e., focused on one content area). The coalitions were used to increase breast cancer screening among traditionally under-screened populations. One of the strengths of the breast health partnerships was that each was created using different partners (from business, health care providers, voluntary health agencies, libraries, senior service programs, media, and elected officials). In addition, each coalition chose its own operating procedures (e.g., deciding when, where, and how frequently to meet). Each of the partnerships was asked to collect information for process as well as outcome evaluation. Although the coalitions were categorical, the author highlights the potential of this coalition to affect other health issues by creating linkages and improving communication among partners.

In the second chapter, Parker et al. describe "non-categorical" coalitions (i.e., focused on broader health issues) developed as part of the North Carolina Community-Based Public Health Consortium. The overall intent of the coalitions was to improve "minority health and to make public health education and public health services more responsive to community needs." The chapter describes the different stages of coalition development and the issues that need to be considered in effective coalition functioning. This chapter also highlights the importance of considering non-categorical coalitions as a way to include community members in prioritizing community issues that need attention. Moreover, non-categorical coalitions are described as advantageous because they decrease the need for individuals and organizations to serve on multiple coalitions.

In the last chapter in this section, Block et al. describe the use of coalitions of community-based organizations in collecting data. The ". . . state and local health departments, hospitals, physician clinics, tribal health services, health planning agency, and health provider educational institutions . . ." jointly identified key factors to be included in the survey. In this instance the coalition was seen as assisting the organizations to collect local data on disease prevalence, health risk behaviors, and health care access that they would otherwise be unable to collect. The use of coalitions for data gathering was seen as setting the stage for future programmatic collaboration.

As you read these chapters, consider the following set of questions:

Objectives and Data Sources

1. For each of the coalitions described, are the objectives and research questions well described? Why is this important?
2. Why would it be important to conduct process as well as impact and outcome evaluations on coalition activities?
3. What existing sources of data might be useful to non-categorical coalitions as they begin to prioritize areas for intervention?

Methods and Strategies

4. What strategies may be most important in each of the coalition stages identified by Alter and Hage (as described in Parker et al.)?
5. How were coalition members recruited for each of the coalitions described?
6. What are the advantages and disadvantages of categorical coalitions?

Dissemination and Implications for Public Health Practice

7. What are the advantages and disadvantages of coalition approaches to program development? To data collection? To policy development?
8. Who should be included in a coalition? What are some ways to recruit members? What are the limitations of "representative membership"? What is the role of community-based organizations? What about community members themselves?
9. What are the advantages and disadvantages of coalitions to address specific issues? What about more coalitions that define their own agendas?
10. To what extent can coalitions increase power of each of the members or member organizations? How might coalitions negatively impact empowerment of disenfranchised populations?
11. What are some caveats to consider in using coalitions as a means to increase diversity (ethnic/racial/political) of input on health changes?

13

Community-Based Breast Health Partnerships

Susan J. True

This chapter discusses the development of Breast Health Partnerships (BHPs) to generate community commitment to and participation in public health efforts to improve access to comprehensive breast cancer screening and early detection services, particularly among underserved, uninsured, or poorly insured low-income women not previously screened. The evolution of New York State's screening program from a facility-based effort to a community-based approach serving women in all 62 counties throughout the state is described.

Breast cancer is a serious health problem in New York State, with more than 10,000 new cases and 3,700 deaths reported each year. A disproportionate number of these deaths occur among low-income women and minorities who, even when they understand the benefits of early detection, may not have access to screening services.

Since 1988, New York State has supported a program of breast cancer screening directed to underserved and uninsured or underinsured women. Twelve projects representing 10 major urban and 2 multicounty rural areas have been funded to provide a comprehensive program of community education, targeted outreach, and breast cancer screening service delivery. Together, these projects screened more than 40,000 women in five years. Sixty percent of these women were age 50 and older, with those 65 and older representing more than 18 percent of the total enrolled. Nearly 51 percent had never had a mammogram before, and an additional 28 percent had not had one in more than a year. More than 30 percent of screened women had no insurance at all, while approximately 44 percent had public or private insurance that did not cover screening procedures. Evaluation of these projects demonstrated that, although the numbers of women screened could be increased with more funding, the demographic profile of clients in any particular program remained stable. This finding suggested the need for more varied outreach strategies and the participation of a wider array of health care facilities and

J Public Health Management Practice, 1995, 1(3), 67–72

providers. The National Breast and Cervical Cancer Early Detection Program administered by the Centers for Disease Control and Prevention provided the impetus for a change in approach as well as the opportunity for New York to expand the screening program to eligible women in all parts of the state. The concept of the community-based BHP was proposed as an innovative approach to maximize resources while expanding the tested and successful aspects of the existing program statewide.

Community-based BHPs are problem-solving groups that work to bring the resources of individual partners "to the table" to overcome obstacles to the recruitment of underserved women and to coordinate the delivery of comprehensive breast cancer screening services. BHPs are based on several important premises: the members of a community are better able to identify barriers to services for the population they represent than anyone else; they are best able to design effective strategies to eliminate these barriers; and they will support interventions they develop to the greatest extent possible. Public health programs that acknowledge the collective wisdom, expertise, and resources of a community can successfully channel local energies toward improving public health. Generating a commitment to change is key, as these screening projects are developing against a backdrop of health care reform focused almost entirely on managing costs while ensuring universal coverage. Issues of universal access, quality assurance, recruitment of the underserved, referral, coordinated follow-up, and surveillance are less frequently a part of this discussion, yet represent essential components of any partnership's plan to coordinate comprehensive breast cancer screening at the community level. In the BHP model, the New York State Department of Health (DOH) is the catalyst for examining local problems related to breast cancer screening and early detection, generating solutions applicable to local needs and circumstances, and identifying the extent to which local resources can support proposed interventions and improvements.

WHY PARTNERSHIP?

Partnership is more than collaboration, more than cooperation, more than combination. A BHP is more than the sum of its partners. Partnerships amplify the work that gets done and, consequently, the benefits that accrue to the community. Partnerships are reciprocal; all partners give and get. Each partner has some resource, skill, or connection that is valuable to the group. Deciding to participate in the BHP signifies a willingness to make that contribution in order to meet the goals of the group. Numerous benefits result from encouraging public and private business, service and social groups, nonprofit agencies and institutions, medical care providers, and interested individuals to participate in the "community of solution":

- each partner brings a different area of expertise or knowledge about a particular clientele, and can adapt strategies accordingly, increasing the likelihood of successful efforts;
- everyone who is interested is welcome to participate, so there is a wide range of human and material resources available and no single agency bears the burden of the work or the responsibility for the success or failure of activities;
- participation from those who are not usually in the health service delivery system may foster creativity and effective new relationships among partners;
- increasing the community's self-reliance through developing significant in-kind components strengthens the community and its ability to compete for private and public dollars in this and other arenas.

GETTING STARTED

Once the decision had been made to pursue the development of BHPs, DOH staff from the Cancer Services Program contacted the DOH or Public Health Nursing Service in each county to request their assistance in convening a meeting of the local agencies and providers most likely to be interested in breast cancer screening. County health units were approached first because it was felt they would be more responsive to this request from the state DOH than any other local organization. From the outset, it was made clear to the local units, most of which are understaffed and overextended, that this was not a new program they were expected or required to organize. Rather, the BHP represents an opportunity for local health units to ensure that a public health need is met, without having full responsibility for the related program. Many, however, have embraced the BHP concept as a way to fulfill their mission to preserve and protect the community's health by assuming a leadership role.

Early meetings provided opportunities to create enthusiasm, assess needs and resources, and bring together an array of potential partners. During these meetings, the natural skills and abilities of certain partners asserted themselves, and decisions about which agencies would play the three primary partnership roles were made. Each BHP completed an application describing the contribution each partner would make, a plan for recruiting eligible women, and their service plan (Figure 1).

HOW ARE BREAST HEALTH PARTNERSHIPS STRUCTURED?

Any organization, group, or individual concerned about breast cancer is welcome to participate in a BHP; partners can be added at any time and may include health care providers, local businesses, agencies such as the American Cancer

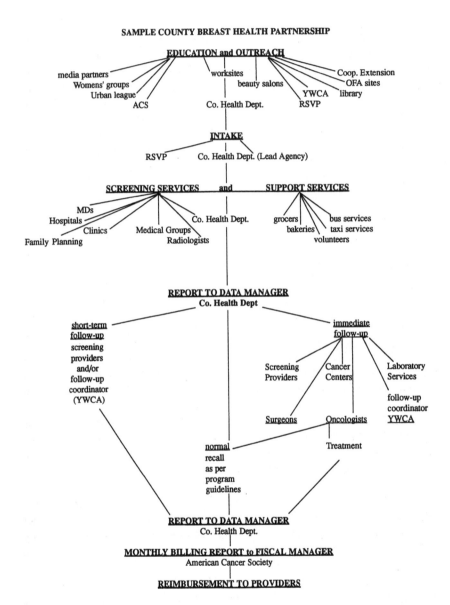

Figure 1. Sample county Breast Health Partnership.

Society and YWCA, libraries, local health departments, senior services programs, media representatives, and elected officials. Each BHP is unique, because it represents local resources responding to local needs. Some are large, some small; some meet regularly, some do most of their planning by phone. Several are formally organized, with bylaws and procedures, whereas others are more informal associations. Some have regularly scheduled screening events; others offer appointments in every week all year long. A few conduct major recruitment campaigns, whereas many rely on existing channels to identify potential clients. In this regard, one hallmark of the program is flexibility.

Although different in the way they get things done, the BHPs share key elements. All are required to:

- provide comprehensive breast cancer screening services to eligible women;
- ensure that women who screen positive have access and support for diagnostic testing, and that those diagnosed with breast cancer are treated, regardless of their ability to pay;
- use the same screening intake form and follow-up form to document the demographic characteristics of their clients, the services provided, and the outcomes for women; and
- negotiate with providers within the same Maximum Allowable Reimbursement Rate schedule.

In addition, all screening projects have access to teaching days to sharpen their skills and to technical advisors assigned regionally to assist them in solving problems.

Each BHP has a lead agency, a data manager, and a fiscal contractor. These roles may be filled by virtually any partner (there are a few restrictions for the fiscal contractor), and may be combined according to the skills and interests of those who come forward to assume them. In the current year (1994–95), the agencies performing these functions do so as their contribution to the BHP.

The lead agency provides a point of contact between the community and the BHP, as well as between the DOH and the BHP. Most often, the phone number published for the BHP is maintained and staffed by the lead agency. County DOHs, YWCAs, and American Cancer Society units have typically volunteered for this role (Table 1).

The fiscal contractor is the legal entity with which the department enters into a contract on behalf of the BHP. It is important that the fiscal contractor have the confidence of all partners, as it is this agency that submits BHP vouchers, receives payments, and distributes funds according to the types of services provided. The

Table 1 Agencies filling primary roles in Breast Health Partnerships

Agency	Lead	Data mgt.	Fiscal
DOH or PHNS	22	17	16
American Cancer Society	11	7	11
YWCA	2	4	5
Hospital	7	11	9
Other health facilities	2	5	3
PP	1	1	1
County office	1	1	1
Medical societies	1	1	1
Office for Aging	1		
DSS		1	1

excellent reputation, credibility, and neutrality of the American Cancer Society has resulted in that agency frequently assuming this function; many DOHs are also fiscal contractors. In some communities, one of the provider partners is also the fiscal contractor; this is a good barometer for the extent to which cooperation rather than competition is at work in the BHP.

The data manager collects the standardized screening intake forms from all partners, reviews them for completeness, batches them, and submits them for data entry to a data management firm working with the statewide program. Incomplete forms are returned to the partners. A billing statement, summarizing the number of each procedure provided, by provider site, is generated by the management firm and sent to the data manager. The data manager reviews the report and forwards it to the fiscal contractor, who uses it to generate reimbursement vouchers. Because the data and fiscal management functions are closely related, some BHPs have one agency serving in both roles.

FUNDING THE BREAST HEALTH PARTNERSHIPS

The BHPs receive funds based on documentation of services provided. Early BHPs participated in a pilot phase when they were asked to recruit and serve eligible women and accept a $55 reimbursement for each screening mammogram provided. As the BHPs gained experience with successful recruitment strategies and coordination of services, and the DOH program became more sophisticated and better funded, a broader array of screening and diagnostic procedures were reimbursable. In addition, we now offer small fees to offset the costs of recruitment and follow-up of suspicious findings.

Repeatedly over the last two years, the BHPs have reported that their work could be made more efficient and effective if dedicated staff were available to support certain activities. As with nearly every other aspect of the BHPs, their needs vary. Some believe the most important assistance would come in the person of a BHP coordinator. Others manage the logistics of the BHP well, but would benefit from having someone to implement specific outreach strategies. Still others are satisfied with all aspects of the BHP coordination and promotion, but need to hire a nurse to perform clinical breast examination, or a person to do follow-up. For the next program year, a funding formula has been developed that will allow some infrastructure building, while continuing to offset the costs of clinical services.

BHP EXAMPLES

Promotion of breast health practices and publicity about the availability of local, coordinated, subsidized services are critical components of a breast cancer screening program, but often represent a large expense. Having both public and private partners can yield interesting solutions to this problem. For example, a community's "pennysaver" newspaper provides one free advertising slot for every certain number purchased. A thriving clothing merchant regularly advertises in this paper. The merchant donates his or her "free" space to the BHP to advertise an educational session about the benefits of screening. The "pennysaver" owner donates his or her time and the skill of his or her staff to design the announcement.

Space, refreshments, and amenities for educational presentations are also routine expenses that the BHP can eliminate through creative partnership. A church donates its community room for an educational session because two Rotarians have agreed to put all the chairs away and clean the floor before leaving. A local grocery store provides cookies and milk. Girl Scouts who routinely meet at the church that night volunteer to set up the refreshments and provide supervision for children of mothers attending the session.

Finally, services must be secured. Because the reimbursement for various screening and diagnostic procedures is fairly low, it is unlikely that a provider would participate for the financial profit generated. There can, however, be other rewards. A private radiology group in a small town has the capacity to increase the number of mammography appointments available each week. BHP promotion of breast cancer screening increases the demand for this service among all women in the area. The radiologists agree to make some proportion of new appointments available to uninsured women referred through the BHP, because the remainder of the new patients might never have come in without prompting by the BHP publicity.

An example of a well-functioning BHP is provided by the Genesee Breast Health Partnership, which sponsored a Women's Health Week in October 1994. Thirty-three partners worked together to make this week a success. Examples include:

- Avon representatives throughout the region put an invitation to screening in each bag of products they delivered;
- The American Cancer Society, Office for Aging, Chamber of Commerce, and Salvation Army distributed flyers or put articles in their newsletters, reaching more than 2,300 individuals and 250 employers and business places;
- *The Daily News* wrote articles about the event, and a radio talk-show hostess invited members of the BHP to be on her show each week for four weeks prior to the event;
- Volunteers taped invitations to the doors of each apartment in the two senior citizen high-rises in the largest town in this rural county;
- The Zonta Club secured donated refreshments and served them at each screening site;
- American Cancer Society volunteers made 100 cloth tote bags, which were filled with donations from various agencies and businesses in the area (Niagara Mohawk, Key Bank, health maintenance organizations, Chamber of Commerce, United Way, and partners); and
- Clients at the Genesee Mental Health Day Treatment Program assembled all the gift bags.

Plans called for 100 women to be screened during this week. One of the facilities at which screening was to have taken place was unavailable at the last minute, and practitioners requested more time with each woman than was originally scheduled, so a total of 58 eligible women were actually screened during Women's Health Week. The remaining women were rescheduled and screened at their convenience. In organizing and implementing this effort, partners gained experience in working together to focus community resources on a tangible activity that everyone could support. They also learned about strategies that were not successful. For example, the invitations taped to doors in the senior citizen residences generated few participants. When the effort was evaluated, partners agreed to contact the building managers to schedule small group educational opportunities for residents, along with a more personal approach to making appointments.

EVALUATION OF THE BREAST HEALTH PARTNERSHIPS

Structural, process, and outcome assessments are all components of the comprehensive evaluation plan for the BHPs. A matrix has been developed to record the participating partners in each BHP; this is being used to determine which new partners should be approached, as well as to compare the relative resources available through each partnership when planning public education, outreach, or service delivery strategies. The number, nature, and location of screening services and diagnostic procedures performed, along with all outcomes and the timeliness of coordinated services, are regularly reviewed based on reports generated by the data management system. In addition, the demographic characteristics and insurance status of women screened are monitored; these data are useful in evaluating the success of outreach strategies. Management reports facilitate troubleshooting within the project, may suggest improvements in referral patterns or additional partners, and ensure fiscal accountability and appropriate stewardship of public funds.

Almost as important as the screening of an underserved population of women is the interaction the BHPs have generated among providers and interested others in their communities. More than 800 partners participate in 48 BHPs. Many of these have not worked together before; partners are finding other areas in which their skills and resources are complementary. BHPs have reported that providers who would not even attend the same meeting in the past now work side by side to arrange referrals for women with findings or to plan new recruitment strategies. These are the changes that will ultimately make the program successful—changes that reflect a new attitude about collaboration and community strength.

•   •   •

With these changes taking place, communities will be better prepared to face the challenges of encouraging all their members to develop healthy lifestyles, including use of preventive care and early detection services. In return for their participation, individual partners get improved communication with peers and connections to people and agencies with whom they might not otherwise interact, enhanced community goodwill, a healthier community, and the potential for more business, more effective achievement of individual goals, and a competitive edge in future endeavors where a cooperative and organized community is advantageous.

14

Coalition Building
for Prevention

*Edith A. Parker, Eugenia Eng, Barbara Laraia, Alice Ammerman,
Janice Dodds, Lewis Margolis, and Alan Cross*

Coalitions generally have been defined as alliances among different sectors, organizations, or constituencies for a common purpose.[1] Coalitions differ from other community groups in that they are composed of individuals representing diverse organizations and community sectors; develop formal working relationships; are relatively durable; are issue oriented, structured, and focused on specific goals external to the coalition; and include collaboration by coalition members on behalf of the organizations they represent and advocacy by these members on behalf of the coalition itself.[2]

In recent years, reports of the use of coalitions in community-based public health have gained in number as have reports of the effectiveness of coalition efforts.[2-4] Coalitions have focused on issues as diverse as tobacco control[5]; alcohol and substance abuse[6]; adolescent pregnancy prevention[7]; cardiovascular disease risk reduction[1,4]; and public health practice and training.[8] McLeroy and colleagues suggest the current popularity of coalitions may "lie" in their democratic appeal. More specifically, they suggest that the appeal of coalitions may lie in (1) the perceived opportunity for broad community involvement in solving local problems and changing community norms; (2) the belief among professionals that coalitions can address community health concerns while empowering or developing capacity in local communities; and (3) the belief that better coordination of services and improved working relationships among organizations will reduce redundancy in community services or administrative costs and thus provide more efficient use of local resources.[3]

Support for the project was provided through the W.K. Kellogg Foundation's Community-Based Public Health Initiative. The authors gratefully acknowledge the contributions of the entire membership of the North Carolina Community-Based Public Health Consortium.

J Public Health Management Practice, 1998, 4(2), 25–36

The impetus behind the formation of most public health coalitions has been to address a categorical health problem.[1,4-7] Despite the suggestion of McLeroy and colleagues of the "democratic appeal" of coalitions, the membership of coalitions reported in the literature rarely included representatives from ethnic or racial minority communities.[3] It appears, therefore, that although promising, the state of the art in coalition building still falls short of being the answer to the Institute of Medicine's call for a new model of public health that allows coalition partners gathered around a table to achieve "policy development and leadership that foster local involvement and a sense of ownership, that emphasize local needs, and that advocate equitable distribution of public resources and complementary private activities commensurate with community needs."[9(p.9)] If the coalition's agenda is organized around attacking categorical illnesses identified by health professionals as priority problems for communities without community input, which is essentially the "old way of doing business," then lack of involvement from underserved communities is not surprising.

This chapter examines the four-year development of a consortium that differs in both its agenda and membership from the many examples described in the literature. The North Carolina Community-Based Public Health Initiative (NC CBPHI) did not take a categorical approach of targeting a specific disease. Instead, NC CBPHI's focus was on building four county-level coalitions at different stages of formation to achieve the following common goals: (1) to improve minority health in four relational African-American communities; (2) to make public health education programs and services more responsive to the needs of these communities; and (3) to ensure a key role for CBO partners in shaping public health services and working with health professionals in their communities.

These goals clearly emphasize the importance placed by NC CBPHI on the *process* of coalition building during its initial four years. For NC CBPHI, the underlying assumption was that the product of a process that could achieve these goals would be indeed a "new" model of public health. Hence, the evaluation findings to be presented are on those factors that affected coalition functioning and success. The factors identified through the NC CBPHI experience are compared to those found by other evaluations of coalition building.

The NC CBPHI was one of the seven national sites funded through the W.K. Kellogg Foundation's Community-Based Public Health Initiative.[10] This initiative grew out of the foundation's concern that public health agencies and academic institutions "should become linked with community-based organization (CBOs) in underserved communities if needed changes in the discipline (as outlined in the 1988 Institute of Medicine Report on the Future of Public Health[9]) are to be achieved and if these changes are to be responsive to society's greatest needs."[10(p.1)] The overall goals of the initiative were to make public health educational programs and services more responsive to the needs of communities and neighborhoods; and to ensure that communities and CBOs play a key role in shaping public health services and in working with health professionals in their community.

Each NC CBPHI coalition included, at minimum, the following organizational partners: a CBO serving minority populations; a county health department; a private, not-for-profit local health center; a school of public health; and a school of medicine. The four county coalitions were linked together through a steering committee representing all 11 organizational partners. The steering committee's governance structure designated six voting members from health agencies and the university respectively, and seven from CBOs. The president and vice president positions alternated between a health agency and CBO representative; the secretary-treasurer position was always held by a university representative. In sum, this steering committee and the four county coalitions comprised the overall NC CBPHI Consortium.

EVALUATION METHODS AND FRAMEWORK

The NC CBPHI employed a multiple case study participatory evaluation design, with each county coalition, the overall consortium, and academic partners respectively serving as single cases. A cross-case analysis of evaluation reports on each of the four county coalitions was conducted to identify the factors affecting coalition functioning and success. These evaluation reports were generated at baseline, Year 2, and Year 3, using the following data sources: in-depth qualitative interviews with 40 coalition members; participant observations of 60 coalition meetings and sponsored events; and review of 20 coalition documents, such as quarterly and annual reports submitted to the steering committee. All in-depth interviews and field notes were transcribed, entered into the Nota Bene[11] text analysis software, and coded using a focused coding method.[12,13] Patterns uncovered in text lines that had been assigned the same code were used to generate themes relevant to the evaluation. The subsequent evaluation reports focused on four broad areas: changes (such as increased community problem-solving capacity) in the community with which each county coalition was working; coalition functioning; changes in health department and academic partners; and accomplishments in reaching minority youth.

To guide the evaluation's examination of coalition functioning, a conceptual framework was needed to reflect the NC CBPHI partners' agreed-upon principles for coalition participation and commitment. These principles included: a specific African-American community in each county would have agreed to participate with a coalition; each organization would carry out the tasks of community-based practice (i.e., action-oriented community diagnosis, needs assessment, and community participation); each organization would commit to implementing the proposal regardless of funding from the Kellogg Foundation; and the "CEO" of each organization would sign a written document agreeing to the above principles.

Given NC CBPHI's intent, as reflected in these principles, to develop partnerships and collaboration across the four county coalitions as well as within each county coalition, Alter and Hage's framework was found to be the most relevant framework for conceptualizing how stages and levels of collaboration might be operationalized in coalition functioning.[14] The first stage of the framework is that of an *obligational* network, in which the collaboration among organizations consists of information exchange and communication and is dependent on personalized communication among staff members (called "boundary spanners"). A shift to the next stage of a *promotional* network occurs when the organizations are willing to contribute individual agency resources to the coalition, dependent in some way on the coalition's collective output, and feeling a normative obligation to comply with the coalition.

In the promotional network stage, coalition members have identified a problem common to the participating organizations and work together on addressing that problem, with each organization playing a defined role. In this stage, organizations still retain their autonomy because the scope of cooperative decision making is well defined and usually limited (in either time or in the amount of resources involved) to the identified problem(s). The organizations, however, do give up some degree of control over their own operations by accepting the actions suggested by a coalition.

A *systemic* network is the final stage in this framework. As a systemic network, a coalition has evolved to address common problems that are so complex that resources from more than the coalition structure are needed and are established. In this stage, organizations relinquish their individual autonomy to the coalition and as a consequence, decision making and assignment of individual organization members are ceded from the individual organization to the coalition.

The stages of coalition building described by both Butterfoss and her colleagues and Florin and his colleagues seem most relevant to Alter and Hage's obligational network stage of development because collaborative ventures may be new to these coalition partners (see Table 1).[2,14,15] At the time when NC CBPHI was funded, two coalitions were judged to be at the obligational network stage because the organizations had no prior experience of working together. Both coalitions were in smaller and more rural counties than the other two coalitions. The third coalition, located in a county with a sizable rural population and a large university, had some organizational partners with a history of limited collaboration (e.g., subcontracts for services, field placements for students) and was judged to be at the promotional network stage. The fourth coalition had a strong history of collaborative projects (e.g., jointly awarded grants, cosponsored conferences) among all its partners and was, therefore, judged to be closest to the systemic network stage.

Table 1 Stages of coalition development compared to stages of interorganizational networking

Stages of coalition development		Stages of interorganizational networking
Butterfoss et al.	Florin et al.	Alter and Hage
1. Formation—Occurs at initiation of funding; recruitment of members; establishing structure and training; task identification	1. Initial mobilization—Recruit participants and engage constituencies 2. Establishment of organizational structure 3. Building capacity for action—Through changes in members attitudes, knowledge, skills; and establishing interorganization linkages with variety of community organizations.	Obligational Network—Collaboration within coalition consists of information obligational and communication
2. Implementation—Needs assessment and program development and implementation	4. Planning for action—Needs assessment; development goals and objectives; program development 5. Implementation—Develop workplan and implement activities	Promotional Network—Organizations still retain autonomy but work together on problem identified as common to all organizations
3. Maintenance—Monitoring and upkeep of membership and planned activities	6. Refinement—Use evaluation data for program refinement and revise strategies accordingly	Systemic Network—Coalition has evolved to address common problems so complex that resources from more than the coalition structure are needed and are thus established. Individual organization autonomy is ceded from the individual organization to the coalition
4. Outcome—Impact that results from deployment of community-wide strategies	7. Institutionalization—of processes for leader succession and recruitment and integration of functions into ongoing missions of existing organizations	

FACTORS AFFECTING NC CBPHI COALITION FUNCTIONING AND SUCCESS

Alter and Hage's framework was applied to the cross-case analysis to examine how the four NC CBPHI county coalitions, at different network stages, developed over a three-year period.[14] The findings revealed six factors that affected coalition functioning and success (see Table 2). These factors were similar to those identified by other studies[2,4,15] and are described below.

Participation in coalition activities was found to be positively related to coalition functioning and success. There appeared to be four specific coalition functions that were affected by members' participation.

Recruitment and retention of coalition members

The four coalitions were successful in establishing a racially and organizationally diverse membership. Some of this success was attributed to the initial design of NC CBPHI, which required each coalition to include a CBO that served a minority and underserved community as well as a health agency and academic institution. However, the coalitions were able to go beyond these initial requirements and recruited members from the business community, county government, and community clergy. For example, the coalition at the systemic network stage had identified economic development as crucial to improve the health status of the minority community they served. The strategy they chose was to support and increase the number of minority-owned businesses in the community. To recruit local businesses to join the coalition, they hosted a series of "breakfast round-

---

Table 2 Identified factors important in successful NC CBPHI coalition functioning

Participation
- Recruitment and retention of coalition members
- Recognition of limitations of "representative membership"
- Continued and active participation of coalition members
- Participation of members' constituent populations

Communication

Mutually agreed upon and recognized governance system
- Role clarification and division of labor
- Agency accountability of organization members and the coalition as a whole
- Operating procedures

Staff–coalition members relationship

Technical assistance and leadership training

Ability to recognize and deal with conflict

tables" for minority business owners to come together and discuss their issues and concerns with the coalition. These breakfast roundtables were held at a minority-owned restaurant in the community and subsidized by a local bank as part of its community service. As the coalition with the strongest history of collaboration among its members, this did not support Herman and colleagues'[16] finding that coalitions built on prior collaborations were less likely to expand past these existing networks. Rather, the NC CBPHI experience corroborated Florin and colleagues' conclusion from studying 35 coalitions organized to prevent substance abuse (i.e., more effective coalitions were those able to recruit members from business, clergy, senior citizens groups, police, volunteer community organizations, parent groups, youth organizations, university, and medical sectors).[15]

Recognizing the limitations of "representative" membership

The question of who represents grassroots community members arose among NC CBPHI coalitions. In the coalition at the systemic network stage, for example, the CBO was an umbrella organization for more than 20 African-American grassroots groups. However, it was described by some coalition members as not necessarily being "grassroots" itself. A member of this CBO in question responded in the following way:

> Are they looking for community people who have the greatest chance of succeeding or are we looking for representatives so that all levels of people are on these boards? . . .Why make the same old community action mistake? Why not respect leadership that has emerged and has the greatest chance of making institutional change; the people who are already affiliated and have experience in managing? . . . Are we building on the strength of the community or the weakness?

A member of this coalition, who was considered more grassroots but was not a member of this particular CBO, perceived another advantage of its participation:

> [This CBO] is not a grassroots organization. . . . That's not all bad because grassroots organizations normally don't have the liaisons to bring in people like . . . the lady from the Children's Defense Fund . . . the thing they [the CBO] have done is connect themselves to other grassroots oriented organizations. So they have the connections and all of the members can benefit from the connections.

All four coalitions recognized that despite their success in establishing diversity in membership, minority communities are, like all communities, not homogenous. Thus, the participation of a minority CBO does not guarantee a membership that represents the heterogeneity of minority communities.

Continued and active participation of coalition members

NC CBPHI coalitions were able to maintain a reasonably active level of participation over the initial three years. As noted earlier, the agreed-upon principles of coalition participation and commitment appeared to partially explain why. Each organization's signed commitment to implementing the project regardless of funding proved crucial to sustaining their active participation. For example, during this three-year period, three county health department directors, who had been actively involved with NC CBPHI from its inception, accepted positions elsewhere. Yet, each health department remained actively involved in the work of the coalition, with other health department personnel moving into coalition and consortium leadership roles.

Other studies have found that a member's perceived costs and benefits were a strong predictor of participation and satisfaction with the coalition.[17-19] Similarly, NC CBPHI found that respecting members' time availability caused perceived benefits from attending meetings to outweigh perceived costs. For example, the four coalitions gave serious attention to determining the best times to hold coalition meetings. One coalition chose 5 PM to ensure that community members with jobs could attend. Another coalition alternated meeting times between evening and daytime hours. The other two coalitions continued with daytime meetings because, they noted, community coalition members were available at those times. Also, coalitions tried to limit their monthly meetings to two hours, recognizing that all members had other time commitments.

Finally, maintaining active membership was also attributed to each coalition's setting aside time to establish a basic level of trust among coalition members, for both individuals and the organizations they represented. The amount of time required varied according to the coalition's network stage. For example, in the coalition that began at the systemic network stage, there appeared from the onset to be a high level of trust among partners that resulted in the ability to disagree without great disruption. The past working relationship between the CBO and the health department was seen as contributing to this trust. As noted by this respondent, "There is a lot of trust and they [coalition members] can fuss. They can really have a fight and move on." In contrast, for a coalition that began at the promotional network stage, the ability to establish enough trust to discuss controversial and sensitive issues did not happen until Year 3.

Participation of coalition members' constituent groups

Those expected to participate in NC CBPHI coalition activities went beyond the actual members of the coalitions. That is, the wider community also needed to participate as change agents to define and effect meaningful changes in how health agencies and universities "conduct business as usual." To achieve this broader participation, the coalitions formed a standing Communications Committee and an ad hoc Video Committee to establish a unified voice communicating common messages on what is NC CBPHI, each coalition's goals and activities, and the importance of participation from all sectors in communities, health agencies, and universities. However, given NC CBPHI's multiple agendas, knowledge of the overall initiative and concepts varied among coalition members. Said one respondent:

> Those types of things have not come out [goals of the project for institutional change]—that the health department is supposed to be changing and that Cooperative Extension is there to help, or the School of Medicine. The community people have seen their involvement. They [coalition partners] come to the meetings but what have they done as far as the community part, you know, being in the community. So they [community members] don't know the key players and what their jobs are or what their part of this is supposed to be about.

A staff member of another coalition questioned the degree of importance to be placed on community members understanding the philosophy behind NC CBPHI, saying:

> I agree with you that people don't hear enough about NC CBPHI within project communities. I don't want to create loyalty to a project, but rather, to what community members could do in the community.

Nevertheless, to communicate the philosophy and goals of NC CBPHI to the wider community, coalitions used different strategies. One coalition used the video to make formal presentations to different county agencies and community groups. A community representative from another coalition made sure that at every community event she attended, she described the philosophy and goals of NC CBPHI and how it related to that particular event. Regardless of the strategy used, most coalitions acknowledged that it takes time and effort for dissemination activities to have an effect.

A particularly innovative strategy used to elicit more participation from health department staff in NC CBPHI was the series of Shared Leadership and Model Development workshops. These workshops brought employees from each of the four coalition health departments together to share and discuss "creating a new model of public health practice." In between workshop sessions, each team of health department participants returned to their agency and worked together on strategies to disseminate the NC CBPHI model into their health department.

Communication emerged as a factor that affected coalition functioning and success. Separate from the previously described communication strategies to elicit participation in NC CBPHI, there were other aspects of communication important to coalition functioning, such as formal and informal channels of communication.[20] NC CBPHI coalitions, for the most part, established good systems of formal administrative communication (i.e., written record of meeting minutes, reminder notices, and coalition announcements). Establishing a climate conducive to good informal and interpersonal communication, however, was more of a challenge.

A conducive climate was defined as one in which agencies communicated in an understandable fashion (i.e., kept professional terminology or jargon to a minimum), solicited and listened to community members' opinions, and respected their input. Coalitions with a prior history of working together appeared to feel more comfortable participating in coalition discussions. Noted one community representative about her coalition:

> Everybody is able to state their opinions, everybody's *opinions counts* . . . . Lots of time, community people feel you have all these agency people here, I may sound stupid. But everybody's made to feel comfortable and allowed to speak our minds. . . . I don't always agree but that's okay too. [We] always come up with an idea that will work for the total group.

The following quotes from another coalition point to the challenge of achieving and maintaining a climate conducive to good interpersonal communication. A new coalition member representing a health agency partner noted that in the three previous meetings, the community member representatives had not said a word. When she asked a community member what the coalition could do so that community members would speak out at meetings, this is the response she received:

> It'd be more easy if they'd [other coalition members] be quiet. The coalition shouldn't speak for us. . . . Listen to community and let community speak for themselves.

This same community member noted her difficulty in understanding the jargon used in a previous coalition meeting:

> Like that budget discussion. She [pointing to the agency representative] said she didn't understand what was going on. If you have a college education and can't understand it, how do you think I can understand it.

A mutually agreed upon and recognized governance system was found to be a crucial factor affecting coalition functioning and success. Although a governance system did not have to be "formally approved," its existence needed to be recognized by all coalition members. For example, three of the four coalitions had governance systems from the initiation of their coalitions, yet formal passage of by-laws in all four coalitions did not occur until well into Year 3. As one coalition member noted:

> Having the governance structure in place, I think, it's an important milestone. With the structure, now moving along as a coalition—not to say

we weren't—but without the governance structure, we had no structure or format. . . . It's hard to make decisions collectively. It's easier to make decisions [with a governance structure], easier to organize the structure of the coalition.

Role clarification and division of labor

A governance structure was found not only to clarify the roles of organizational partners in a coalition, but also the roles of coalition staff. A member of the coalition that began at the obligational network stage described the effect of a governance structure on role clarification:

One thing would be establishing governance so we now have officers and a distribution of responsibilities in decision making instead of decision making resting with one agency.

Even with governance systems in place, coalitions found they had further work to do on role responsibilities and accountability. Coalitions scheduled retreats that included issues of roles and division of labor on the agenda. One coalition divided into a committee structure, with individual committees focusing on health, economic development, and leadership development. This helped to define member roles and diminish the potential for turf battles among organizational partners.

Accountability of organizational members and the coalition as a whole

When a governance structure was not in place, coalitions were less able to act on issues of organization accountability. One member, whose coalition was late in adopting a formal governance structure, noted:

They've been the silent partner since the inception of the grant. We had high expectations, but they have not been met. Having no governance in place, how do you hold [organizations] accountable when there is no definition of what they were to do?

The ability to hold organizational partners accountable for their agreed upon actions appeared easier to accomplish for those coalitions at the systemic and promotional network stages. In the coalition at the systemic stage, one respondent noted: "We know the partners well enough, so if something is going wrong, we can raise our concerns." The coalition at the promotional network stage was able to renegotiate a contract with an organizational partner who was not making a full contribution to the coalition.

Establishing a climate that ensured a coalition's accountability as a whole was also an important task. For example, in many of the NC CBPHI coalitions, members noted that coalition follow-up on ideas discussed could have been better. Although this was assumed to be an integral part of staff's duties, the coalitions needed to establish a procedure:

> We need to translate what has come out of meetings into action plans . . . to write goals or make changes at the health department or police department.

Another accountability procedure needed was around attendance. In one coalition, late arrivals of members became such a problem that meetings routinely began 10 to 15 minutes late. The coalition chair noted in frustration, "You can only scold people so much about being late."

Operating procedures

Even seemingly simple coalition functions, such as scheduling meetings, were found to be affected by governance structures. Hence establishing rules of operation about decision-making procedures and general meeting norms was essential to coalition functioning. Coalitions needed to decide if they were operating on a consensus or a majority rule system; if they wanted an executive committee to discuss issues in detail and then bring suggestions to the larger coalition or have general coalition discussions to decide all issues; and how they would ensure a proper balance between process and task functions.

For NC CBPHI coalitions, a major challenge was achieving a balance between administrative and programmatic tasks. Members in some coalitions were concerned that community partners were becoming frustrated with the lengthy discussions of administrative tasks. Interestingly, one CBO representative expressed a different opinion, suggesting that community involvement in administrative decisions was important to maintaining the community's trust in the coalition because these decisions often involved the transfer of resources. In an attempt to strike a balance, all coalitions established an executive committee and two coalitions alternated the focus of monthly meetings between administrative and programming decisions.

Staff–coalition members relationship emerged as a factor affecting all coalitions. No matter the network stage, staff supervision and role delineation arose for each coalition to address. Balancing staff autonomy with coalition input was a challenge described by several coalition members, such as this:

> I suppose the coalition could be more directive and maybe the staff could bring things to the coalition more. But it's a real hard thing to work out because the coalition only meets once a month and the program needs to go on a daily basis. We have talked about that a little bit in the past, about how to really work that since this is a real. . . . We're

trying to make it a coalition program so that all the partners are involved. I think we've been fairly successful at that. We don't have it all down yet. . . . I think the coalition expects staff to direct it—that's just my sense. . . . A lot is left to staff, but I think that's appropriate.

The coalition's role in supervising staff was sometimes unclear because staff were employees of one particular agency and thus guided by that agency's personnel policies. To overcome this challenge, coalitions used different strategies. In one coalition, staff who were employees of the health department were directly supervised by health department staff, but all coalition members were encouraged to participate in this employee's annual performance review. In another coalition, the health department director was responsible for staff's administrative oversight, days off, training, and travel while the coalition was responsible for staff's program activity oversight (i.e., what the staff would actually be doing). Nonetheless, even when the relationship between staff and coalitions was articulated, issues of staff accountability and autonomy remained unresolved. Coalition members remained reluctant to address any dissatisfaction they had with staff performance, in part, because there was no one direct supervisor.

Opportunities for staff training and development were affected by the relationship between staff and coalition members. Because many of the staff were relatively young in their careers, continuing education was crucial for staff development. To respond to this need, the academic partners offered workshops and seminars on community organizing, grant writing, and other topics.

Technical assistance and leadership training for each coalition as a whole were needed and desired to improve coalition functioning, but never implemented. As suggested by Florin and colleagues, coalitions can build their capacity for action by building the capacity of their members.[15] Although NC CBPHI did include some leadership training in the retreats and annual meetings organized as well as during a national networking conference it hosted, these exposures were not tailored to the specific needs of each coalition. To ensure that all coalition members were "singing from the same hymn book" (as expressed by one member), training was needed on content areas, such as what is public health and what are public health agencies mandated to do; and skills areas, such as program planning, group facilitation, and community organizing. As noted by an evaluation staff member observing a coalition discussing its concern about community mobilization strategies:

While it is staff and residents' council members who will primarily implement these strategies, the presence of the whole coalition [at a training] will ensure that all members understand the complexity of mobilization activities.

Ability to recognize and deal with conflict was the final factor identified as affecting coalition functioning. Some coalitions were reluctant to admit that conflict or tension was present. One coalition member noted that when tension builds up between coalition partners during meetings, this tension is not directly addressed at the meetings but "behind closed doors." For this particular coalition, which was at the obligational network stage, the introduction of a governance system enabled them to recognize and manage conflict. The coalition at the promotional network stage used focused retreats to address conflict. Not surprisingly, the coalition at the systemic network stage seemed most able to recognize and address tensions when they arose. As one coalition member said:

> The coalition functions on a consensus model and is still in a phase of, the feeling of, well, we're going to make this work. And so there's willingness to kind of, hear other people's ideas. . . . I'm not aware of people being so set in a "This is the way we need to do it and if you don't do it this way, you know, I'm going to oppose what you're suggesting." That kind of conflict is not happening. And it's not to say that there is mindless consensus . . . there is discussion, good discussion. Hard questions are asked.

NC CBPHI coalitions experienced less conflict over budget matters than other studies of coalitions.[4] This appeared to have been due, in large part, to making the hard decisions *before* being funded. That is, the university was designated by the partners to serve as the fiscal agent for the overall consortium, and it then channeled funds through annual subcontracts to each coalition's designated fiscal agent. Each coalition was required to submit an annual work plan with a proposed budget, and quarterly reports on progress and expenditures for review by the consortium's Program and Finance Committee. The two coalitions for whom the health department served as the fiscal agent experienced some conflict over financial management matters. To address the disagreements, one coalition held a focused retreat that resulted in the establishment of a petty cash account to allow more flexibility in spending. The other passed a set of bylaws that assured the coalition's role in controlling the budgeting process.

DISCUSSION AND IMPLICATIONS FOR PUBLIC HEALTH PRACTICE

The four NC CBPHI coalitions differed in both their agenda and membership from the many examples described in the literature by taking a noncategorical approach and focusing on improving minority health and making public health education and public health services more responsive to community needs. A cross-case analysis of the four coalitions revealed six factors that affected coalition functioning and success, no matter the stage of development.

These factors suggest that the process of coalition building can be positively influenced by: (1) facilitating active participation of coalition members and the wider community; (2) ensuring a system for both formal and informal communication among organizational partners; (3) establishing a governance system and rules for operation as soon as possible; (4) clarifying division of labor between coalition members and staff, task definition for coalition staff, and supervisory responsibilities for staff; (5) identifying training needs and securing technical assistance and skills training for all coalition members, including staff; and (6) establishing mechanisms to anticipate and manage conflict. Practitioners working with coalitions should consider these, as well as factors identified by others, in designing and implementing coalition activities. Broader implications for public health practice are proposed below.

The NC CBPHI coalitions made a special effort to both involve minority community members as coalition members and undertake a noncategorical health approach to enable community members involved with the coalitions to address issues they considered to be important to minority health. This facilitated active community participation because it allowed organizational partners to tap into already existing community areas of activation. It also reduced excessive time demands that can be placed on community members when multiple "disease-centered" coalitions are created and community members are recruited to join each separate coalition. Hence, if possible, public health practitioners should promote coalitions that are noncategorical and allow community members to determine the issues upon which the coalition will focus. Further, practitioners considering coalition building as an intervention strategy should make every effort to recruit a diverse membership that draws from a range of sectors and reflects heterogeneity within minority communities.

It is important for public health practitioners to realize that establishing trust and building partnerships does take time. For coalitions with no or little history of previous collaboration, it required as much as three years for trust to be established, governance to be decided upon, and members to feel comfortable raising issues related to accountability or conflict. Thus, it is equally important for funding institutions to be patient when interested in seeing the results from a project taking a coalition-building approach.

The NC CBPHI experience is finding that even those communities with little history of collaboration among agencies and between agencies and minority community members can establish a partnership representing a "new model of public health." No matter their initial stage of network development, each coalition was able to contribute to their communities' health and well being. A variety of successful projects were implemented, which included construction of a playground at a housing community, establishing a free-standing neighborhood center offering health and economic development services and leadership training, organizing citizen drug patrols in a rural community to reduce trafficking of crack, and a "teens in power" program. Given a noncategorical approach, most of the initial projects were not health specific but focused on meeting urgent perceived needs of the community. However, as the coalitions evolved over time, they have all moved to health-specific projects. For example, one of the coalitions that began at the obligational network stage is conducting a community-based diabetes education program and has acquired additional funding to expand its self-monitoring center. Previous projects for this coalition included community leadership training, access to water and sewage, and the construction of a community park.

Alter and Hage noted that one sign of a coalition's movement from an obligational to a promotional or systemic network is its ability to acquire additional funding for the coalition.[14] NC CBPHI coalitions were all able to accomplish this. One coalition secured a position for one staff member by gaining the county commissioners' commitment to fund it permanently. In another coalition, successful grants were written to the local city government for youth activities. Matching funds were acquired from a municipality for a private foundation grant to renovate and expand a neighborhood park. Responsibilities for grant writing varied by coalition, but in most cases the coalition staff person took the lead in writing, receiving assistance from the coalition's representative for the academic partner and the consortium's program manager.

•   •   •

Coalition and community members cited NC CBPHI as an example of how agencies can collaborate with community groups as equal partners. Further, the relationship established among the agencies was considered by many to be a model to other agencies on how "people can work together across agency and organizational lines." A community member noted: "There is a feeling that we are equal partners and what we said mattered from the outset, how we felt about things, that it was not just an honorary seat." Challenges still remain in interpersonal communication between coalition partners as they continue past the initial funding period and into their fifth year of collaboration. NC CBPHI coalitions are demonstrating that agency–academic–community partnerships can activate community groups from different parts of a county to affect meaningful changes.

REFERENCES

1. V.T. Francisco et al. "A Methodology for Monitoring and Evaluating Community Health Coalitions." *Health Education Research* 8, no. 3 (1993): 403–416.

2. F.D. Butterfoss et al. "Community Coalitions for Prevention and Health Promotion." *Health Education Research* 8, no. 3 (1993): 315–330.

3. K.R. McLeroy et al. "Community Coalitions for Health Promotion: Summary and Further Reflections." *Health Education Research* 9, no. 1 (1994): 1–11.

4. C.A. Smith et al. "Cardiovascular Risk Reduction in Rural Minority Communities: The Bootheel Heart Health Project." *Journal of Health Education*, 1997: in press.

5. T. Rogers et al. "Characteristics and Participant Perceptions of Tobacco Control Coalitions in California." *Health Education Research* 8, no. 3 (1993): 345–358.

6. K.L. Kumpfer et al. "Leadership and Team Effectiveness in Community Coalitions for the Prevention of Alcohol and Other Drug Abuse." *Health Education Research* 8, no. 3 (1993): 359–374.

7. J.B. Nezlek and J. Galano. "Developing and Maintaining State-Wide Adolescent Pregnancy Prevention Coalitions: A Preliminary Investigation." *Health Education Research* 8, no. 3 (1993): 433–448.

8. J. Miller. Public Health Partnerships Shape the Future. *WKKF International Journal* 4, no. 1 (1992).

9. Institute of Medicine. *The Future of Public Health*. Washington, D.C.: National Academy Press, 1988.

10. W.K. Kellogg Foundation. *Grantmaking Initiative Announcement for Community-Based Public Health*. Battle Creek, Mich.: Author, 1990.

11. The Technology Group, Inc., Nota Bene, version 4.0. Baltimore, Md.: 1993.

12. M.Q. Patton. *Qualitative Evaluation and Research Methods*. Newbury Park, Calif.: Sage, 1990.

13. A. Strauss and J. Corbin. *Basics of Qualitative Research: Grounded Theory Procedures and Techniques*. Newbury Park, Calif.: Sage Publications, 1990.

14. C. Alter and J. Hage. *Organizations Working Together: Coordination in Interorganizational Networks*. Newbury Park, Calif.: Sage Publications, 1992.

15. P. Florin et al. "Identifying Training and Technical Assistance Needs in Community Coalitions: A Developmental Approach." *Health Education Research* 8, no. 3 (1993): 417–432.

16. K.A. Herman et al. "Evolution, Operation and Future of Minnesota SAFPLAN: A Coalition for Family Planning." *Health Education Research* 8, no. 3 (1993): 331–344.

17. R. Rich. "The Dynamics of Leadership in Neighborhood Organizations." *Social Science Quarterly* 60, no. 4 (1980): 570–587.

18. J. Prestby et al. "Benefits, Cost, Incentive Management and Participation in Voluntary Organizations: A Means to Understanding and Promoting Empowerment." *American Journal of Community Psychology* 18 (1990): 117–149.

19. S. Norton et al. "Perceived Costs and Benefits of Membership in a Self-Help Group: Comparisons of Members and Nonmembers of the Alliance for the Mentally Ill." *Community Mental Health Journal* 29, no. 2 (1993): 143–160.

20. N.M. Clark et al. "Sustaining Collaborative Problem-Solving: Strategies from a Study in Six Asian Countries." *Health Education Research* 8, no. 3 (1993): 385–402.

15

The Bridge to Health Project: A Collaborative Model for Assessing the Health of a Community

*Derryl E. Block, Jennifer Peterson, Michael Finch,
Ann M. Kinney, Paul Miller, and James Cherveny*

The Bridge to Health Project was designed to gather population-based health status data about approximately a half million residents in a primarily rural region in northeastern Minnesota and northwestern Wisconsin. Seventy organizations participated in this project. These organizations represented state and local health departments, hospitals, physician clinics, tribal health services, health planning agencies, and health provider educational institutions. The lessons learned from this project may aid similar initiatives in other communities and regions.

IN THE BEGINNING

Early in 1994, St. Mary's Medical Center, a not-for-profit hospital in Duluth, Minnesota, made the decision to incorporate information about the region's health status into its strategic planning database. Using the Healthy People 2000 Consensus Set of Health Status Indicators[1] as a guide, it became apparent that data on several important indicators were not available.

Although there were several sources of existing data, most noticeably vital statistics and the Behavioral Risk Factor Surveillance System,[2] there was a data gap concerning local information related to disease prevalence, health risk behaviors, and health care access. Additionally, even existing data were not adequate for analysis of small areas as was the desire in this project. Because the region is considerably more rural and older than either state that the Medical Center serves, there was uncertainty about how well the existing data portrayed the region's health status. The need to collect local data to get an accurate picture of the health of this population was apparent.

J Public Health Management Practice, 1998, 4(3), 43–49
© 1998 Aspen Publishers, Inc.

Because health status assessment is a core function of public health, the Medical Center first approached public health representatives to verify the need for data on lifestyle factors. Public health planners confirmed that local data were lacking, and agreed to become partners in planning a collaborative survey that would involve other health organizations throughout the region.

The wisdom of involving other stakeholders proved critical to the success of the project. First, many organizations needed local health status data for planning. Various viewpoints from the health care field provided a broad perspective to the survey. The involvement of representatives and local care providers throughout the region encouraged greater local participation and more ownership of the process by those who need to base programs and services on these data. Increased local involvement may have produced greater response rate. Finally, a positive experience collaborating on the survey process set the framework for cooperation in future projects.

Principles from community development theory were utilized in planning the process that would be used to construct and administer the survey.[3,4] A grassroots participatory process was designed to include key stakeholders, primarily health organizations, in the 16-county region. All participants were viewed as equal partners. Because the Medical Center provided both staff and financing for the project, it decided to aggressively pursue strategies to attenuate its power in the decision-making process.

Some other decisions were made, early in the process, before inviting participants:

1. The process would be inclusive of all local health providers and others interested in the project. State health departments would be encouraged to be involved due to their expertise and available resources related to health status.
2. An experienced consultant would be hired to facilitate, not lead, the process.
3. The resulting data would be nonproprietary and available to any interested party.
4. St. Mary's Medical Center would provide staff support (a project coordinator, a research manager, and research assistants) as well as funding for the project. The budgeted amount for non-personnel expenses was $60,000.
5. Sponsoring organizations would be invited to contribute in-kind support. Financial contributions would be welcomed, but not required for participation in the project.

Initial collaborative steps

It was essential to build support for the collaborative effort prior to the first meeting. Much time was devoted to contacting key stakeholders to inform them of the project and listen to their concerns. Potential barriers to the project's success were identified and addressed early in the process. Examples of barriers included perceptions that health status assessment was a public health and not a hospital function, competitive issues among providers, decision-making procedures within the collaborative group, and accessibility to the survey data that would be collected.

A key step in the early phases of the process was the development of a set of ground rules for participation. For instance, the group decided that participating organizations would have an equal voice in the decision making and that participants could attend any meetings. Additionally, decisions would be made by a consensus of those present. Consensus was defined as, "I can live with the decision." Additionally, it was decided to rotate locations for meetings.

Three work groups were established: (1) a *data team* to determine the methodology of the survey and design the survey tool; (2) a *communication team* responsible for formal internal communications among participants, as well as external communications such as logo development, media relations, and press conferences; and (3) a *steering committee,* a final decision-making body, receiving recommendations from the other two work groups. Participants could be members of any or all work groups. A professional facilitator aided the work groups in reaching consensus during their first few meetings.

Methodology

A representative sample and a high response rate were deemed critical to the success of the project. In the two years prior to this project, at least four other regional efforts were undertaken in the state of Minnesota to measure health status: none of these yielded participation rates of more than 30 percent (personal communication, Ann M. Kinney, Research Scientist, Minnesota Department of Health, March 4, 1995). To aid in research design and methodological decisions, and to supplement the existing expertise of the group, an academic researcher was engaged.

The data team agreed upon 18 geographical regions of interest. These included two metropolitan areas, the remainder of the two counties within which these metropolitan areas fall, and 14 adjacent counties, all of which are classified as rural. Power calculations were performed, and the goal of achieving a representative sample of 300 returned surveys from each of these 18 geographical regions was formulated. A random sample of households with telephones in each of the 18 geographical regions was purchased from Survey Sampling Inc. of Fairfield, Connecticut.

After reviewing existing instruments for measuring health status, participants decided to develop a customized instrument of their own. Given the broad range of interests of the group, a multivoting prioritization process was used to determine the topics to be included. Participants were sent a list and description of health indicators considered for study. They were asked to select and prioritize eight items. The results of the voting process were compiled and returned to the group for consensus. An instrument consisting of 119 items was developed by the data team.

The Medical Outcomes Study[5,6] instrument was reviewed, and items were chosen to represent eight domains of health status (physical functioning, role limitations due to physical health, bodily pain, general health perception, role limitation due to emotional health, and general mental health). Additionally, standard wordings of questions were chosen from the Minnesota Behavioral Risk Factor Surveillance Survey[7] as well as the Minnesota Health Care Insurance and Access Survey.[8] Most items were derived from existing instruments where reliability and validity had already been assessed. The instrument was pretested prior to administration.

A mixed mail/phone survey methodology was utilized.[9] The process involved four phases: (1) an initial mailing of the survey; (2) a postcard reminder 10 days later; (3) a second survey mailing seven days subsequent to the postcard to those who failed to respond to the mailed survey and reminder postcard; and (4) telephone interview of those who failed to respond to the second survey mailing.

Communication decisions

An important consideration for increasing response rate was to create a neutral image for the project. The chosen name for the project, Bridge to Health Survey, did not identify any particular sponsoring organization. All presentations and publications about the project, including the face sheet of the survey instrument itself, contained a list of the 70 sponsoring organizations. A special toll-free telephone line was installed by the Medical Center for the data collection period. Subjects who had questions could call the "Bridge to Health Hotline" for clarification. To maintain neutrality and to dispel the idea that this was a marketing survey, completed questionnaires were returned to a local university address.

INITIAL RESULTS AND PLANS FOR DISSEMINATION

The survey was conducted during a 10-week period in the fall of 1995. Of an initial sample of 11,360 adults, 2,882 could not be contacted because of wrong addresses, no phones, or because they were deceased. Of the 8,478 who were considered reachable, 5,438 (64%) responded. It was recognized that approximately 15 to 20 percent of the sample list would be unusable because of out-of-date phone numbers and addresses. After the mail portion of the survey was completed, it was apparent that one quarter of the sample was not usable. This required that the initial sample be supplemented with a second sample surveyed only by telephone, resulting in an extra 791 telephone surveys being conducted with people who had never received the mailed written version of the survey. Thus, the total sample was 6,229 subjects with 4,801 filling out questionnaires, and 1,428 having phone interviews. Of these, 6,034 surveys were deemed usable for analysis (4,737 mailed questionnaires and 1,297 phone interviews).

A survey report with regional level results was developed,[10] and in mid April 1996 a conference was held to alert regional providers and planners about the existence of the data. A public use data file was also developed. The collaborating organizations are planning interventions based on the survey data with the purpose of improving the health of the region.

LESSONS LEARNED

The project has been very successful thus far; a public use data set was created and is being used by members of the health care community. Two studies have been conducted to date using these data, one exploring barriers to care in this population, and one looking at alcohol consumption among mothers. Participants and others in the region are using the data set to answer questions specific to their areas of interest. For example, county specific data have been requested and generated to help agencies in their health planning. The participating organizations that collaborated on this project have forged new collaborative relationships. Based on the data, a region-wide emphasis on tobacco prevention is being planned and Bridge to Health members collaborated on a grant application to further this project. In addition, other regions in the state and across the country have requested information and seek to emulate the Bridge to Health process.

We have learned several lessons that we believe are essential to the success of this project. These lessons (not necessarily in any order) concern the importance of (1) sound survey methodology, (2) role clarification and staff support, (3) effective group process and structure, and (4) the homegrown nature of the project.

Sound survey methodology

The first lesson involved the use of sound survey methodology. The Bridge to Health participants debated and then agreed upon the importance of collecting data that were valid, salient, and representative of the health status of the people of the region. Once the decision to make the survey scientifically sound was made, other decision points became clear. For instance, the discussion about the number and type of geographic areas of interest to be surveyed led to a discussion of sample size. Participants stopped expecting that the survey would glean representative ZIP code-specific data as originally intended. Because a good response rate was deemed imperative, the questionnaire and methodology were designed with that in mind.

Role clarification and adequate staff support

The second lesson involved the clarification of participants' roles. The lead facilitator had a background in community development. She suggested that the group develop ground rules, allowed enough time for participants to discuss and come to their own conclusions, and helped keep the group on task. During various stages of the group process, members assumed different roles. For example, one member consistently pressed for the inclusion of questions relating to poverty. Another member was concerned with keeping the group on task and pressed for closure on issues. Knowing and trusting each other helped participants recognize and utilize the special skills and talents within the group.

Humor erupted spontaneously both with "sick" medical humor and in relation to the process. For instance, in pretesting the instrument, one rural respondent indicated that she restricted her neighborhood activities because of not feeling safe due to bears. When the issues of safety and violence was discussed, particular Bridge to Health Project members would say "Don't forget the bears!"

The group included seasoned practitioners, administrators, and planners who were attracted to a quality outcome. The participants had credibility: the credibility of knowing the community, and the credibility of being able to discern quality research. Most participants concentrated on giving suggestions based on knowledgeable opinions, clarifying meanings, and decision making.

Other important roles were filled by university researchers and representatives of the state health departments. Their research expertise helped ensure sound methodology. Also important were the competencies of the Medical Center research department in sampling, instrument construction, surveying, and analyzing a large data set.

There was a division of labor between the paid staff of the Medical Center and representatives of other organizations. Technical support, such as gathering resources and mailing minutes and agendas, was the Medical Center staff's responsibility. All participants utilized their individual expertise through designing the questionnaire and providing suggestions about survey methodology. The Medical Center staff assigned to the project had technical expertise in survey layout, coding, mass mailings, and data analysis. Therefore, the larger group did not have to be concerned with time-consuming technical tasks such as designing a questionnaire that could be scanned.

It is important to note that in the Bridge to Health Project the technical experts were blended into the process. Other communities without research experts readily available might decide to contract for technical assistance from an outside organization after the planning stage is completed.

Process

The third lesson was that fostering collaboration between organizations and obtaining quality survey data could not have been achieved without a well-organized process. This process can be conceptualized in three stages: *initial planning*; *group process leading to the generation of data*; and *transition to utilizing the data to improve health.*

The Medical Center was the major organizer in the *initial planning* stage of the project. This phase involved initial definition of the scope and structure of the project, provision of background research, contribution of monetary and personnel resources, and selection and invitation of participants. The Medical Center's donation of staff time and monetary support was crucial to the success of this undertaking. Monetary resources paid for sample list, survey printing and mailings, telephone interviews, consultant fees, refreshments, and mailings to the Bridge to Health Project participants.

Decisions were made early about what organizations would be invited to participate. In this project, health care organizations with broad bases of interest were initially invited, including public health, tribal health, hospitals, and clinics. Participants were also asked to suggest other groups to invite. However, this snowball process of inviting participation did not ensure representation from consumer and advocacy groups. In retrospect, including the viewpoints of these groups would have been advantageous.

The second stage was the *group processes leading to the generation of survey data.* These included the identification and resolution of critical issues regarding methodology, achieving consensus, facilitating internal and external communication, and designing the survey tool. Open communication was essential to the process. Ground rules were established and group norms developed for interaction and decision making. Agendas and meeting minutes from each work group were sent to all participants, and anyone could comment on or question any part of the process. Decision aids were used to enhance communication during particularly sensitive parts of the process. For instance, when the data team decided which questions would be included in the instrument, a list of questions used in other surveys, arranged by subject, was distributed to participants. This helped the participants come to conclusions much faster. A typical comment was, "I want this question to be asked, but I don't like the wording of any of the examples so let's try to develop our own wording." When it was impossible to develop the wording of a question, the group decided to exclude the topic from the questionnaire.

The third stage was the *transition to data utilization to improve health.* This stage is taking place as this manuscript is written. A regional conference was held to launch the survey report. A public use data set with documentation was produced and made available to the general public. A computer facility and programming staff were made available by St. Mary's Medical Center to assist organizations that do not have the requisite skills in performing custom analyses of the data. The Minnesota Center for Health Statistics also identified a staff member to provide customized statistical analysis. Contact has been made with a local college and university to encourage students in various disciplines to use the data set for their course work and for their own research. Most importantly, the coalition of organizations is continuing to meet to plan interventions based on the data to improve health in the region.

Homegrown nature of the project

The fourth important lesson points to the benefits of engaging the end users in the process. For organizations to develop collaborative relationships, individuals from these organizations need to work together toward a common goal. The Bridge to Health Project provided the framework for these organizations to collaborate.

Before involving other organizations, the Medical Center first considered the use of a consulting firm to collect regional health status data. After interviewing national consulting firms, it was apparent that utilizing an outsider's template for data collection would not necessarily be appropriate for this region, and would not foster collaboration.

The authors believe that Bridge to Health Project participants "bought into the process" because their participation (i.e., goal setting, choosing the methodology, developing the instrument) determined the outcomes. The group made the decisions, not the Medical Center nor any other participant organization. Because the process was "homegrown" it appears that participants shed some organizational turf issues, and felt ownership and personal commitment to the project. The list of survey sponsors displayed on the questionnaire attested to the ownership that participants felt toward the project. In an attempt to better understand collaborative functioning, a survey of participants in the Bridge to Health collaborative is planned.

ENVIRONMENTAL FACTORS

Certain environmental factors may have contributed to the success of this collaborative. The health care environment and the timing for the Bridge to Health Project were conducive to the success of this collaborative effort. This region is labeled "outstate" in both Minnesota and Wisconsin. Being away from centers of political decision making might facilitate communities to reclaim their power.

There are also important market forces that are motivating health care organizations to focus on health status improvement. This region is moving into a managed care environment. While about 75 percent of the state of Minnesota market is presently managed care, only about 18 percent of this region's health care market is managed care.[11] A capitated prepaid managed care program for medical assistance recipients has been instituted in a number of counties in the Minnesota region. It is important for organizations to have good morbidity data when bidding for capitated health care programs. As mentioned above, there was doubt as to whether state level morbidity data were valid for this specific region.

Concurrent with cutbacks in government spending, there is a supportive atmosphere for local data collection efforts. This kind of regional data collection can help state departments of health gain access to local level data that they cannot afford to collect. Governmental institutions need collaboration and local efforts to fulfill their mandates. Thus, collaboration is growing in importance. There is legislation in Minnesota mandating collaboration plans between public health and managed care organizations.[12]

•   •   •

This process may not be applicable in all settings. The success of this project may be a function of the culture of cooperation that is inherent in this region, the organizational culture of the sponsoring Medical Center, and a serendipitous coming together of talented people with compatible personalities. However, much of what was learned from this project is transferable to other communities or regions planning similar projects.

REFERENCES

1. U.S. Department of Health, Education and Welfare. "Consensus Set of Health Status Indicators for the General Assessment of Community Health Status—United States." *Morbidity and Mortality Weekly Report* 40 (1991): 449–451.

2. Remington, P.L., et al. "Design, Characteristics, and Usefulness of State-Based Behavioral Risk Factor Surveillance: 1981–87." *Public Health Reports* 103 (1988): 366–375.

3. Bracht, N., and Kingsbury, L. "Community Organization Principles in Health Promotion: A Five-Stage Model." In *Health Promotion at the Community Level*, ed. N. Bracht. Newbury Park, Calif.: Sage Publications, 1990: 66–86.

4. Green, L.W. *Community Health.* 6th ed. St. Louis: Times Mirror/Mosby College, 1990.

5. Ware, J.E., Jr., and Sherbourne, C.D. "The MOS 36-Item Short-Form Health Survey (SF-36): Conceptual Framework and Item Selection." *Medical Care* 30 (1992): 473–483.

6. Ware, J.E., et al. "Comparison of Methods for the Scoring and Statistical Analysis of SF-36 Health Profile and Summary Measures: Summary of Results from the Medical Outcomes Study." *Medical Care* 33 (1995): AS264–AS279.

7. Minnesota Department of Health. *Behavioral Risk Factor Surveillance in Minnesota, 1986–1992.* Center for Health Statistics, Minnesota Department of Health, Minneapolis, Minn.

8. Call, K.T., et al. *Minnesota Health Care Insurance and Access Survey, 1995.* Minneapolis: Institute for Health Services Research, School of Public Health, University of Minnesota, August 1996.

9. Dillman, D. *Mail and Telephone Surveys: The Total Design Method.* New York: John Wiley & Sons, 1978.

10. Bridge to Health Collaborative. *Bridge to Health Survey: Northeastern Minnesota and Northwestern Wisconsin Special Health Study Survey.* St. Mary's Medical Center, Duluth, Minn., 1996.

11. Minnesota Department of Health. *Minnesota Health Care Market Report 1995.* Minnesota Department of Health, Health Policy and Systems Compliance Division, St. Paul, Minn., 1995.

12. Local Public Accountability and Collaboration Plan, Minnesota Statute 62Q.075 (1996).

PART V

Evaluation

In the fifth section, the importance of program evaluation in public health practice is illustrated. Evaluation involves systematic approaches to determine
whether program objectives are being met (summative evaluation). In addition,
formative evaluation helps program managers assess whether the program is being implemented successfully. Evaluation is an essential part of public health as
practitioners and policy makers are called upon to document successful programs
and make careful use of limited public health resources.

The first chapter by Goodman offers a rationale for evaluation of community-
based interventions and provides five principles that are essential for sound evaluation. These five areas include: (1) assessment of program theory, (2) tailoring of
evaluation instruments to the individual community, (3) a use of both quantitative and
qualitative methods, (4) use of concepts from social ecology and social systems, and
(5) involvement of local "stakeholders" (i.e., citizens and local leaders). For each of
these five principles, Goodman furnishes a set of tools (e.g., questionnaires, participatory planning approaches) and also provides entry points into a rapidly growing and
widely dispersed literature on evaluation of community interventions.

Foley et al. describe the evaluation of an intervention in East Harlem, New
York, designed to increase immunization coverage among children. The "Hope
for a Million Kids" campaign featured door-to-door canvassing. Their evaluation
included three aspects: (1) semi-structured interviews with key planning and
implementation personnel, (2) an assessment of the number of children reached by
the intervention, and (3) a retrospective analysis of costs. Although they estimated
that more than 50,000 families were reached, based on vouchers, 211 children
were immunized as a result of the event at a cost of $594 per immunized child. The
authors note that the implementation of the New York City Immunization Registry may provide benefits in the future.

As you read these chapters, consider the following set of questions:

Objectives and Data Sources

1. How does one go about developing program objectives prior to program evaluation?
2. What types of data are routinely used for evaluating public health programs and policies?
3. In the chapter by Foley et al., are these sources routinely available and used to document immunization rates?
4. In a program evaluation, how would quantitative data differ from qualitative data?

Methods and Strategies

5. What are the differences between process, impact, and outcome evaluation?
6. If an intervention involves coalitions, how might they be involved in the development of evaluation strategies?
7. As illustrated by Foley et al., what are the challenges in planning a health fair that involves numerous health services providers?

Dissemination and Implications for Public Health Practice

8. When an evaluation is completed, how should its findings be disseminated? Can the early involvement of stakeholders assist in this dissemination?
9. Should the evaluator be part of the program being evaluated or an "outside" expert?

16

Principles and Tools for Evaluating Community-Based Prevention and Health Promotion Programs

Robert M. Goodman

This chapter is written as an overview and practical guide for the evaluation of community-based disease prevention and health promotion programs. More detailed accounts of evaluation issues and technical approaches for evaluating community programs can be found elsewhere.[1-4] The present chapter first offers a rationale for evaluating community-based programs and an introduction to evaluation approaches, then enumerates five selected principles that are contemporary to community evaluation. At the end of each principle, an annotated reference list is provided that contains tools for applying the principle to community evaluation.

A RATIONALE FOR EVALUATING COMMUNITY-BASED HEALTH PROMOTION PROGRAMS AND INTRODUCTION TO EVALUATION APPROACHES

An underlying premise of community health promotion is that well-planned local initiatives can produce desired social and health results. Steckler et al.[5] maintain that community health promotion is founded on democratic principles, and citizen participation is integral to community health promotion if community members are to take ownership for local health concerns. Thompson and Kinne maintain that "proponents of community approaches . . . recognize that local values, norms, and behavior patterns have a significant effect on shaping an individual's attitudes and behaviors."[6(p.45)]

Without sufficient evaluation, the effectiveness of a community program cannot be assured. Other reasons that often are given for evaluation include requirements by funding agencies for programs to be accountable, information on what programs work and how, and ethical considerations that programs are of benefit to clients and are cost effective.[1-3,7] Skillful evaluation can facilitate the ongoing improvement of program efforts; gaining of community support, grant money, and

J Public Health Management Practice, 1998, 4(2), 37–47
© 1998 Aspen Publishers, Inc.

donations; overcoming resistance to the program, detecting unforeseen challenges and side effects of the program; identifying intermediate successes; and increasing program responsiveness and accountability to community stakeholders.[8]

Program evaluation is divided into two general types: formative and summative.[9,10] Formative evaluation focuses on program development and summative on program results. Formative evaluation is frequently associated with process evaluation. The former examines the *acquisition and development* of necessary resources and structures to implement program activities effectively, including the hire or assignment of staff with the appropriate skills to the program, purchase of needed equipment and materials, allocation of program space, and development of activity protocols. The latter examines the *actual implementation* of the program, including the degree and quality of program delivery; for instance, does the program reach the appropriate audience, do sufficient numbers of individuals receive the program, is the program delivered in a consistent manner, are accurate records maintained?[3,11] Summative evaluation is often divided into near-term impacts and final outcomes.[12] Impacts usually are changes in the knowledge, attitudes, and behaviors of the program's target audience. If a program produces such impacts, then the likelihood increases that desired outcomes will result, including lower risk of disability or death.

In the last decade, evaluation approaches, in general, have developed in sophistication,[3] but evaluations of complex community efforts have experienced relatively fewer innovations.[13] In recent years, community health initiatives have become more comprehensive and complex, and evaluators are challenged to capture their rich nature.[14–16] Community initiatives often have broad and multiple goals that require complex interactions, multiple levels of intervention that occur in diverse settings, and multiple change strategies that require broad and repeated exposure. Frequently, community initiatives are purposely flexible and responsive to changing local needs and conditions; therefore, evaluation formats must be able to adapt in the middle of the assessment process. The responsibility for program implementation is likely to be shared by many community organizations and individuals; therefore, evaluation should be sensitive enough to reflect these complex working arrangements. Community health promotion may center on elusive concepts like community empowerment, ownership, leadership, and capacity building that are difficult to measure. Community programs often take many years to produce results; therefore, evaluators must maintain ongoing and harmonious relationships with community constituents.

In sum, adequate evaluation of complex community initiatives requires multiple data collection and analysis methods extended over long periods of time. In so doing, evaluators face significant challenges in developing adequate sampling, measurement, design, and implementation strategies with enough conceptual and methodological integrity to justify the effort.[17,18] Further, evaluators must be sensitive to and wise about local political realities and competing interests of different program stakeholders. Also, evaluators must be interpersonally skilled to interact effectively over the long haul with program representatives.[19]

CONTEMPORARY PRINCIPLES IN COMMUNITY EVALUATION

The five principles that follow address both formative and summative aspects of evaluating community health initiatives. Taken as a whole, the principles can help the evaluator address the complexity of community programs. Table 1 provides a summary of the principles and describes the tools available in the literature to assist with the application of each principle. The table is meant to augment the "Practical Tools" sections that appear at the end of each principle.

Principle 1: Evaluation of community programs should include an assessment of program theory

A common theme in the contemporary evaluation literature emphasizes the requirement that community health promotion programs should have theories of causation that guide their intervention strategies.[7,19–21] These theories are sometimes referred to as theories of action,[22] or logic models.[7] Kumpfer defines logic models as a ". . . a fancy term for what is merely a succinct, logical series of statements that link the problems your program is attempting to address, how it will address them, and what the expected result is."[7(pp.7,8)] Patton[22] describes a theory of action as a construction of means-ends hierarchy that constitutes a comprehensive description of the program. Weiss[16] describes program models as a series of micro-steps that contain important assumptions such as: training will lead to more skilled staff; information will reach target audiences; when informed, target audiences will attend programs. Micro-steps may be constructed as a series of "if . . . then" statements. For instance, Figure 1 is an example of a logic model taken from a program that activates community coalitions to reduce and prevent the abuse of alcohol, tobacco, and other drugs. If/then statements applied to this program include: *if* a local lead agency organized an ad hoc committee of leaders, *then* they will form multisectoral committees; *if* the committees are formed, *then* they will conduct needs assessments within their respective sectors; *if* needs assessments are conducted, *then* the chairpersons of each committee will consolidate the assessments; *if* the assessments are consolidated, *then* a comprehensive community plan will result; *if* a plan is produced, *then* it will guide plan implementation; *if* the plan is implemented, *then* the program will result in improved community health indicators.

Table 1 A summary of evaluation principles and tools

Principle	Tools	Description
1: Evaluation of community programs should include an assessment of program theory	Logic models	A diagram that illustrates the sequencing of program activities that should occur for planning, organizing, implementing, and producing desired results (see Figure 1). References 7, 19, and 21 should be obtained for step-by-step instructions for constructing a logic model.
2: Evaluation instruments that are used to measure community programs must be contoured to each individual community	Questionnaires and surveys	These instruments are often used at the beginning and then at later points in the program's life to determine whether the desired changes have occurred over time. The instruments also can be used just at one point in time to determine the status of the community when the instrument was administered. Whether applied at one point or several, the instrument is administered to individuals. The individual results are usually aggregated for statistical analyses. Reference 30 should be obtained for step-by-step instructions for developing questionnaires/surveys that can be contoured to a particular program's needs.
	Social indicators	Unlike questionnaires and surveys, social indicators do not depend on individual respondents, but often are based on data collected by government and other organizations, for instance the number of drunk driving arrests in a community. Social indicators generally are used over time to compare changes over time. For instance, do the rates of arrest increase, decrease, or remain constant over the course of the program's implementation? References 13, 26, 29, and 31 should be obtained for numerous illustrations of the types of social indicators that often are useful in evaluating community health initiatives.
3: Evaluation approaches used should be guided by the questions asked and often require both a quantitative and qualitative orientation	Experimental and quasiexperimental evaluation designs	These designs are often used to enable statistical comparisons between communities receiving a program and communities without the program to assess program effectiveness in producing desired results. Reference 3 is an introductory text that provides a detailed yet straightforward understanding of these designs, which can become quite complex.
	Qualitative designs	Unlike experimental designs, qualitative designs are not generally formulated for statistical comparisons, but provide for in-depth probing of a program's receptivity in a community.

continues

Table 1 Continued

Principle	Tools	Description
		Interviews with program stakeholders, reviews of program materials, and observations of program activities are the main methods used in these designs. Reference 33 is an introductory text that provides the essential components for developing program case studies, a qualitative design that often employs interviews, observations, and document reviews.
4: Evaluation should be informed by social ecology and social system concepts	Ecology and system designs	These designs combine principles from both experimental and qualitative designs in order to provide a comprehensive assessment of complex community programs. The designs are sensitive to a program's current stage of development and shift measurement strategies at each developmental stage, for instance from the program planning stage to program formation and implementation. Also, the designs include measurement strategies that are meant to be comprehensive, accounting for program effects on individuals, social networks, community organizations, social trends, and policy. Reference 14 should be obtained for a more detailed elaboration of ecology-informed designs. The reference also includes several measurement strategies and instruments for different developmental stages and social levels. Other references are described at the end of Principle 4 that should be obtained for more in-depth and technical approaches.
5: Community evaluation should involve local stakeholders in meaningful ways	Participatory planning	Participatory planning tools help to stimulate and reinforce community member involvement in the formulation and implementation of the evaluation in order to assure community problem solving for program improvement. Reference 58 should be obtained for a four-step approach for program and evaluation planning that is nontechnical and developed for lay community members to implement, including goal setting, and process, outcome, and impact assessments.

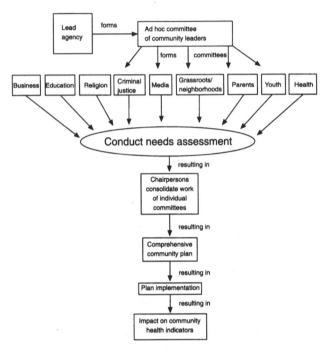

Figure 1. A logic model for a community coalition to address alcohol, tobacco, and other drug abuse.

Logic models should be developed well in advance of program formation and implementation. By so doing, the evaluator can work with the program stakeholders to explore the assumptions upon which the cause and effect relationships are based to ensure that time, effort, and expense are not wasted on programs with weak conceptual foundations and links. The theory of action can assist community stakeholders in developing consensus regarding the assumptions underlying the program, in assuring that the intervention is targeted at the problem of concern, and in making explicit how program activities are linked to produce the desired outcomes.[16,22] The models can help in defining the resources that are required for each stage of a program's development, thus enabling program stakeholders to consider whether sufficient resources can be obtained in advance of program implementation. Thus, logic models serve as program planning as well as evaluation tools. Further, models are templates for comparing how consistent the desired program (as reflected in the model) is with the program that is implemented.[7,16]

Evaluations that illustrate such consistencies may have more influence on both policy and popular opinion.[16] For many of these reasons, Patton[22] maintains that one of the first responsibilities that the evaluator has is to help program stakeholders identify and fill in the gaps in the program's theory of action. The Practical Tools section suggests several useful references for developing logic models.

Practical Tools. Kumpfer and colleagues[7] provide an approach to developing logic models, discuss evaluation design questions, and provide an extensive listing of evaluation instruments and measures for the practitioner. Scheirer[21] devotes an entire volume of the journal to the use of program templates that are similar to logic models. The templates are composed of lists of components of effective practice, intended program elements and what the program actually produced, and are a basis for judging and improving a program's formation and implementation. Goodman and Wandersman[19] incorporate the use of logic models into FORE-CAST, a system of formative evaluation. They present a step-by-step approach to developing models and using them to identify whether a complex community program is developing according to the model.

Principle 2: Evaluation instruments that are used to measure community programs must be contoured to each individual community

By developing a theory of action, program stakeholders construct their own unique blueprint for their community program. It may be similar to program models in other locales, but, first and foremost, the model should reflect the realities that are unique to the community in which it is implemented. Just as theories of action are unique, other types of evaluation instruments, like surveys and health status indicators, must be carefully adapted to fit the realities of each community.

The tension between the desirability of using a tried and tested measure as opposed to one contoured specifically to each program is evident in the community evaluation literature. For instance, Kumpfer[7] maintains that standardized evaluation instruments should be sought out, but she also notes that locating such measures can be frustrating as the instruments must conform to the language skills, age appropriateness, cultural relevance, and attention span of local audiences. Padilla and Medina[23] assert that cultural sensitivity should span the entire evaluation process including the adaptation, translation, and administration of measures, along with the analysis, scoring, and interpretation of results. Without such cultural adaptations, biases may occur that can lead to misinterpretation of a program's results.[24] In order to reduce culturally induced bias, Suzuki et al.[25] offer the following suggestions: develop alternative measures and procedures for diverse populations, understand the norms of ethnic groups to which evaluations are applied, increase collaboration with bilingual and bicultural professionals in developing evaluations, increase racial and ethnic community involvement in the assessment process, and consult the literature and research available regarding multicultural assessment procedures.

Sometimes community programs try to use standard measures that are compiled by governmental agencies to compare their program to national or statewide standards. For instance, a program may compare its status on drunk driving arrests, birth outcomes, and tobacco consumption with other communities, or with state and national averages. But highly aggregated data may not be pertinent to local community level evaluation because the data may not reflect the realities of different locales.[26] For instance, national data may show declines in drug use, whereas local data might indicate drug use is increasing.[26] Hayes and Willms[27] suggest that funders or evaluators can be misguided in requiring selected indicators for monitoring community progress, because such requirements can stifle community initiative and ownership if local groups perceive that the project is being wrested away from them due to outside and inappropriate requirements.

Another type of measurement problem due to aggregating data occurs when individuals are asked questions about the community in which they live, or the organization in which they work. Cheadle et al.[13] note that most measures of community are really taken at the individual level and then aggregated. For instance, to identify whether organizations in the community become more aware of a health promotion effort or more active in that effort, individuals (usually administrators) in the organization may be surveyed to provide a surrogate measure for organizational change. Although this can provide useful information for some purposes, it may be misleading when examining health promotion program impacts and outcomes.[28] To address this issue, some advocate for the use of indicators that can be derived from observations of the community or organizational environment. Such indicators might include the number, type, or visibility of no smoking signs in a work place; more media attention as reflected in the number of column inches devoted to a health issue in the local newspaper; supermarket sales records for specific products, such as cigarettes; or the amount of space devoted to a product, for instance the percent of low fat products as compared to fast food (and fat containing) products.[13,29] As with surveys, questionnaires, and health status measures, environmental indicators should be contoured to be relevant to the particular community and program under study.

One important conclusion that may be drawn from Principle 2 is that questionnaires, surveys, and environmental indicators developed in other locales, and standard indicators should be used with caution. This is not to say that measurement instruments and indicators should be disregarded, but they should be adapted and interpreted in light of local realities. Thus, the tools presented below should not be viewed as "gold standards." They may best be considered points of departure that require modification to fit local conditions.

Practical Tools. DeVellis[30] provides a user-friendly set of steps for developing your own surveys or questionnaires including: determining what you want to measure, generating questions, determining formats for measures, having experts review the items, validating the items, pilot testing the instrument, and revising it based on feedback from experts and the pilot test. Gruenewald et al.[26] suggest several social indicators for measuring the larger level impact that programs have on communities. Also, they provide a systems approach similar to the construction of logic models that can help in identifying appropriate social indicators. Coulton[31] identifies several social indicators that are relevant for community programs that focus on child well-being. Cheadle et al.[13] and Wagner et al.[29] offer lists of environmental indicators that can supplement individual level measures in evaluating a complex community-based program. Suzuki et al.[32] edit a volume of papers that discuss issues and techniques for rendering measurement as culturally sensitive and relevant.

Principle 3: Evaluation approaches used should be guided by the questions asked and often require both a quantitative and qualitative orientation

Principle 2 illustrates that a good measure is hard to find. Moreover, given the complexities of community health initiatives, one good measure is hardly enough. The techniques that the evaluator uses should be like the wardrobes of the rich and famous: abundant, elegant, and diverse enough to fit all occasions. The elegant evaluator should be able to fashion evaluation strategies that are tailored to the specific evaluation questions and concerns of a community project. In developing the widest array of possible evaluation strategies, the elegant evaluator should be versed in both quantitative and qualitative approaches. Yin[33] points out that when a program evaluation focuses on questions that ask who, what, where, and how much, often these lead to quantitative inquiry. When the questions are posed as why or how, then qualitative methods often are most appropriate. Deciding upon what evaluation questions are important may be the best guide for suggesting which method is choice.

Quantitative approaches are frequently linked to experimental and quasiexperimental designs. The former require that potential program recipients be randomly assigned to the program or to a control group that does not receive the program. Quasiexperimental designs deliberately (not always randomly) match program recipients with others who do not receive the program. Quantitative approaches typically use statistical techniques to judge whether program recipients benefit from the program in contrast to controls or comparisons. Qualitative approaches seldom use randomization and often do not have comparison groups. These approaches focus on the program itself, using detailed observations of activities and events, interviews with program stakeholders, and review of program documents to judge program results.[34]

Some argue that quantitative and qualitative approaches are not easily used in combination.[35] Similarly, some debate whether any approach to evaluation other than experimental designs can be definitive.[36–38] Others argue that qualitative approaches are superior because validity is enhanced when stakeholders are sought out to share a range of perspectives regarding program benefits and challenges.[39,40] Steckler and colleagues offer a pragmatic view regarding the combination of qualitative and quantitative methods. They write that

> . . . health education and health promotion programs are complex phenomena which require the application of multiple methodologies in order to properly understand or evaluate them. . . . Today, the issue no longer is whether to use quantitative or qualitative methods, but rather how they can be combined to produce more effective evaluation strategies.[34(p.4)]

This moderate view seems most appropriate for community evaluation. In fact, qualitative techniques are often embedded in experimental designs. For instance, if a statistical analysis of a program's outcomes indicates that the program produced no significant result when compared with a control group, then qualitative techniques, like interviews with program stakeholders or program document reviews, may help to explain why the program was not effective. Conversely, quantitative techniques are often embedded in qualitative evaluation designs. For instance, interviews may be analyzed by counting the number of times different respondents express a program-related concern, thereby providing an indication of the magnitude of each concern that is expressed. Thus, it is important to recognize that although quantitative and qualitative evaluation *designs* have the different orientations that are noted above, *within* either design, the *methods* used to evaluate a program may be both qualitative and quantitative.[41]

Practical Tools. Windsor et al.[3] offer one of the more straightforward explanations of different experimental and quasiexperimental designs and apply them to the evaluation of health promotion programs. The text also provides several qualitative approaches. Many works are available on qualitative methods, but Yin[33] offers a good overview, providing a step-by-step approach for doing qualitative case studies. He offers practical guidelines for asking qualitative evaluation questions, determining which methods to employ, structuring an evaluation protocol, and gathering and analyzing qualitative data.

Principle 4: Evaluation should be informed by social ecology and social system concepts

Recently, evaluators have emphasized that the assessments of complex community programs be based on ecological and systems principles.[26,42,43] Social ecology and systems theories accentuate the individual, social, and environmental dynamics that underlie human behavior.[26,44] According to these theories, complex health issues such as substance abuse, teen pregnancy, violence, or chronic disease should be viewed as interwoven into the social fabric. Programs that address such issues effectively often intervene at different levels simultaneously to influence individual knowledge, attitudes, and behavior; social support systems and networks; community capacity to mobilize effective initiatives; coalitions of cooperating organizations; and alliances that affect politics and policy through media and lobbying.[1,45] Consequently, the assessments of programs that concern socially imbedded problems should take into account the multiple levels at which they occur, including: intrapersonal, interpersonal, organizational, community, and public policy.[43]

A growing body of evidence suggests that effective community programs not only intervene across several strata of the social ecology, but also develop in stages including: beginning mobilization, establishing organizational structure, building capacity for action, implementing, refining, and maintaining the program.[46] Each stage may be conceptualized as an intermediate outcome for the program. If a stage is not fully nurtured, a program can fail to thrive.[47,48] The evaluator can assist in nurturing community programs from one stage to the next by tailoring evaluation methods for feedback during each stage. If a program does not achieve its long-term outcomes, knowing which intermediate outcomes were not met can help identify the weak links in a complex community initiative.[13]

The importance of the ecological and systems perspectives is that evaluation should be conceptualized across two dimensions: first, the multiple social levels at which interventions are directed (intrapersonal, interpersonal, organizational, community, and public policy); and second, the stage of program development (initial mobilization, establishing organizational structure, building capacity for action, implementing, refining, and institutionalizing). Such criteria pose unique challenges for evaluation because more traditional approaches may not be sufficient for assessing complex interventions. For instance, randomized controlled designs may be impractical, expensive, and unwieldy. Evaluating program effectiveness may require increased reliance on case methods and other qualitative approaches, and the judicious combination of these methods with experimental and quasiexperimental designs.[34] Thus, Principle 4, which advocates for complex, ecology-based evaluations, extends from Principle 3, which advocates for the astute combination of both qualitative and quantitative approaches.

Practical Tools. Goodman et al.[14] demonstrate how an ecological assessment is accomplished in assessing community efforts to combat substance abuse. They also discuss several useful evaluation tools that may be adapted to other programs. Parcel and colleagues[49–51] and Steckler et al.[52] provide examples of staged approaches to the evaluation and measurement of health promotion programs in schools. They can serve as models for understanding how the evaluation method can shift when moving from one program stage to the next. Also, they provide measurement tools that may be adapted to each stage of the evaluation. In a more general vein, Nelson[53] provides a useful manual that contains checklists for evaluating all aspects of school health programs including assembling an evaluation team strategically, posing important questions, contouring evaluation to both implementation and outcomes, developing objectives for the evaluation, providing instruments for evaluation, and providing references for other organizations that might be helpful in constructing evaluations. Muraskin[54] provides a general "how to" manual for designing and implementing evaluations that include practical advice for approaching the entire evaluation process. Fawcett and colleagues[8] provide a manual for evaluating community programs in cardiovascular disease. The manual explains ways to design process, intermediate, and long-term outcome measures. The manual is particularly useful for developing community-based monitoring systems for process evaluation and provides other measurement instruments for community-based outcomes. King et al.[55] offer a thorough listing of elements that may be considered when evaluating program implementation that include elements of the program's context; its origins and history; its rationale, goals, and objectives; aspects of program personnel, program participants, budget and administrative arrangements; materials and facilities, program activities, measurement and data collection procedures.

Principle 5: Community evaluation should involve local stakeholders in meaningful ways

Principle 5 brings the chapter full cycle back to its introduction, which suggests that citizen participation is a foundation of community programming. When involving community members in the development and implementation of the evaluation, the evaluator acts as a coach, collaborator, and builder of capacity. These roles facilitate program development as well as evaluation. If program stakeholders perceive the evaluation as an integral part of the program, it can enhance community understanding, stakeholder commitment, and utilization of results; be perceived as a cost-cutting measure; and a bridge between different cultural groups that may participate. In general, the distance between the evaluator and community is reduced when local stakeholders are involved in the evaluation in meaningful ways.[17]

When the evaluator becomes actively engaged with community groups, an array of skills become important that are informed more by community development than by evaluation technology *per se*. The community engagement process requires skills in effective interpersonal communication, team building, group process and negotiation, teaching skills, political acumen, and the ability to gain cooperation and trust. Some evaluation approaches, such as participatory evaluation, incorporate these skills into the evaluation process.[1] In participatory evaluation, community constituents help define the evaluation questions, often participate in data gathering, and use the data analysis as feedback for suggesting program improvements. A recent approach to qualitative evaluation, called empowerment evaluation, supports community groups in developing skills for self-evaluation and consciousness-raising.[56] Empowerment evaluation is designed to ". . . help people help themselves and improve their programs using a form of self-evaluation and reflection. Program participants conduct their own evaluations and typically act as facilitators; an outside evaluator often serves as a coach or an additional facilitator depending on internal program capabilities."[56(p.5)]

Empowerment evaluation has generated controversy. Some criticize it for being inappropriate as an approach to evaluation.[57] According to this point of view, empowerment is viewed as a worthy goal, but the clients of an evaluation are not considered expert enough to conduct a skillful, objective, and technically worthy evaluation. Moreover, allowing clients to select criteria for evaluation, collect data, and write, edit, and disseminate reports leaves room for significant bias to infiltrate the evaluation process.[57]

The criticisms of empowerment evaluation notwithstanding, its orientation is quite compatible with community development practices that are aimed at citizen participation and ownership. Although it is unlikely that lay citizens can develop the expertise of a professional evaluator without considerable training, increasing community members' capacity to be wise consumers of evaluation and to interact with and conduct some aspects of the evaluation can pay dividends for current and future community health initiatives. Therefore, supporting evaluations that build community member skills for self-assessment seems to be a worthy goal. The tools that follow offer methods for interacting with community groups in order to build their capabilities in program evaluation.

Practical Tools. Linney and Wandersman[58] produced a manual that facilitates citizen involvement in planning community programs, developing community plans, and evaluating program activities. They provide an extensive list of measurement tools for both process and outcome evaluation. Fetterman et al.[56] provide a rationale for citizen empowerment approaches to evaluation. Their edited volume contains a section titled "Workshops, Technical Assistance, and Practice," which includes tools for actively engaging the community in the evaluation process. Of particular note are chapters by Dugan,[59] who identifies evaluator tasks for building community capacity across the program stages, and Butterfoss et al.,[60] who offer self-assessment tools for conducting community needs assessment, developing a quality plan for the program, and assuring that the elements are in place for program implementation.

•   •   •

The five principles that are presented above constitute important aspects of contemporary evaluation of community programs. Selected references are provided along with each principle for those who may want more practical guidance. Given the complexity of community health promotion programs, it is unlikely that their evaluations can be conducted effectively without rigor and sophistication. This chapter suggests that such demands should not deter the practitioner from attempting to import the principles into evaluation efforts. To the contrary, the practitioner is encouraged to learn by doing; to become more skilled at applying each principle through trial, midcourse correction, and retrial. Because instruction in evaluation usually is part of the curriculum of many university programs, practitioners may be able to identify experts in their communities who are willing to consult in the development of program logic models, measurement instruments, multiple methods, ecology and systems approaches, and community involvement. The program practitioner may be wise in taking such a collaborative approach. After all, few complex community health initiatives can be implemented by one person, and to do justice to the program, its evaluation often should be a shared effort. The task of evaluating may require considerable effort, but without such effort how can we assure that program operations are effectively developed and implemented, and that they produce the desired results? Given the enormous amount of effort that practitioners usually devote to the development and delivery of community health initiatives, it simply is prudent that evaluation be used to inform program refinements and other improvements with the goal of optimizing effectiveness.

REFERENCES

1. B.A. Israel et al. "Evaluation of Health Education Programs: Current Assessment and Future Directions." *Health Education Quarterly* 22, no. 3 (1995): 364–389.

2. L.W. Green and F.M. Lewis. *Measurement and Evaluation in Health Education and Health Promotion.* Palo Alto, Calif.: Mayfield, 1986.

3. R. Windsor et al. *Evaluation of Health Promotion, Health Education and Disease Prevention Programs.* Mountain View, Calif.: Mayfield, 1994.

4. T. Koepsell. "Epidemiologic Issues in the Design of Community Intervention Trials." In *Applied Epidemiology,* eds. R.C. Brownson and D.B. Petitti. New York: Oxford University Press (1998): 177–212, in press.

5. A. Steckler et al. "Health Education Intervention Strategies: Recommendations for Future Research." *Health Education Quarterly* 22, no. 3 (1995): 307–329.

6. B. Thompson and S. Kinne. "Social Change Theory: Applications to Community Health." In *Health Promotion at the Community Level,* ed. N. Bracht. Newbury Park, Calif.: Sage Publications, 1990.

7. K.L. Kumpfer et al. *Measurements in Prevention: A Manual on Selecting and Using Instruments to Evaluate Prevention Programs.* U.S. Department of Health and Human Services, Center for Substance Abuse Prevention, Technical Report 8. Rockville, Md.: Government Printing Office, 1993.

8. S.B. Fawcett et al. *Evaluating Community Efforts to Prevent Cardiovascular Diseases.* Atlanta, Ga.: Centers for Disease Control and Prevention, National Center for Chronic Disease Prevention and Health Promotion, 1995.

9. M. Scriven. "The Methodology of Evaluation." In *Perspectives of Curriculum Evaluation*, eds. R.W. Tylor et al. Skokie, Ill.: Rand McNally, 1967.

10. M. Scriven. "Beyond Formative and Summative Evaluation." In *Evaluation and Education: A Quarter Century*, eds. G.W. McLaughlin and D.C. Phillips. Chicago: University of Chicago Press, 1991.

11. J.E. Veney and A.D. Kaluzny. *Evaluation and Decision Making for Health Services*, 2nd ed. Ann Arbor, Mich.: Health Administration Press, 1991.

12. P.H. Rossi and H.E. Freeman. *Evaluation: A Systematic Approach*. Newbury Park, Calif.: Sage Publications, 1989.

13. A. Cheadle et al. "Environmental Indicators: A Tool for Evaluating Community-Based Health-Promotion Programs." *American Journal of Preventive Medicine* 8, no. 6 (1992): 345–350.

14. R.M. Goodman et al. "An Ecological Assessment of Community Coalitions: Approaches to Measuring Community-Based Interventions For Prevention and Health Promotion." *American Journal of Community Psychology* 24, no. 1 (1996): 33–61.

15. A.C. Kubisch et al. "Introduction." In *New Approaches to Evaluating Community Initiatives: Concepts, Methods, and Context*, eds. J.P. Connel et al. Washington, D.C.: The Aspen Institute, 1995: 1–21.

16. C.H. Weiss. "Nothing As Practical As Good Theory: Exploring Theory-Based Evaluation for Comprehensive Community Initiatives for Children and Families." In *New Approaches to Evaluating Community Initiatives: Concepts, Methods, and Context*, eds. J.P. Connel et al. Washington, D.C.: The Aspen Institute, 1995: 65–92.

17. P. Brown. "The Role of the Evaluator in Comprehensive Community Initiatives." In *New Approaches to Evaluating Community Initiatives: Concepts, Methods, and Context*, eds. J.P. Connel et al. Washington, D.C.: The Aspen Institute, 1995: 201–225.

18. C. Jackson et al. "Evaluating Community-Level Health Promotion and Disease Prevention Interventions." *New Directions for Program Evaluation*, no. 43 (1989): 19–32.

19. R.M. Goodman and A. Wandersman. "FORECAST: A Formative Approach to Evaluating the CSAP Community Partnerships." *Journal of Community Psychology*, CSAP special issue, (1994): 6–25.

20. H.T. Chen. *Theory-Driven Evaluations*. Newbury Park, Calif.: Sage Publications, 1990.

21. M.A. Scheirer. "A User's Guide to Program Templates: A New Tool for Evaluating Program Content." *New Directions for Evaluation*, no. 72 (1996).

22. M.Q. Patton. *Utilization-Focused Evaluation*, 2d ed. Beverly Hills, Calif.: Sage Publications, 1986.

23. A.M. Padilla and A. Medina. "Cross-Cultural Sensitivity in Assessment Using Tests in Culturally Appropriate Ways." In *Handbook of Multicultural Assessment: Clinical, Psychological, and Educational Applications*, eds. L.A. Suzuki et al. San Francisco: Jossey-Bass, Publishers, 1996: 3–28.

24. M.A. Keitel et al. "Ethical Issues in Multicultural Assessment." In *Handbook of Multicultural Assessment: Clinical, Psychological, and Educational Applications*, eds. L.A. Suzuki et al. San Francisco: Jossey-Bass, Publishers, 1996: 29–48.

25. L.A. Suzuki et al. "Multicultural Assessment: Present Trends and Future Directions." In *Handbook of Multicultural Assessment: Clinical, Psychological, and Educational Applications*, eds. L.A. Suzuki et al. San Francisco: Jossey-Bass, Publishers, 1996: 673–684.

26. P.J. Gruenewald et al. *Measuring Community Indicators: A Systems Approach to Drug and Alcohol Problems*. Applied Social Research Methods Series, Vol. 45. Thousand Oaks, Calif.: Sage Publications, 1997.

27. M.V. Hayes et al. "Healthy Community Indicators: The Perils of the Search and the Paucity of the Find." *Health Promotion International* 5, no. 2 (1990): 161–166.

28. A. Steckler et al. "Some Thoughts on Collecting and Analyzing Organizational Level Data." *Health Education Research* 12, no. 3 (1997): i–iv.

29. E.H. Wagner et al. "The Evaluation of the Henry J. Kaiser Family Foundation's Community Health Promotion Grant: Design." *Journal of Clinical Epidemiology* 44, no. 7 (1991): 685–699.

30. R.F. DeVellis. *Scale Development: Theory and Applications.* Applied Social Research Methods Series, Vol. 26. Newbury Park, Calif.: Sage Publications, 1991.

31. C.J. Coulton. "Using Community Level Indicators of Children's Well-being in Comprehensive Community Initiatives." In *New Approaches to Evaluating Community Initiatives: Concepts, Methods and Context,* eds. J.P. Connel et al. Washington, D.C.: The Aspen Institute, 1995: 173–199.

32. L.A. Suzuki et al., eds. *Handbook of Multicultural Assessment: Clinical, Psychological, and Educational Applications.* San Francisco: Jossey-Bass, Publishers, 1996.

33. R.K. Yin. *Case Study Research: Design and Methods.* Beverly Hills, Calif.: Sage Publications, 1984.

34. A. Steckler et al. "Toward Integrating Qualitative and Quantitative Methods: An Introduction." *Health Education Quarterly* 19, no. 1 (1992): 1–8.

35. N.W. Blaikie. "A Critique of the Use of Triangulation in Social Research." *Quality & Quantity* 25 (1991): 115–136.

36. R.F. Boruch. "The Future of Controlled Randomized Experiments: A Briefing." *Evaluation Practice* 15, no. 3 (1994): 265–274.

37. R.F. Boruch and W. Wothke, eds. "Seven Kinds of Randomization Plans for Designing Field Experiments." In *Randomization and Field Experimentation.* San Francisco, CA: Jossey-Bass, Publishers, 1985: 95–113.

38. E. Suchman. *Evaluation Research: Principles and Practice in Public Service and Social Action Programs.* New York: Russell Sage Foundation, 1967.

39. E.G. Guba and Y.S. Lincoln. *Fourth Generation Evaluation.* Newbury Park, Calif.: Sage Publications, 1989.

40. Y.S. Lincoln. "Tracks Toward a Postmodern Politics of Evaluation." *Evaluation Practice* 15, no. 3 (1994): 299–309.

41. C.S. Reichardt and T.D. Cook, eds. "Beyond Qualitative Versus Quantitative Methods." In *Qualitative and Quantitative Methods in Evaluation Research.* Beverly Hills, Calif.: Sage Publications, 1979: 3–13.

42. M. Shinn, ed. "Special Issue: Ecological Assessment." *American Journal of Community Psychology* 24, no. 1 (1996).

43. K.R. McLeroy et al. "An Ecological Perspective on Health Promotion Programs." *Health Education Quarterly* 15 (1988): 351–377.

44. J.P. Connel et al. "How Do Urban Communities Effect Youth? Using Social Science Research to Inform the Design and Evaluation of Comprehensive Community Initiatives." In *New Approaches to Evaluating Community Initiatives: Concepts, Methods, and Context,* eds. J.P. Connel et al. Washington, D.C.: The Aspen Institute, 1995: 93–125.

45. R.A. Winett et al. *Health Psychology and Public Health.* New York: Pergamon Press, 1989.

46. P. Florin et al. "Identifying Technical Assistance Needs in Community Coalitions: A Developmental Approach." *Health Education Research* 8 (1993): 417–432.

47. R.M. Goodman et al. "Mobilizing Organizations for Health Enhancement: Theories of Organizational Change." In *Health Behavior and Health Education: Theory, Research, and Practice*, 2nd ed., eds. K. Glanz et al. San Francisco: Jossey-Bass, Publishers, 1996.

48. R.M. Goodman et al. "Evaluation of The Heart To Heart Project: Lessons from a Community-based Chronic Disease Prevention Project." *American Journal of Health Promotion* 9, no. 6 (1995): 443–455.

49. G.S. Parcel. "Diffusion Research: The Smart Choices Project." *Health Education Research* 10, no. 3 (1995): 279–281.

50. S.G. Brink et al. "Diffusion of an Effective Tobacco Prevention Program. Part I: Evaluation of the Dissemination Phase." *Health Education Research* 10, no. 3 (1995): 283–295.

51. G.S. Parcel et al. "Diffusion of an Effective Tobacco Prevention Program. Part II: Evaluation of the Adoption Phase." *Health Education Research* 10, no. 3 (1995): 297–307.

52. A. Steckler et al. "Measuring the Diffusion of Innovative Health Promotion Programs." *American Journal of Health Promotion* 6, no. 3 (1992): 214–224.

53. S. Nelson. *How Healthy is Your School?: Guidelines for Evaluating School Health Promotion.* Kent, Ohio: American School Health Association, 1986.

54. L.D. Muraskin. *Understanding Evaluation: The Way to Better Prevention Programs.* Washington, D.C.: Government Printing Office, 1993.

55. J.A. King et al. *How to Assess Program Implementation.* Newbury Park, Calif.: Sage Publications, 1987.

56. D.M. Fetterman et al., eds. *Empowerment Evaluation: Knowledge and Tools for Self-Assessment and Accountability.* Thousand Oaks, Calif.: Sage Publications, 1996.

57. D.L. Stufflebeam. "Empowerment Evaluation, Objective Evaluation, and Evaluation Standards: Where the Future of Evaluation Should Not Go and Where It Needs to Go." *Evaluation Practice* 15, no. 3 (1994): 321–338.

58. J.A. Linney and A. Wandersman. *Prevention Plus III: A Four-Step Guide to Useful Program Assessment.* Rockville, Md.: U.S. Department of Health and Human Services, Office for Substance Abuse Prevention, 1991.

59. M.A. Dugan. "Participatory and Empowerment Evaluation: Lessons Learned in Training and Technical Assistance." In *Empowerment Evaluation: Knowledge and Tools for Self-Assessment and Accountability*, eds. D. Fetterman et al. Newbury Park, Calif.: Sage Publications, 1996.

60. F.D. Butterfoss et al. "The Plan Quality Index: An Empowerment Evaluation Tool For Measuring and Improving the Quality of Plans." In *Empowerment Evaluation: Knowledge and Tools for Self-Assessment and Accountability*, eds. D. Fetterman et al. Newbury Park, Calif.: Sage Publications, 1996.

17

Evaluation of a Children's Immunization Program: Process, Outcome, and Costs

Mary E. Foley, Pierre Kory, and Gerry Fairbrother

Recent immunization rates for the population as a whole have increased.[1,2] However, in many urban areas immunization rates are much lower than for other parts of the United States.[3] School-aged children are now appropriately immunized with the recommended doses of three critical vaccines: four doses of diphtheria, tetanus, pertussis (DTP) vaccine, three doses of oral polio vaccine, and one dose of measles vaccine.

But immunization levels of preschool-aged children (19–35 months) are only 78 percent for the same vaccination series.[4] The problem of underimmunization of children has been addressed in a variety of ways, including urging primary care physicians to screen for absent or tardy age-appropriate immunization at every possible entry point into the sociomedical system and media campaigns, as well as community outreach efforts and events.

Community outreach efforts have been successful in raising community awareness through mass immunization campaigns. How successful these mass campaigns have been in increasing the immunization coverage rates of targeted children is less clear. Little is reported in the scientific literature, and reports outside the peer-reviewed literature show mixed results.[5–7] An evaluation of New York City's Immunization Day in 1993[8] reported a lack of political will and social mobilization—the hallmarks of successful immunization campaigns in developing nations—and a low turnout for the event. Recently released data from the National Immunization Survey, a household immunization survey, showed an overall statewide coverage for New York State of 79 percent ± 4.2 for four or more doses of diphtheria and tetanus toxoids and pertussis vaccine/diphtheria and tetanus toxoids (DTP/DT), three or more doses of poliovirus vaccine, and one or more doses of measles-containing vaccine (MCV) for children aged 19 to 35 months[4]; citywide coverage for New York City showed 81 percent ± 6.2 for the same anti-

J Public Health Management Practice, 1998, 4(4), 97–105

gens at any age for 1995.[4] However, geographical pockets of underimmunization still exist.

HOPE FOR A MILLION KIDS IMMUNIZATION EVENT

Hope for Kids (HFK), a volunteer organization devoted to better health for children, has successfully utilized community outreach techniques in tandem with special neighborhood events as the impetus for community mobilization. Hope for a Million Kids Immunization Outreach project is an annual national initiative designed to increase immunization coverage for children. A major component of this project is the involvement of the traditional health care system and the strengthening of community linkages to health care services. In the spring of 1996, HFK organized a national effort, "Hope for a Million Kids," planned as the child immunization project for National Immunization Week, April 20–27, 1996. The goal of this project was to provide a million children with educational information and opportunities for vaccination. In New York City, HFK invited the Child Vaccination Program (a joint project of the Children's Defense Fund, New York City's Department of Health (DOH), and the Chase Manhattan Bank), the Manhattan Borough President's Office, East Harlem health care providers, community-based organizations, local elected and community leaders, and many other agencies to collaborate in a communitywide campaign to increase age-appropriate immunizations in the East Harlem neighborhood of New York City.

More than 3,000 HFK volunteers canvassed the neighborhoods of East and Central Harlem, for two days, door-to-door, to provide education about immunizations. A Health and Human Services Street Fair (Health Fair), preceded by a Volunteer Kick-Off Rally, was held prior to the immunization week. Two local hospitals, a medical center, and four community-based neighborhood health organizations provided sites and personnel for administering immunizations and enrolling the family in ongoing health care services during the Immunization Event week.

This chapter evaluates the communitywide immunization campaign's efforts (Immunization Event), including assessment of the planning and coordination efforts, the success of the HFK volunteers in reaching their goal of 100,000 children, the number of immunizations administered resulting from the outreach efforts, and estimates of costs associated with the event.

METHODS

A complete evaluation of the Immunization Event derives from three distinct sources: (1) semistructured interviews of 12 key planning and implementation personnel; (2) an assessment of the number of children reached through outreach efforts, both during the health fair and at immunization sites; and (3) a retrospective analysis of costs.

Documentation of planning and implementation

Members of the research team conducted face-to-face, open-ended, semistructured interviews of 12 event organizers and lead personnel on the three planning subcommittees. These interviews were designed to facilitate discussion about the planning and implementation process, resources required and used, perceived strengths and limitations of the event, and recommendations for strategies in conducting future Immunization Events. Information was also gathered about social mobilization, community outreach, political involvement, publicity, and other key issues related to the planning process. Each interview took about 45 minutes, and responses were recorded verbatim on the surveys.

Children reached

Hope for Kids canvassers recorded names, addresses, and the number of children in each family encountered in the door-to-door outreach effort. Health information packets containing a map of providers, schedules of immunizations, flyers on the importance of immunizations, and other health-related information, were distributed to the head of the family. The number of children in the household comprised the number of "children reached." At registration tables set up at the entrance to the health fair site, information about the number of adults, number and ages of children, and ZIP codes was collected. Hourly raffles of various prizes provided incentives for registration at the event. At the immunization sites, HFK volunteers distributed surveys to parents. The surveys included questions about the number of children brought in for immunizations; dates of birth; sources of information about the free immunizations; whether they had a free voucher for the immunizations and how they obtained it; site of their children's primary care; when they take their children for health care; and if they had the children's immunization cards with them. Survey data were entered into Epi Info software (version 5), and frequencies and percentages were calculated.

Additional data were collected on the number of immunizations administered to parents with vouchers. Health care provider sites kept a daily count of immunizations administered by ages of these children throughout the Immunization Event week. At the end of Immunization Event week, the number of immunizations by child's age and by immunization site were calculated for those with vouchers.

Analysis of costs

Costs for the HFK door-to-door educational outreach, preparation and implementation of the Kickoff Rally and Health Fair, and the services and personnel costs during the Immunization Event week were itemized and tallied. All costs incurred were identified primarily through interviews with the event planners. A retrospective examination of financial records for the event from various agencies supplemented information from these interviews. Interviewees calculated the number of persons from their agency and the number of hours per week that key persons, staff, and volunteers contributed to the planning and staffing for the event. Salary estimates for DOH employees were obtained directly from the DOH. Salaries of employees from other agencies involved were estimated based on job titles and knowledge of salaries in not-for-profit organizations in New York City. Hourly wages were calculated by dividing the annual salary by 1,820 (52 weeks × 5 days × 7 hours per day), a common method used to calculate hourly wages. We used the July 1, 1996, federally negotiated fringe benefit rate of 28.1 percent, which approximates the fringe rates of involved agencies.

RESULTS

Planning for Hope for a Million Kids Immunization Outreach and Health Fair

Planning spanned approximately four months, from January until April 1996, and was led by a planning committee for the last two months. Major components of this phase included community mobilization and recruitment of health care provider sites. The planning effort was carried out by a community planning committee, which was divided into three working subcommittees: Health and Human Services Providers, Outreach and Mobilization, and Entertainment and Logistics. Committee members attended two-hour weekly meetings in addition to the time devoted to carrying out assigned tasks.

Public sector support for the event was in the form of donated printed materials and human resources; financial support had to be raised from private sources. Ultimately, more than $100,000 in private funds and materials was donated.

Planning for such an event is time consuming. During the approximately four-month preparatory period, nearly 1,800 hours were spent by staff in planning for the health fair; about 600 hours were spent in planning the door-to-door canvassing. Overall, time allotted for the planning process was deemed adequate by most planners who were interviewed after the event. However, some felt more time was needed: "Another four to five weeks would have made it much less stressful." Comments from some of those interviewed suggested that more time could have been spent specifically to mobilize media coverage. Others felt that more time should have been devoted to fund-raising, thereby lessening the amount of donated supplies and human resources.

Community outreach

Community outreach and organization is a key component of an immunization campaign and a determinant of whether community members will participate and be immunized. All individuals interviewed agreed that community outreach and involvement was the strong point of the event. Some interviewees indicated that the planning process would now serve as a community organization model for future events. The event also provided an opportunity for networking among the principals in the many diverse organizations. Many used the planning meetings to bolster outreach databases in their organizations. For example, more than 100 individuals from at least 50 different citywide and key local organizations had attended planning meetings and 31 health and human service organizations provided information and services at the health fair.

Recruitment of health care provider sites

The East Harlem Community Health Committee, Inc. (EHCHC) is a 20-year-old membership organization of consumers, community health centers, hospitals, social service providers, government agencies, and other community-based agencies. It is a forum for provider agencies and consumers to collaborate, plan, exchange ideas, and work together to improve health care in the community. One subcommittee of the EHCHC, the Pediatric/Child Health subcommittee, supported the Immunization Event and devoted many of its meetings to the activities involved in planning and implementing the event. It is noteworthy that all of the local East Harlem institutional providers, who are also active in the EHCHC, participated in the planning process and many served as vaccination sites during the following week: Boriken Neighborhood Health Center, East Harlem Health Center, Mount Sinai Medical Center's Adolescent Health Center and Pediatric Primary Care Clinic, Settlement Health and Medical Services, North General Hospital, Metropolitan Hospital, and the DOH's Child Health and School Health Clinics (CHC).

Identification and immunization of children

On the day of the health fair and the next day, more than 3,000 Hope for Kids volunteers canvassed the neighborhoods of East and Central Harlem, door-to-door, to provide education about immunizations and other health-related topics. The volunteers exceeded their target of reaching 100,000 children by reaching a full 120,000. More than 2,000 people attended the health fair. Registration data at the health fair indicated that at least 562 children attended the fair. Planners say that this is an undercount due to flaws in the registration forms and the registration process at the fair: some forms were incomplete or improperly filled in by parents or guardians, and forms were available in English only; thus, those with no or marginal English literacy skills were not counted. Finally, to maintain quality control, all forms should have been completed by a staff person.

Parent survey findings

During the subsequent week, 149 parents brought young children to designated immunization sites (or health care facilities) in East Harlem and completed a survey. Survey findings indicate that parents brought between one and five children to receive immunizations. A majority of the respondents stated that they came to the immunization sites for a previous appointment (44.4%). However, more than one-third of the survey respondents (36.2%) stated that they came to the immunization sites with a voucher for free shots. Parents learned about the free immunizations in many ways. As displayed in Table 1, the most popular source of information about the free immunizations was from the HFK volunteers (26.8%).

Table 1 Sources of information about the Immunization Event

Information source	N	(%)
HFK*	40	(26.80)
HFK + Fair	9	(6.00)
HFK and other source(s)†	13	(8.70)
Day Care/Head Start	1	(0.67)
School	8	(5.40)
MD	1	(0.67)
Friend	4	(2.70)
Friend and other source(s)†	5	(3.30)
Flyer	2	(1.30)
Community agency	4	(2.70)
Fair + Other	6	(4.00)
Other	36	(24.20)
No answer	20	(13.40)
Total	149	(100.00)

*HFK = Hope For Kids Volunteer
†Other source(s) may also include newspaper and religious organization

Many parents (30%) bring their children to the physician for regular checkups or routine physicals; 11 percent bring children to the physician for a regular check-up or routine physical examination and for shots. A majority of respondents (73.8%) had their child's immunization card with them.

Children immunized

Tally sheets of numbers of children immunized, as a result of the health fair and door-to-door outreach, were maintained at the immunization sites. As can be seen in Table 2, a total of 211 children immunized that week came with vouchers for free immunizations. Fifty-seven (27%) were 0 to 11 months old. A majority of children were immunized at Metropolitan Hospital (43%). At two sites no immunizations were administered.

Costs

Planning activities incurred personnel costs for both the health fair and the door-to-door canvassing, as well as expenses related to Planning Committee meet-

---

Table 2 Number of children immunized by age and site as a result of Hope for a Million Kids Immunization Event

| | Age | | | | |
Site	0–11 mo	12–24 mo	2–4 years	5+ years	Total
Settlement Health and Medical Services	9	11	8	3	31
Metropolitan Hospital	33	15	12	32	92
Boriken NHC*	14	6	24	27	71
East Harlem CHC†	1	2	7	2	12
North General Hospital	0	2	1	2	5
Mt. Sinai's Adolescent Health Center	0	0	0	0	0
Mt. Sinai's Pediatric Primary Care Clinic	0	0	0	0	0
Total	57	36	52	66	211
Percent Total	(27.0%)	(17.1%)	(24.6%)	(31.3%)	(100%)

*NHC = Neighborhood Health Center
†CHC = Child Health Clinic
Note: Numbers for Metropolitan Hospital that originally indicated all children vaccinated were adjusted to reflect children vaccinated with vouchers.

ings. Total planning time was calculated to be 2,394 hours contributed. The total costs associated with planning was $67,013. Implementation costs included personnel costs for health fair coordination, security, staffing tables, and coordinating community canvassers. Expenses for implementation, and for such items as furniture rentals, buttons and T-shirts for the volunteers, refreshments, permits, and insurance, totaled $46,868. More than 400 hours (412) were calculated for implementation activities. A fringe rate of 28.1 percent was included for all personnel costs. Total direct costs of $113,882 combined with overhead of 10.15 percent brought the total cost estimate for the event to $125,441.

Table 3 displays the principal activities and associated costs for planning and implementing the Immunization Event. Planning costs accounted for 58.8 percent ($67,014 × ±10.15% overhead = $73,815.92 / $125,441) of the total cost; implementation costs accounted for 41.2 percent of the total costs. Together, planning and implementation costs, excluding volunteer activities and donations, was $125,441. Thus, for the 211 children immunized as a result of the HFK Event, the cost per child was $594.50 ($125,441/211 children). If the cost of time contributed by volunteers (estimated at $122,549), and donations (estimated at $95,650) are added, altogether, the value for planning and implementation costs, volunteer hours, and donations amounted to $343,640 ($218,199 + $125,441). Using this figure, for 211 children immunized, the cost per child immunized ($343,640/211 children) was $1,629. The cost of vaccines was not included in these figures, as no tally was kept of the type of immunization given to each child by the research team.

DISCUSSION

This report describes the process, outcome, and costs of an education and outreach effort to increase awareness of the health care needs of children, and to provide immunizations to children during a week-long campaign in the Central and East Harlem communities in New York City. The Immunization Event aimed to reach 100,000 children with information about immunizations and other health issues. The health information dissemination activities of the event, undertaken by the Hope for Kids volunteers, was laudatory. More than 50,000 families and 120,000 children in East and Central Harlem neighborhoods were reached. However, the low turnout of children immunized with vouchers in the subsequent week at the various designated immunization sites was disappointing. It is possible that the number of immunizations administered increased over the weeks subsequent to the event, but this was beyond the scope of the study.

Planning and coordination processes

The planning process for the event, although arduous, was reportedly a positive experience. It served to bring together a broad array of city and community-based

Table 3 Major cost areas of Hope for a Million Kids Immunization Event

Principal activities	Hours contributed	Total cost of time contributed
Planning		
Personnel costs		
Health Fair planning	1,789	$47,165.56
Door-to-door canvassing planning	605	$19,096.28
Expenses		
Planning committee meetings		$752.00
Total planning	2,394	$67,013.84
Implementation		
Personnel costs		
Health Fair coordination	207	$1,242.21
Security	42	$1,034.84
Staffing tables	138	$3,246.25
Coordinating canvassers	25	$570.24
Expenses		
Rent tables and chairs		$764.70
Health care folders		$19,000.00
Volunteer buttons		$1,224.00
Volunteer T-shirts		$16,000.00
Refreshments		$200.00
Children's entertainment		$1,000.00
Banner		$200.00
Decorations		$300.00
Sound equipment rentals		$2,000.00
Permits (sound and street)		$46.00
Insurance		$40.00
Total implementation	412	$46,868.24
Total direct costs		$113,882.08
Overhead (10.15%)		$11,559.03
Total cost		$125,441.11

Note: all personnel costs include a fringe rate of 28.1%.

health and human service providers. New relationships developed during this collaborative initiative that may be further strengthened in the planning of future immunization or health care events. The success in this phase of the event was due in part to the efforts of staff of the Child Vaccination Program (CVP)—one of the main partners in the Hope for a Million Kids Event. Their experience in local community organizing, as well as their earlier outreach efforts in the East Harlem community, were key factors. Invitations were sent to more than 300 East Harlem groups for the first planning meeting and the CVP made presentations and enlisted the endorsement of key East Harlem entities: the Community School and Planning Boards, the Health and Education/Youth Committees; New York City Housing Authority Jefferson Housing Management, and its Tenant Association President. In addition, the NYC Community Development Agency and the Agency for Child Development hosted meetings to enlist all their East Harlem-funded programs, including the Day Care and Head Start programs. The effort to mobilize public and volunteer organizations and agencies was one of the most successful aspects of the event.

Costs

The cost of immunization per child for the event was excessive—about $594. This figure would be even higher if other costs were considered: costs of vaccines administered, associated storage costs, and cost of vaccines wasted due to lack of administration. These costs are considerably higher than those reported in a mass immunization program in New York in 1993 of about $279 per immunized child, and sharply contrast with the cost per visit to immunize a child routinely at a child health clinic in New York City of $75 to $115.[8] High costs associated with this event can be attributed to the paucity of immunizations that were actually administered as a result of the event. It should be noted that along with the high financial cost associated with each immunization administered, the "opportunity costs" were also significant. For example, several key leaders took considerable time out of their regular jobs to work on the event. As a result, important work was neglected or postponed. Moreover, time and energy expenditures invested in the planning and implementation phases of the event by staff were considerable. Taking into account the thousands of hours invested by the volunteers, the total input associated with such low turnout is staggering. Simply put, the "cost" per child immunized is unacceptably high. The actual number of immunizations administered as a result of the event would have to be greatly increased for the Immunization Event to be considered a success. In short, the high cost of the event was matched by very low benefit. However, because the administering of immunizations was not the only goal of the campaign, it should not be judged solely on this basis. Several unmeasurable benefits, such as public, widespread knowledge of immunization schedules and the importance of immunizations, along with a knowledge of the area health care providers and institutions, could result in an increase in immunization coverage over the longer term.

Immunization days or other mass activities alone will rarely lead by themselves to sustainable programs.[9] To maintain continuous age-appropriate immunization status, it is critical to link the family to primary health care service programs.[10] In this respect, one goal of immunization campaigns should be to establish the process of obtaining childhood immunizations as the first visit expected at a continuous source of health care. The Hope for a Million Kids Immunization Event advanced toward this goal by encouraging participants to register for continuous care at the site administering the immunization.

Given the success of the door-to-door awareness campaign, the low turnout for immunizations is troubling. Some staff who were interviewed suggested that a continuous radio and print media blitz in addition to the Health Fair and Rally Kick Off was needed. This might have served to maintain a high level of awareness and, thus, provided needed cues to action in the targeted population of East Harlem. Some members of the EHCHC noted a deficit in sustained educational efforts in the community regarding immunizations for preschool children. Immunization coverage of a population is a function of three interlocking domains: (1) health-seeking behaviors on the part of parents of young children; (2) barriers to care; and (3) provider practices that inhibit appropriate immunizations.[11] However, low turnout rates for mass immunization programs is a familiar story in the United States, especially in the absence of an epidemic. A successful community-based immunization program must include an accessible system of comprehensive primary health care, coordination between pediatric and public health practitioners, community surveillance of immunization status, an interactive information system containing the immunization status of each child that is accessible to all providers, and incentives to families to seek preventive health services for immunization beginning in the second month of life.[12]

This evaluation is limited in several ways. (1) The exact number of children attending the health fair is not certain due to problems with completion of registration forms. (2) Because not all parents of children vaccinated during the subsequent week in East Harlem facilities completed the survey, generalizations of information from these surveys are cautioned against. (3) It is possible that door-to-door contacts raised awareness about immunizations, resulting in improved compliance with regularly scheduled immunization visits and other positive changes in parental behaviors. However, these results were not able to be measured. (4) There is no way to determine how many of the 211 children vaccinated subsequent to the event would have been vaccinated anyway.

Two recent developments in the health care delivery system are likely to have an impact on the immunization rates for preschool children. The first is the recent establishment of the New York City Immunization Registry that will provide a systematic method of maintaining child immunization data in East Harlem. Birth record data were loaded into the registry beginning in early 1997.[13] Data from this system will automatically be transferred to the central immunization registry. Efforts are underway to use the Electronic Birth Certificate to capture the hepatitis B vaccine administered in the nursery and the providers' medical record number, which will link to future submissions. Ultimately, all providers will be able to access the registry to obtain data on individual patients. In addition to tracking childhood preventive services, the system will also enable public health officials to obtain community-level, population-based immunization coverage information. The second factor is the nation's recent five-year budget plan that allocates $24 billion to extend health care coverage to uninsured children.[14] Coverage includes hospital and physicians' services, laboratory services, X-rays, regular checkups, and immunizations for children. The extent to which these funds will impact health care of currently uninsured children and, in particular, immunization rates, has yet to be determined.

In conclusion, immunizations are the most basic of all preventive health care strategies, and are a unique component of preventive health services and childhood health needs. However, we are still far from achieving the national goal of *Healthy People 2000* of full immunization coverage for 90 percent of children who receive the basic immunization series by age two.[15] Health fairs and community outreach are appropriate to raise public awareness about the need for age-appropriate immunizations. However, because health fairs are so labor intensive they are not an efficient method of raising immunization rates and should not be implemented every year. The implementation of a system of immunization registries may obviate the need for offering immunizations at such events in the future.

REFERENCES

1. Centers for Disease Control and Prevention. "Vaccination Coverage of 2-Year-Old Children—United States, 1993." *Morbidity and Mortality Weekly Report* 43 (1994): 705–709.

2. Centers for Disease Control and Prevention. "State and National Vaccination Coverage Levels among Children 19–35 Months—United States, April–December, 1994." *Morbidity and Mortality Weekly Report* 44 (1995): 613–623.

3. E.R. Zell et al. "Low Vaccination Levels of U.S. Preschool and School-Age Children." *Journal of the American Medical Association* 271 (1994): 833–839.

4. Centers for Disease Control and Prevention. "National, State, and Urban Area Vaccination Coverage Levels Among Children Aged 19–35 Months—United States, January–December, 1995." *Morbidity and Mortality Weekly Report* 46 (1997): 176–182.

5. Atlanta Project. Immunization/Children's Health Initiative. *A Report of the Atlanta Project, A Program of the Carter Center.* Atlanta, Ga.: Carter Center, 1994.

6. R.J. Miller. *Example of Public Outreach Program: Kansas.* 28th National Immunization Conference, Fourth Plenary Session, Charlotte, N.C.: June 1994.

7. S.S. Hutchins, et al. *The Role of a Mass Vaccination Day in a Measles Outbreak.* 19th Annual Meeting of the American Public Health Association. Session 2207, Atlanta, Ga.: APHA, 1991.

8. G. Fairbrother and K.A. DuMont. "New York City's 1993 Child Immunization Day: Planning, Costs and Results." *American Journal of Public Health* 85 (1995): 1662–1665.

9. Joint World Health Organization/UNICEF Statement. *Planning Principles for Accelerated Immunization Activities*. Geneva, Switzerland: WHO, 1995.

10. C.K. Mitchell and S.M. Franco. "Factors Associated with Improved Immunization Rates for Urban Minority Preschool Children." *Clinical Pediatrics* 34 (1995): 466–470.

11. F.T. Cutts et al. "Causes of Low Preschool Immunization Coverage in the US." *Annual Review of Public Health* 13 (1992): 358–398.

12. National Advisory Committee. "The Measles Epidemic: The Problems, Barriers, and Recommendations." *Journal of the American Medical Association* 226 (1991): 1547–1552.

13. G. Fairbrother et al. "Design Issues for a Big City Immunization Registry." *American Journal of Preventive Medicine* 13, suppl. 1 (1997): 26–31.

14. Balanced-Budget Bill Extends Health Care to Children. *The Nation's Health* August 1997, 1–5, passim.

15. U.S. Department of Health and Human Services. *Healthy People 2000: National Health Promotion and Disease Prevention Objectives*. DHHS Pub. No. (PHS) 91-50212. Washington, D.C.: DHHS, 1990.

PART VI

Opportunities and Future Challenges

The last section presents some of the opportunities and future challenges that academicians, practitioners, and community members face in conducting community-based research.

The first chapter, on the *Guide to Community Preventive Services,* describes the rationale for, the goals of, and the methodology used in developing this new resource. The *Guide* will provide information on intervention effectiveness related to how to change risky health behaviors, specific diseases, injuries, and impairments. In doing so, the *Guide* also addresses the changes that need to occur in the conditions that influence public health (e.g., ecosystems and access to health care) and policy development, and the role of private health care systems in creating changes in behaviors, conditions, and policies. The *Guide* will also address the development and monitoring of community health improvement programs. As such, the *Guide* has the potential to provide information on the most current trends, innovative methodologies, and suggestions for evaluation of community-based research. This effort is being overseen by a 15-member, nonfederal task force, and the full *Guide* will be published in the year 2000.

The second chapter, by Holtgrave and Valdiserri, provides an example of how community-based programs can be both grounded in previous research findings and responsive to those most affected by program activities and policies. The involvement they describe includes the development of program priorities, coalition development, and building of community assets. They also highlight the importance of process, impact, and outcome evaluation activities. Holtgrave and Valdiserri add to the material already presented by acknowledging the need to address the dynamic nature of planning objectives within community-based programs, and providing an example of bringing grantees together to learn from each other in the spirit of cooperation rather than competition.

McAfee and Thompson provide us with some issues to consider in thinking about the role of managed care in community-based prevention programs. They help to reframe some of the current thinking by suggesting the use of the term health improvement organization rather than health maintenance organization. The authors also encourage medical care organizations to reassess their role in developing and implementing policies that promote health. In doing so they remind us that the boundaries between public health and medical care are changing. For example, current trends have medical care organizations, not public health, providing services for the traditionally underserved. In addition, more physicians and medical personnel are being trained in public health, and more public health practitioners are being employed within medical care environments. McAfee and Thompson note the tension in managed care between those who want to apply the standard that prevention ". . . must end up saving money" versus those willing to spend reasonable amounts of money to add years of quality life for enrolled individuals.

In the last chapter in this section, Brownson and Bal discuss the implications of bringing together state, federal, and local constituencies in working on cancer control and prevention. They reiterate some common themes presented throughout this book, including the importance of coalition building and the use of data for planning and evaluation of programs and policies. They also raise some critical points to consider in thinking about the future of community-based research, including the concern of overwhelming individuals and organizations by creating too many categorical coalitions, and the promise of the Internet for dissemination of data and sharing of programs. Finally, they challenge academicians, practitioners, and community members to become flexible enough in our definitions and our approaches to meet the ever-changing health needs of communities.

As you read these chapters, consider the following set of questions:

Objectives and Data Sources

1. How can community-based prevention programs incorporate state-of-the-art findings and approaches, yet retain responsiveness to the setting and community of interest?
2. How can the information presented in the *Guide to Community Preventive Services* be used by local community coalitions in developing programs and policies?
3. Within the field of HIV/AIDS prevention and control, which data sets are essential in developing community-based efforts?

Methods and Strategies

4. What are some specific ways that managed care organizations can influence the development of preventive health programs and policies? How can private-public partnerships assist in these efforts?
5. What are some alternatives to multiple categorical coalitions?

Dissemination and Implications for Public Health Practice

6. Holtgrave and Valdiserri point to the opportunities of bringing multiple grantees together. How can the lessons learned from these gatherings be passed on to other gatherings of grantees in a way that not only provides information but also enhances the integration of learning and reciprocal learning across funding streams?

18

Development of the *Guide to Community Preventive Services*: A U.S. Public Health Service Initiative

Marguerite Pappaioanou and Caswell Evans, Jr.

In 1994, the Public Health Service (PHS) determined that developing the *Guide to Community Preventive Services* (the *Guide*), which was based on the best available scientific evidence and current expertise regarding effective population-based preventive strategies, would be an important contribution to practitioners and providers of population-based preventive health services in the United States. The PHS asked the Centers for Disease Control and Prevention (CDC) to convene a nonfederal task force and to coordinate strong federal leadership and involvement in developing and publishing the *Guide*. The Director of CDC appointed a 15-member, independent, nonfederal task force on Community Preventive Ser-

---

Address inquiries on the Task Force and on the development of the *Guide* to the Community Preventive Services Guide Development Activity, Division of Prevention Research and Analytic Methods, Epidemiology Program Office, CDC, Mailstop D-01, 1600 Clifton Rd., Atlanta, GA, 30333, Phone: 404-639-4301; Fax: 404-639-4816. Address inquiries on the implementation of the *Guide* to the Public Health Practice Program Office, Mailstop K-39, CDC, 4770 Buford Highway NE, Atlanta, GA 30333: Phone: 770-488-2460; Fax: 770-488-2474.

The authors acknowledge the contributions of the Task Force on Community Preventive Services (Appendix 1) and of the many persons who were responsible for developing and launching this important initiative, including Drs. Phil Lee, J. Michael McGinnis, C. Earl Fox, and the Public Health Functions Working Group, Department of Health and Human Services, Office of the Secretary; Drs. David Satcher, Claire Broome, Dixie Snider, Alan Hinman, Edward Baker Jr., Steven Thacker, Jeffrey Harris, Randy Gordon, Ray (Bud) Nicola, Donna Stroup, Steven Teutsch, and the CDC Work Group on Community Preventive Services, Centers for Disease Control and Prevention; and Dr. Lloyd Novick and Mr. Ron Bialek, Council on Linkages Between Academia and Public Health.

J Public Health Management Practice, 1998, 4(2), 48–54

vices that, over a four-year period, will develop a *Guide to Community Preventive Services.* The Task Force met for the first time in August 1996.

This chapter presents an overview of the Task Force on Community Preventive Services and the development of the *Guide,* including background leading to the *Guide's* development, the primary target audience, purpose, general scope, and content of the *Guide,* and the general process and methods being used to develop evidence-based chapters in the *Guide.*

BACKGROUND

The *Guide to Clinical Preventive Services,* first issued by the U.S. Preventive Services Task Force (USPSTF) in 1989[1] and revised in 1996,[2] has served as an important guide to practitioners to use when considering which clinical preventive services to provide to their patients. The USPSTF conducted a rigorous review of evidence on the effectiveness of more than 100 interventions to prevent 70 illnesses and conditions. Based on this evidence, the USPSTF made recommendations on the provision of primary and secondary prevention services (e.g., screening, immunization, chemoprophylaxis, and counseling) to patients in clinical settings.

In developing the *Guide to Clinical Preventive Services,* the USPSTF considered population-based (e.g., community, occupational, school-based) preventive services outside its scope. However, since its publication, practitioners and providers of preventive health services in both the public and private sectors have expressed a need for similarly developed, evidence-based recommendations upon which they can make informed decisions for selecting, funding, and implementing population-based (community) preventive health services. During 1991–1992, a pilot effort was undertaken at CDC to assess the feasibility of developing analytic frameworks and synthesizing evidence on population-based interventions in public health. In discussions during 1994, the Public Health Functions Working Group, Department of Health and Human Services, crystallized ideas on how to meet those needs and considered the prospects for developing a guide that would synthesize and present information on the effectiveness of population-based public health interventions. During 1994–1995, the Council on Linkages between Academia and Public Health Practice, with support from the Kellogg Foundation and in collaboration with federal, state, and local public health agencies, carried out a more detailed and comprehensive study that assessed the feasibility and benefits of developing evidence-based practice guidelines for public health practices and tested a methodology for evaluating scientific evidence on which guidelines for public health practices could be built. The Council concluded that public health practice guidelines that are based upon scientific evidence and empirical information are feasible and "the potential benefits of public health practice guidelines are immediate and far reaching."[3,4]

Based on the success of the *Guide to Clinical Preventive Services* and supported by findings of the Council on Linkages feasibility study, the PHS's Public Health Functions Work Group decided to initiate the development of the *Guide to Community Preventive Services*. The two guides will complement each other by strengthening our nation's capacity to meet our health promotion and disease prevention objectives and ensuring improved health outcomes for all.

PRIMARY TARGET AUDIENCE AND PURPOSE OF THE *GUIDE TO COMMUNITY PREVENTIVE SERVICES*

The Task Force expects that the *Guide* will enjoy a rich and diverse readership. The primary target audience of the *Guide* is persons involved in the planning, funding, and implementation of population-based services and policies to improve health at the community and state level. The purpose of the *Guide* is to provide information needed by this audience for informed decision making on the most relevant, effective, and cost-effective public health strategies, policies, and programs for their communities.

PROCESS TO DEVELOP THE *GUIDE*

The 15-member independent, nonfederal Task Force on Community Preventive Services (Task Force), appointed by the Director of CDC (Appendix 1), meets approximately quarterly. (Meetings are announced by public notice in the Federal Register and are open to the public.) Task Force members have expertise in multiple disciplines (e.g., infectious disease, chronic disease, environmental health, maternal and child health, mental health, and substance abuse), and represent different public health perspectives (e.g., state and local health departments, managed care, behavioral and social sciences, communications sciences, epidemiology, academia, decision and cost-effectiveness analysis, information systems, primary care, and management and policy). The 15-member Task Force is complemented by the active participation of four consultants to the Task Force who have had previous experience with other guidelines efforts, federal agency liaison members, and liaison representatives from professional groups involved in public health (Appendix 2).

TIME LINE TO DEVELOP THE *GUIDE*

The first meeting of the Task Force was held in August 1996. Individual components of the *Guide* will be published as they are completed; the projected completion date for the entire *Guide* is July 1, 2000.

CONTENT AND SCOPE OF THE *GUIDE*

The Task Force has developed a working table of contents for the *Guide* based on the following criteria: the *Guide* will (1) coordinate with Healthy People 2000 (2010) Priority Areas; (2) allow for breadth of scope; (3) address risk behaviors with the most impact on health; and (4) address major causes of ill health among children and young adults.

The Task Force has proposed that the following sections comprise the *Guide*: (1) background about the Task Force on Community Preventive Services, the *Guide to Community Preventive Services*, and the purpose and target audience of the *Guide*; (2) methodology; (3) changing risk behaviors; (4) reducing specific diseases, injuries, and impairments; (5) changing ecosystems (including environmental concerns); and (6) crosscutting public health activities. The Task Force also has determined that the following additional subject areas will be addressed by the *Guide*: (1) determinants of public health, (2) access to health care, (3) policy development, (4) developing a community health improvement program, (5) performance indicators to monitor community health, and (6) the role of private health care systems in improving community health.

The final complete set, order, and composition of sections has not been determined. Additional subject areas may be identified. (The Task Force continues to refine the *Guide's* table of contents and methods used in its development. For continually updated information, see the home page on the Task Force on Community Preventive Services and the *Guide* at the following Internet address: http://web.health.gov/community/guide/.)

METHODS TO DEVELOP THE *GUIDE*

The Task Force also is determining the most appropriate methods to (1) search for evidence on the effectiveness and cost-effectiveness of population-based interventions, (2) assess the quality of that evidence, and (3) translate the evidence into recommendations. Chapter development teams, comprising subject-matter experts from a variety of perspectives (e.g., program managers, local and state health officials, managed care organizations, community groups, and academicians), are formed for each chapter being developed. Briefly, these teams

- Develop a proposed approach to the organization of the chapter.
- Use predetermined criteria for selecting topics, subtopics, and interventions to be assessed in the chapter.
- Develop logic and analytic frameworks that describe key relationships among determinants, population-based interventions, and outcomes being evaluated in the chapter.

- Develop strategies for the consistent and systematic retrieval of evidence.
- Review and rate the quality of evidence from individual studies, taking into account study hypothesis, population and setting, definitions of exposure and outcomes, follow-up/completion rates, bias, data analysis, and confounding.
- Develop evidence tables that synthesize the body of evidence for review by the Task Force.
- Use an explicit process determined by the Task Force for translating the evidence into recommendations.
- Draft the chapter. Once chapters are drafted, they will be field tested for content and format before being finalized and published.

For the *Guide to Clinical Preventive Services*, the USPSTF considered results from randomized controlled trials, controlled trials, cohort or case-control studies, multiple time series, uncontrolled experiments, and opinions of respected authorities. In making recommendations, they assigned greater weight to evidence resulting from well-designed studies; for example, their strongest recommendations were reserved for clinical preventive services supported by data from randomized controlled trials.[1,2] Because evidence from randomized controlled trials likely will be less prevalent for many population-based interventions, the Task Force is addressing the need to determine how evidence from published quantitative and qualitative studies, unpublished evidence (e.g., evaluation reports carried out by state health departments), and potentially, expert opinion, will be translated into recommendations for the *Guide to Community Preventive Services*.

FIELD TESTING AND IMPLEMENTATION OF THE *GUIDE*

As initial chapters of the *Guide* are drafted, they will be field-tested to obtain early feedback and input from the primary target audience on content and format—a process essential to ensure optimal usefulness to end users. Sections of the *Guide* will be made available in both printed and electronic form as they are completed.

PROVISION OF SUPPORT TO THE TASK FORCE

CDC is providing institutional and staff support to the Task Force (Appendix 3) by convening meetings of the Task Force; coordinating support from federal agencies, state and local health departments, professional organizations, academic institutions, managed-care organizations, public health practitioners, and other health partners in the development and implementation of the *Guide*; and developing an electronic database of the *Guide* and supporting evidence.

REFERENCES

1. U.S. Preventive Services Task Force. *Guide to Clinical Preventive Services: An Assessment of the Effectiveness of 169 Interventions*. Baltimore: Williams & Wilkins, 1989.

2. U.S. Preventive Services Task Force. *Guide to Clinical Preventive Services,* 2nd ed. Baltimore: Williams & Wilkins, 1996.

3. Council on Linkages between Academia and Public Health Practice. *Practice Guidelines for Public Health: Assessment of Scientific Evidence, Feasibility and Benefits*: *A Report of the Guideline Development Project for Public Health Practice.* October 1995.

4. L.F. Novick. "Public Health Practice Guidelines: A Case Study." *Journal of Public Health Management Practice* 3, no. 1 (1997): 59–64.

APPENDIX 1

TASK FORCE ON COMMUNITY PREVENTIVE SERVICES

Caswell Evans, Jr., DDS, MPH, Assistant Director, Health Services and Director, Office of Public Health Initiatives, Los Angeles County Department of Health Services, Los Angeles, California; and Project Director and Managing Editor of the Surgeon General's Report on Oral Health (Chairperson)

Jonathan Fielding, MD, MPH, MBA, Professor of Health Services and Pediatrics, School of Public Health, University of California, Los Angeles, California (Vice-Chair)

Ross C. Brownson, PhD, Professor, St. Louis University School of Public Health, St. Louis, Missouri

Patricia Buffler, BSN, PhD, MPH, Dean, School of Public Health, University of California, Berkeley, California

Mary Jane England, MD, President, Washington Business Group on Health, Washington, D.C.

David Fleming, State Epidemiologist, Portland, Oregon

Mindy Fullilove, MD, Associate Professor, Clinical Psychiatry and Public Health, New York State, Psychiatric Institute and Columbia University, New York City

Fernando Guerra, MD, MPH, Director of Health, San Antonio Metropolitan Health District, San Antonio, Texas

Alan Hinman, MD, MPH, Task Force for Child Survival and Development, Atlanta, Georgia

George Isham, MD, Medical Director and Chief Health Officer, HealthPartners, Minneapolis, Minnesota

Garland Land, MPH, Director, Center for Health Information, Management, and Epidemiology, Missouri Department of Health, Jefferson City, Missouri

Charles Mahan, MD, Dean, College of Public Health, University of South Florida, Tampa, Florida

Patricia Dolan Mullen, DrPH, Professor of Behavioral Sciences and Health Education, School of Public Health, University of Texas, Houston, Texas

Susan Scrimshaw, PhD, Dean, School of Public Health, University of Illinois, Chicago, Illinois

Robert S. Thompson, MD, Director, Department of Preventive Care, Group Health Cooperative of Puget Sound, Seattle, Washington

CONSULTANTS TO THE TASK FORCE ON COMMUNITY PREVENTIVE SERVICES

Robert Lawrence, MD, Associate Dean, Office of Professional Education Programs, School of Hygiene and Public Health, Johns Hopkins University, Baltimore, Maryland

Michael McGinnis, MD, Scholar in Residence, National Academy of Sciences, Washington, D.C.

Lloyd F. Novick, MD, MPH, Commissioner, Onondaga County Health Department, Syracuse, New York

Sylvie Stachenko, MD, MSc, Director, Division of Disease Prevention, Health Canada, Ottawa, Ontario, Canada

Steven M. Teutsch, MD, MPH, Senior Research Scientist, Outcomes Research and Management, Merck & Co., Inc.

APPENDIX 2

PARTNER FEDERAL AGENCIES SUPPORTING THE TASK FORCE*

Agency for Health Care Policy and Research
Food and Drug Administration
Health Care Financing Administration
Health Resources and Services Administration
Indian Health Service
National Highway and Traffic Safety Administration
National Institutes of Health
Office of Disease Prevention and Health Promotion
Office of Population Affairs
Substance Abuse and Mental Health Administration

PARTNER INSTITUTIONS AND ORGANIZATIONS SUPPORTING THE TASK FORCE

American Association of Health Plans
American College of Preventive Medicine
Association of State and Territorial Health Officials
Association of State and Territorial Directors of Health Promotion and Public Health Education
Association of Schools of Public Health
Association of Teachers of Preventive Medicine
American Public Health Association

---

*As specific topics are selected for inclusion in the *Guide,* those federal agencies responsible for or involved with preventive services in that area become actively involved.

Center for the Advancement of Health
Council on Linkages between Academia and Public Health
Environmental Council of the States
Institute of Medicine
National Association of County and City Health Officials
National Association of State Alcohol and Drug Abuse Directors
National Association of State Mental Health Program Directors
National Association of Local Boards of Health
Public Health Foundation

APPENDIX 3

CDC STAFF COORDINATING SUPPORT TO THE TASK FORCE IN THE DEVELOPMENT OF THE *GUIDE*

Community Preventive Services Guide Development Activity, Division of Prevention Research and Analytic Methods, Epidemiology Program Office, CDC
Marguerite Pappaioanou, DVM, PhD, Chief
April Dixon, Secretary
Julie Ann Wasil, Management Analyst
Peter Briss, MD, Senior Scientist
David Hopkins, MD, MPH, Preventive Medicine Resident
Michael Maciosek, PhD, Prevention Effectiveness Fellow
Benedict Truman, MD, MPH, Senior Scientist
Stephanie Zaza, MD, MPH, Senior Scientist

CDC STAFF COORDINATING SUPPORT TO THE TASK FORCE IN THE IMPLEMENTATION OF THE *GUIDE*

Division of Public Health Services, Public Health Practice Program Office, CDC
Ray (Bud) Nicola, MD, MHSA, Director
Deanne Johnson, Program Manager
Kathy Grooms, Program Analyst
Mark Oberle, MD, MPH, Senior Medical Officer

19

HIV Prevention Community Planning: A National Perspective on Accomplishments, Challenges, and Future Directions

David R. Holtgrave and Ronald O. Valdiserri

Human immunodeficiency virus (HIV) prevention programs that do not meet the needs of affected communities are doomed to failure, and are a waste of scarce, public resources. Centers for Disease Control and Prevention (CDC) and its prevention partners have long recognized this point. For years, CDC has encouraged state, local, and territorial health department grantees to obtain community input when planning HIV prevention programs.[1] There are 65 such grantees (the states, the District of Columbia, the U.S. Territories, and six cities with direct funding mandated by Congress). These grantees received HIV prevention cooperative agreement funding of approximately $175 million (M) in fiscal year (FY) 1994.

Although grantees did obtain community input in the past, it was done in widely varying ways.[2] Further, in FYs 1993 and earlier, Congress required that approximately $102M (71 percent of the total cooperative agreement in FY 1993) be spent on HIV counseling, testing, referral, and partner notification services. Such requirements were a disincentive for community level planning. Therefore, in order to invigorate grantees and communities to work together in close partnership to plan HIV prevention programs, CDC undertook a substantial revision in the process of planning and prioritizing these programs.

A supplemental guidance outlining this process was developed in collaboration with a wide variety of prevention partners (e.g., national minority organizations, associations of health officials, other professional organizations, and many others).[3] The new process requires that each grantee identify HIV prevention priorities through a participatory process. Beginning in January 1994, each grantee must convene at least one community planning group. The community planning groups must represent the local epidemic in terms of affected communities, and also pos-

J Public Health Management Practice, 1996, 2(3), 1–9

sess behavioral, evaluation, and epidemiological science expertise. Each group is cochaired by a health department representative and a community representative elected by the group.

The major tasks of the community planning process are to assess the HIV prevention needs in the grantee's jurisdiction, develop or review a jurisdiction-specific epidemiological profile of the HIV epidemic, prioritize unmet HIV prevention needs, and prioritize the interventions using a number of parameters including a scientific soundness and cultural relevance. This prioritization is then provided to the grantee who uses it to allocate resources among new and existing HIV prevention activities, and to develop an application to CDC for continuation funding. The community planning group is given an opportunity to review the application and to write a letter of agreement (concurrence) or disagreement (nonconcurrence) with the application based on how well the application operationalizes the plan. This letter is included with the grantee's application to CDC. More extensive introductions to the principles and procedures of community planning are available.[4-6]

To specifically support the community planning activities, CDC provided to its 65 grantees $12M in new funding in FY 1994. CDC also provided technical assistance in diverse areas related to the implementation of community planning (described later). In FY 1995, Congress provided an additional $44M to CDC for supplemental cooperative agreement awards to state and local health departments. These funds were competitively awarded and concentrated on two major categories: $39M to address high-priority, unmet HIV prevention needs identified through the community planning process; and $5M to expand, strengthen, and further evaluate HIV prevention community planning. Hence, new resources were made available to support HIV prevention community planning and unmet needs identified through that process.

OVERVIEW

After one year's experience with HIV prevention community planning, it is important to take stock of the process and consider progress to date. In this chapter, we take a national perspective and review the major events of year one, including programmatic challenges that have been met, as well as those that remain to be addressed. We also review the major directions of HIV prevention community planning as year two begins.

METHODS

In order to proactively manage the HIV prevention community planning process, careful evaluation is necessary—both process and outcome.[5] A variety of formal evaluation methods are being used to assess the progress made in community planning. These methods include case studies, tracking specific budget expenditures, assessment of five core process objectives (see box), and grantee level evaluations. A detailed description of these methods is available elsewhere.[5] Other, less formal, yet important, sources of information are available as well (e.g., the varying personal perspectives of key participants in HIV prevention community planning and a detailed timeline kept by CDC staff). Progress-to-date on the collection of formal and informal evaluative information was reviewed in a recent meeting (December 5–7, 1994) in Atlanta. We draw on our knowledge of these implementation and evaluative activities, as well as knowledge gained from our own direct participation in the implementation of HIV prevention community planning. We acknowledge that there is a wide range of other participants in, and observers of, the community planning process, each of whom has a unique voice and perspective to share.

YEAR ONE EVENTS

Supplemental guidance

For several years, CDC has encouraged its 65 health department grantees to utilize community input in planning HIV prevention programs, yet substantial barriers resulted in less than satisfactory outcomes.[1,2] In 1994, CDC received specific resources from Congress to support HIV prevention planning. Further, information and assessments from a variety of diverse sources supported the need for extensive improvements in the manner in which HIV prevention priorities were identified.[6] In the last half of 1993, CDC drafted a guidance for grantees outlining a more participatory, less federally mandated way of identifying HIV prevention

---

Core Objectives for Year One of HIV Prevention Community Planning

- Ensure that the nomination for community planning group membership is an open process.
- Ensure that the community planning group reflects in its composition the characteristics of the current and projected epidemic in its jurisdiction.
- Base prioritization of needs on epidemiologic profile, resource inventory, gap analysis, and research on target populations.
- Base prioritization of interventions on list of unmet needs, effectiveness, cost-effectiveness, theory, and community norms and values.
- Develop the HIV prevention funding application based on the community plan.

Source: Reprinted with permission from *Public Health Reports,* 1995, U.S. Public Health Service, Department of Health and Human Services.

priorities.[2,3] This supplemental guidance was drafted with extensive input from a broad array of HIV prevention partners. These partners included representatives of health departments, national minority organizations, community-based organizations, advocacy groups, and many other professional organizations.

The guidance was finalized and distributed to health department grantees in December 1993 for immediate implementation of the process beginning in January 1994. Rather than mandate a single standardized process in each of the 65 jurisdictions receiving funds, CDC afforded grantees the flexibility to configure a process based on local circumstances and realities. However, all grantees had to adhere to 13 guiding principles outlined in the supplemental guidance. For a more complete description of these principles, see Valdiserri et al.[6]

Community planning began

With the supplemental guidance issued, HIV prevention community planning began officially in January 1994. One major facilitating factor for the implementation of community planning was the removal of the Congressional requirement that a majority of this funding be spent on HIV counseling, testing, referral, and partner notification services. Another facilitating factor was supplemental funding specifically earmarked for planning. The supplemental planning awards to grantees ranged in size from $15,000 to $350,000 and totalled $12M.

In 1994, every one of the 65 HIV prevention grantees used these supplemental funds to implement the HIV prevention community planning process. By October 3, 1994, each grantee had to submit to CDC its application for continuation funding for FY 1995 based on the results of the 1994 community planning process. The continuation application included a report on FY 1994 activities, a detailed community-based plan for FY 1995 HIV prevention programs, and a letter from the community planning group indicating agreement or disagreement with the grantee's operationalization of the comprehensive HIV prevention plan. This continuation application also included some information used by CDC to help evaluate the community planning process at a national level (discussed further later). Twenty-seven grantees requested extensions, ranging from one to three months, for submission of their community-based plan; one of these requests was made even though the planning group disagreed with the request. Of the 38 continuation applications that did not request a planning extension, all contained a letter of agreement (or concurrence) from the associated community planning group.

Technical assistance network established

Because of the highly complex and novel nature of HIV prevention community planning, it was clear at the outset that a great deal of technical assistance would be required by grantees during year one. Grantees were permitted to use some of their community planning funds to purchase technical assistance. However, CDC decided that it was also necessary to have technical assistance available at a national level.

In the winter and early spring of 1994, CDC established a technical assistance network that could provide assistance in the following areas: (a) supporting the representation, inclusion, and participation of affected communities in the process; (b) HIV prevention needs assessment; (c) HIV epidemiology; (d) HIV prevention behavioral science and evaluation; and (e) conflict management. Partners involved in the provision of technical assistance in year one included the following organizations: the National Association of People with AIDS, the National Council of La Raza, the National Minority AIDS Council, the National Native American AIDS Prevention Center, the National Organization of Black County Officials, the United States-Mexico Border Health Organization, the National Alliance of State and Territorial AIDS Directors, the Council of State and Territorial Epidemiologists, and the Academy for Educational Development.

Because of the limited time frame and urgency for developing the technical assistance network to support community planning implementation, CDC primarily relied on two extant mechanisms for providing funding to these technical assistance providers. The first mechanism was by competitively supplementing awards to organizations with existing cooperative agreements with CDC. The second was the use of task-order contractors. These contractors bid for the right to provide work for CDC (within defined content-area boundaries and time constraints); then, when CDC needs rapid assistance in a given area, it may call upon its task-order contractors.

In year one, the first technical assistance activity was the development (in approximately eight weeks) of several written technical assistance documents covering the topics described earlier. These documents were assembled into a binder and distributed to all grantees. CDC and the Academy for Educational Development (AED) worked in partnership to develop this binder of technical assistance materials.[7] The purpose of the binder was to rapidly provide initial technical information that could be used to start the planning process and that could be used as templates for modification to local circumstances. The binder was not intended as definitive or final technical information, but was intended as a starting point. Throughout the year, several mailings to grantees covered specifics of these technical topics in greater detail (e.g., one mailing expanded upon earlier technical assistance about possible priority setting methods).

Information, networking, and training

Several large-scale meetings on community planning were held throughout the first year to promote information sharing, networking, and technical skills training among key participants and opinion leaders in the community planning process. Two meetings were sponsored by the National Alliance of State and Territorial AIDS Directors (NASTAD) and attended by health department AIDS directors (January 6–7, 1994, and April 25–26, 1994). These meetings focused on grantee implementation issues, including technical aspects of establishing community planning groups. CDC sponsored two meetings in the summer of 1994 (June 6–7 and July 12–13) whose audiences were the cochairs of the recently convened community planning groups. These cochair meetings focused on all aspects of HIV prevention community planning, with a special emphasis on priority-setting methodologies. The Division of Sexually Transmitted Diseases/HIV Prevention, National Center for Prevention Services, CDC, sponsored a meeting with all of its grantees in August 1994; several sessions during the week-long program featured community planning. Again, a major goal of these meetings was to foster peer-to-peer discussions and networking among those implementing community planning in the field.

Three other series of meetings on HIV prevention community planning also took place in year one. One series of meetings (September 17, 1993; November 30, 1993; May 3, 1994; September 12, 1994; December 5–7, 1994) allowed governmental and nongovernmental consultants to provide ongoing feedback to CDC on the community planning progress throughout year one. These meetings included a wide variety of prevention partners from health departments, professional organizations, national minority organizations, and community-based organizations, among others. Early meetings focused on discussions related to the guidance, and latter meetings on anticipated changes in year two and beyond.

Another set of meetings provided training for CDC project officers who work closely with health department grantees and who were charged with assisting grantees in the implementation of community planning. Training topics included Orientation to Community Planning (March 1–2, 1994) and Needs Assessment Methodologies (March 23–24, 1994).

A third series of meetings and conference calls were devoted to the coordination of technical assistance services. Technical assistance services covered a variety of topics and were delivered by multiple technical assistance service providers (as well as CDC staff). Therefore, it was necessary to establish excellent communications among all parties so as to minimize overlap, address unmet needs, ensure quality of services, troubleshoot, and optimize the complementary nature of the various services and providers.

Evaluation methods selected and implemented

As briefly noted earlier and described in detail by Holtgrave et al., CDC developed an evaluation strategy to measure the progress of community planning in year one.[5] Each grantee was asked to do a self-evaluation of the community planning process in their jurisdiction, thereby providing information to help them manage their process. However, 65 self-evaluations do not make for a national evaluation. In order to identify areas of community planning in need of support and attention by CDC, technical assistance providers, and grantees, several methodologies (and contractors) were selected.

First, CDC, in conjunction with NASTAD, selected five core objectives to track national implementation of community planning (see box). Grantees each reported on these five core objectives to CDC in their October 3, 1994, continuation application, and the information is being summarized across grantees by the AED. Second, CDC developed tabular formats that grantees used to report on their planned programmatic expenditures by intervention type and population. Over time, budget data collected using these tables will allow some measure of whether community planning will lead to different levels of investment in certain programs (relative to previous years). CDC, NASTAD, and AED are working in partnership to summarize year one budget information.

Third, CDC, the U.S. Conference of Mayors, and Battelle Memorial Institute are conducting case study evaluations of a total of 11 grantees' community planning processes. The case study methodology allows for a detailed, qualitative assessment of important barriers and facilitating factors in the community planning process, and complements the more quantitative evaluation methods described earlier. With the input gained from a national meeting on community planning held in Atlanta from December 5–7, 1994, CDC is currently finalizing its choices for evaluation methods to be used in years two and beyond for community planning assessment.

With private funding, the AIDS Action Council has embarked upon an independent evaluation of the community planning process. Case study methods are being used to understand qualitatively the implementation of HIV prevention community planning in several grantees' jurisdictions.

DIFFICULTIES ENCOUNTERED

Time pressure

Virtually everyone involved with HIV prevention community planning complained of the crushing time pressure in the process. Grantees and community planning groups had approximately eight months to form, work on needs assessments and epidemiological profiles, prioritize unmet needs, consider evidence on the relative effectiveness of different types of interventions, prioritize interventions to address unmet needs, and review the health department's application. CDC staff had only six to eight weeks to develop the technical assistance network and evaluation strategy described earlier. Technical assistance providers had an even shorter time to develop their services and begin service provision. Now we enter into year two of community planning, and long-range technical assistance and evaluation plans must be rapidly finalized.

Because time pressure is a central, chronic characteristic of HIV prevention community planning, it is important to describe its genesis. Community planning activities begun in FY 1994, by definition, can have no impact on prioritization and resource targeting until FY 1995. That is, plans developed in year one of community planning do not impact funding applications (i.e., spending decisions) until year two of community planning. Hence, to allow more time for the start-up phase of community planning would have meant that the earliest possible impact would have been in FY 1996. The choice was, therefore, to either put community planning on a very fast timeline, or to put it on a slower timeline. Because of the urgency of the AIDS epidemic, the former option was chosen. Yet it was recognized by CDC and its partners early on that the fast time frame possibly would mean a suboptimal process in at least the first year.

Stretching the limits of available resources

Although $12M in funding was made available to the 65 grantees specifically to support community planning activities, several grantees voiced concern that planning resources were stretched to the limit. Community planning is a resource intensive activity. It requires significant fiscal and human resources to staff the planning process, travel community representatives to the meetings (especially in rural areas), and in some cases reimburse people for time taken off work to participate in the process. At CDC, too, staff took on community planning responsibilities usually in addition to their other job duties. Although the evaluation activities implemented were multiple and intensive, there were calls for even more detailed evaluative work. The demands of HIV prevention community planning are stretching the limits of available and redirected human and fiscal resources.

Additionally, community planning is stretching the capabilities of some governmental systems to hire and reimburse key participants in the planning process. For instance, some grantees were unable or slow to hire important staff members to implement the planning process. A hiring freeze hampered CDC's ability to staff the community planning process at an optimal level. Grantees' governmental regulations sometimes also place limits on whether and how much community planning group members can be reimbursed for their time. This is an important barrier, especially for (potential) participants who are members of affected communities, but who do not work professionally in the HIV prevention arena; current staff of HIV prevention service provisions and other organizations sometimes can participate in planning activities as part of their jobs.

Finally, grantees have state or local regulations that they must follow in the letting of subcontracts or cooperative agreements within their jurisdictions. Developing and implementing a community-based plan requires a great deal of contractual flexibility—perhaps more than some grantees currently enjoy.

Bringing science into the process

In November 1994, several teams reviewed in great detail the applications of 16 randomly selected grantees. Two of the teams focused on, respectively, the use of epidemiology and behavioral science information in the community planning process. These teams reported their findings at the December 5–7 meeting. Both groups observed and cited difficulties in merging scientific information in the community planning process (of course, there were some exceptions). Difficulties arose in defining, identifying, and bringing to the planning table scientific expertise. For instance, a frequently cited difficulty was the translation of epidemiological information into a format that was both understandable and usable by community planning group members. Successful use of epidemiological information in community planning requires at least the following: (a) the existence of data that matches planning groups' information needs; (b) epidemiologists who can provide such data, translate it into understandable terms, and listen to planning group members for further information needs; and (c) planning group members who are willing to build and maintain a dialogue with epidemiologists so as to gain the data-based information, and to clearly articulate current and future information needs.

As another example, in some cases little identifiable behavioral science expertise was brought into the planning process; in at least one other case, a relatively large proportion of the community planning group claimed behavioral science expertise even though it was not apparent that they had extensive formal training or experience in the area. Some areas did incorporate behavioral and social science into the planning process by having scientists as members of the group, and by inviting scientists to give presentations.

Challenges also arose in using scientific information in priority setting. The guidance encouraged grantees and community planning groups to define the theoretical, effectiveness, and cost-effectiveness bases of their programs. Some grantees did this explicitly in their continuation applications; others noted that they had done so, but did not provide details. It was apparent that attempts had been made to identify relevant scientific literature. However, challenges were met in translating the research literature for use in local community planning efforts. That is, if one identifies a study on the effectiveness of street outreach programs for injection drug users, which was conducted in a particular city, then how much should this guide a community planning group in another area of the country (perhaps grappling with other populations)? This question is one of external validity, and one with no easy answers. At the December 5–7 meeting, calls were issued for intensified (yet, perhaps more streamlined or "user-friendly") technical assistance in these areas.

Priority setting challenges

In order to set priorities among unmet HIV prevention needs and interventions to meet those needs, community planning groups had to consider several factors. The supplemental guidance suggested that at least the following factors be considered: documented need; effectiveness; cost-effectiveness; theoretical basis; consumer values, norms, and preferences; availability of other resources; and other factors of local importance. Some of these factors involve scientific information; others involve value judgments. Hence, community planning groups were faced with making challenging judgments based on both science and subjective values. This was one source of difficulty in priority setting.

A second challenging area was the identification and implementation of a group decision-making process. In other words, groups had to decide how they would make choices. A third area of difficulty was the process of defining key terms. For instance, how is a group to prioritize needs if no common definition of a "need" is agreed upon?

A fourth challenge was the use of explicit, quantitative decision-making rules, which was a new type of decision-making strategy for many persons. A fifth area was the behavioral and epidemiological data requirements imposed by decision-making models. Although dozens of studies are available that demonstrate that HIV prevention programs can change high risk behaviors, we still do not have complete answers to the more complex question of "what works best, for whom, in what settings, and for how long?"[8–11] Hence, lack of an ideal database creates uncertainty. Community planning is inherently an exercise in decision making under uncertainty—yet it is uncomfortable to recognize and make explicit that uncertainty. Large segments of time during the cochairs' meetings last summer were devoted to the topic of priority setting, as was a special technical assistance mailing in August 1994.

TRAJECTORY INTO YEAR TWO AND BEYOND

Dynamic version of community planning objectives

In the first year of community planning, groups had to be formed. However, this does not mean that the groups are composed already for year two. Some community planning groups may have turnover of up to 50 percent of their members. Hence, replacement members must be identified, approved by the planning groups, brought into the process, and achieve parity (i.e., equal partnership and ability to participate in the planning process) while at the same time not alienating or boring current members. Other people may hear about the community planning process and wish to become involved. In some instances, the requests for inclusion at the table may outstrip spaces available (i.e., planning groups should be inclusive but cannot function if unmanageably large). Additionally, possible future policy decisions (e.g., a possible movement toward public health block grants) could impact and make even more complex the HIV prevention community planning process. Hence, "static" issues from year one of community planning now become "dynamic" issues as we enter years two and beyond.

Emphasis on scientific technical assistance

The integration of scientific information into the community planning process in year one posed major challenges. Hence, an area for increased emphasis in year two of the community planning process is enhanced technical assistance in the use of epidemiological and behavioral science experts and expertise. Of course, this is not meant to inappropriately impose science on the process, but rather to provide key information and allow the community planning group to incorporate the information as appropriate in its deliberations. A central challenge, of course, is balancing the need to use the latest scientific findings (e.g., about intervention effectiveness and epidemiology) while at the same time providing the community planning group the freedom it needs to also consider consumer needs, values, and preferences. Some of this technical assistance will have to focus on issues of external validity. Also, the scientific community should listen to the information needs of the community planning groups. If a major purpose of applied HIV prevention research is to help inform judicious selection of the most promising interventions by community planning groups, then the information needs of the planning groups must be heard.

Evaluation methods refined

As the information from the formal evaluation activities is reviewed, decisions will have to be made as to whether the methods used yielded sufficient actionable information so as to manage the community planning process at both the grantee and national level. At the December 5–7 meeting, it was suggested that CDC include a small number of additional objectives in the set of core objectives (e.g., measuring in more detail whether trained behavioral and social scientists participated in the community planning process). Participants in that meeting also recommended that CDC continue its use of qualitative evaluation methods and strengthen its quantitative evaluation strategies (one example involved the quantitative comparison of epidemiological data with representation of specific population groups on community planning groups). Further, it was suggested that CDC make better use of the self-evaluations being conducted by grantees. Finally, a recommendation was made that CDC finalize a multiyear evaluation plan and select a contractor to begin the evaluation work for year two and beyond.

Proactive technical assistance

In year one of the community planning process, the written technical assistance materials were proactive; the interactive (e.g., telephonic) technical assistance was primarily reactive to requests. In years two and beyond, strategies must be developed to make all technical assistance more proactive. That is, some assessment will have to be made of each grantee's technical assistance needs, and strategies identified for meeting each of those needs. Waiting for grantees and community planning groups to identify their own technical assistance needs and ask for specific types of assistance appears to be insufficient.

Barriers to the accessing of technical assistance must also be broken down. For instance, one identified barrier is the perception that those grantees requesting technical assistance are doing poorly. One solution is more proactive technical assistance described earlier. If all grantees are receiving some form of technical assistance, then the stigma of receiving such services is removed. Of course, a remaining challenge will be the balancing of funding technical assistance services through the grantee or CDC; that is, intensified efforts must be made to determine the optimal mix of grantee- and CDC-purchased technical assistance. In fact, a recurrent theme of the December 5–7 meeting was that technical assistance must be moved ever closer to the local level.

• • •

Year one of HIV prevention community planning has met with some substantial challenges. Although the process is alive and thriving, it must be nourished to survive. Hence, in year two we must intensify and make more proactive technical assistance efforts, as well as fine-tune evaluation activities to ensure that the necessary information is available for managing the community planning process. Additionally, more work is needed in building the extremely important bridge between community planning groups and behavioral and epidemiological science.

Still, as we plan for year two and beyond, we must not forget the major accomplishments of year one of HIV prevention community planning. The very heart of the process for planning HIV prevention programs in this country was fundamentally changed, and changed, we believe, for the better.

REFERENCES

1. Centers for Disease Control and Prevention. "Cooperative Agreements for Human Immunodeficiency Virus (HIV) Prevention Projects, Program Announcement and Availability of Funds for Fiscal Year 1993." *Federal Register* 57 (September 4, 1992): 40675–40683.

2. Valdiserri, R.O., and West, G.R. "Barriers to the Assessment of Unmet Needs in Planning HIV/AIDS Prevention Programs." *Public Administration Review* 54, no. 1 (1994): 25–30.

3. Centers for Disease Control and Prevention. *Supplemental Guidance on HIV Prevention Community Planning for Noncompeting Continuation of Cooperative Agreements for HIV Prevention Projects.* Atlanta, Ga.: CDC, 1993. (Available from the National AIDS Clearinghouse, 1-800-329-1652.)

4. Holtgrave, D.R. "Setting Priorities and Community Planning for HIV Prevention Programs." *AIDS & Public Policy Journal* 9, no. 3 (1994): 148–152.

5. Holtgrave, D.R., et al. "Methodological Issues in Evaluating HIV Prevention Community Planning." *Public Health Reports* (1995), forthcoming.

6. Valdiserri, R.O., Aultman, T.V., and Curran, J.W. "Community Planning: A National Strategy to Improve HIV Prevention Programs." *Journal of Community Health* 20, no. 2 (1995): 87–100.

7. Academy for Educational Development, and Centers for Disease Control and Prevention. *Handbook for HIV Prevention Community Planning.* Washington, D.C.: AED, 1994.

8. Choi, K.H., and Coates, T.J. "Prevention of HIV Infection." *AIDS* 8 (1994): 1371–1389.

9. Holtgrave, D.R., et al. "An Overview of the Effectiveness and Efficiency of HIV Prevention Programs." *Public Health Reports*, 110, no. 2 (1995): 134–146.

10. Kelly, J.A., et al. "Psychological Interventions to Prevent HIV Infection are Urgently Needed: New Priorities for Behavioral Research in the Second Decade of AIDS." *American Psychologist* 48 (1993): 1023–1034.

11. Holtgrave, D.R., and Qualls, N.L. "HIV Prevention Programs." *Science* 266 (October 7, 1994): 16.

20

Improving Community-Based Prevention by Transforming Managed Care Organizations into Health Improvement Organizations

Tim McAfee and Robert S. Thompson

Any discussion of community-based prevention would be incomplete without addressing some of the potential effects that may result from two trends in health care delivery. First, during the past decade a growing cadre of physicians and other health care professionals trained in public health theory and practice have been developing prevention infrastructures within nongovernmental health systems caring for a defined population such as health maintenance organizations (HMOs) or managed care organizations (MCOs). These individuals attempt within these systems to apply public health principles to the improvement of preventive care for the population.[1] Second, in the past several years there has also been a shift at the local and state level toward public health departments partially or completely divesting themselves of the business of providing direct patient care. The provision of care to populations such as the poor, historically treated by governmentally sponsored and administered agencies, is giving way to care provided by a range of MCOs reimbursed via capitation agreements with local or state agencies.[2] Because of these two trends, rapid membership turnover, and increasing recognition of the influence of environmental, political, and social forces on disease outcomes, these systems also have an increased interest in efforts to improve the health of the entire community.

In this chapter we provide an overview of capacities for prevention improvement within nongovernmental health systems, particularly relating our experience at Group Health Cooperative of Puget Sound (GHC), a consumer-governed health improvement organization with more than 650,000 members, 6,000 employees, 900 physicians, and a 20-year track record of consciously attempting to improve the quality of preventive services for its members.[3] We also address ways in

J Public Health Management Practice, 1998, 4(2), 55–65

which governmental and academic public health can facilitate prevention improvement in these nongovernmental health systems.

WHAT'S IN A NAME?

Unlike the old days of fee-for-service medicine, most people in the United States now have their health care services provided by an entity that combines some of the functions of an insurer and a deliverer of care for a defined population of people. Although in this chapter we usually use the phrase "managed care organization" (MCO), there is not a consensus on the best name for these entities. Several decades ago, it was "health maintenance organization," or HMO, that was associated initially with closed staff-model systems where physicians were salaried employees of the health plan or an affiliated physician group. But as these systems expanded and new systems were created that included independent providers who accepted patients on a capitated basis, the term managed care organization was introduced. Although this term is currently the most popular, it has a top-down, screw-tightening sound to it that many organizations feel does not accurately describe their work or structure. The descriptive name that our organization uses is "health improvement organization" (HIO), to indicate that we are not only about the business of maintaining health or managing health care, but are actually committed to *improving* the health of our members and the community through a collaborative process. In our case this includes having a board of directors elected by health plan members who hire the CEO and work with medical staff and administration to help ensure that our improvement goals reflect the desires of those we serve. At the individual level, this means using a shared decision-making model to approach complex issues such as hormone replacement therapy, PSA testing, and priority-setting in chronic illness care.[4] GHC also defines itself partially in terms of what it is not—it is not in the business of micromanaging the day-to-day practice of medicine. However, the term "health improvement organization" has not spread widely. Other names used include "integrated health systems," which may allow multiple insurance products, and simply "health plans," indicating any entity that takes responsibility for coordinating and improving the delivery of care.

NONGOVERNMENTAL CAN STILL BE PUBLIC-HEALTH ORIENTED

Many MCOs are creating centers of responsibility for population-based and preventive care improvement. In some organizations these exist as separate departments, and in others are embedded within the mission of quality improvement or other departments. This trend is most consistent within the not-for-profit organizations, but can also be found in for-profit organizations. Many of the individuals working in these capacities received formal public health academic training and some have worked in governmental health agencies previously. They tend to think of themselves as public health workers who happen to work on public health improvement within MCOs.

The past decade has seen the rise of some trends within large health care systems that are in alignment with the values of public health. For instance, there has been a major organizational commitment to the values of quality improvement and population-based medicine. Some of the same forces involved in the "industrialization" of medicine have helped foster these trends, but it also has been an independent force. As companies have desperately looked at ways to decrease premiums while simultaneously trying to improve the quality of care or service, one approach has been to attempt to continuously examine and measure the processes of care, and empower the teams that participate in the processes to systematically examine and improve these processes. This has resulted in drastic decreases in average length-of-stays in hospitals, and guidelines to attempt to better align the practice of medicine with evidence for effectiveness. Unfortunately, rapid across-the-board downsizing to drastically decrease costs has sometimes hampered efforts to improve quality and service, although studies of small area variation within and between plans suggest that approximately 30 percent of costs may be avoided by decreasing variation without threatening quality.[5]

Increasingly, large health care organizations are also beginning to develop infrastructures to monitor and analyze the causes of morbidity and mortality in their populations. Although they are not yet as sophisticated in this realm as most health departments, the need to know what is causing illness and disease, and hence expense, in their populations has led to the development of more sophisticated tracking and monitoring systems.

ECONOMIC AND STRUCTURAL FACTORS IMPACTING PREVENTION EFFORTS

Increasingly, health systems are driven by the bottom line: profit or margin. Ten years ago the majority of health systems were locally based and not for profit, but this has shifted dramatically toward national companies evolving ever-more-complex relationships, including publicly traded for-profits accountable to their shareholders to extract the highest profit margin possible from the "business" of health. Even within the world of not-for-profit health systems such as Group Health, Kaiser-Permanente, HealthPartners, and Harvard-Pilgrim Community Health Plan, increasing attention is being paid to driving down costs and business-oriented strategies in order to survive in what is now clearly a highly competitive volatile marketplace. The phrase cost per-member-per-month (pmpm) has become a steady drumbeat. Not-for-profits are also linking together to create larger regional and national organizations capable of competing with the national for-profits. Group Health, for instance, is affiliating with Kaiser. However, it is important for leaders in governmental public health to recognize that there are important differences between the for-profit and not-for-profit sectors of MCOs.

The difference is the bottom line: for-profits deliver health care services in order to make money for their shareholders. Not-for-profits make money in order to deliver health care services.[6] Many, but not all, of the horror stories about MCOs manipulating physicians have emanated from the for-profit publicly traded sector, such as gag rules on physicians around noncovered services, financial incentives for providing less care,[7] and even frank fraud.[8] There is a rich literature describing improvements in important health care outcomes in staff-model HMO settings in areas such as breast cancer survival,[9] prostate cancer survival,[10] immunization rates,[11] and overall performance.[12] However, these studies were done when not-for-profit HMOs predominated. The generalizability of these improvements to publicly traded for-profits has not yet been rigorously studied.

Whether for-profit or not-for-profit, MCOs are increasingly driven by the bottom line of "what will result in fast cost savings or rapid increases in membership?" when deciding what areas of possible improvement to focus on. Although prevention has often claimed to deliver actual cost savings, the arenas where we can truly deliver on this promise are few and far between. Most preventive services cost money to deliver years of life saved. Even ones where there is clear payoff in terms of decreased utilization of services, this decrease more often comes years after the intervention, such as smoking cessation programs that pay for themselves in four or five years by decreasing hospital utilization.[13] Unfortunately, with both the rapid cycle time for membership in MCOs (many plans roll over 20% of membership/year) and the focus by MCO planners on short-term cost decreases that can be measured in months not years, prevention is not objectively a major part of the equation.

Prevention improvement efforts that are generated by cost containers tend to run more toward what we shouldn't do than what we should. For example, in the heart disease prevention arena the emphasis will be on controlling access to the cholesterol-lowering statin drugs, rather than increasing exercise or improving diet.

To overcome this tendency, we believe it is critical that there be a recognizable organizational division for prevention within MCOs, and that this division work tirelessly to maintain pressure to consider improving preventive services as seriously as improving therapeutic services. Some of the approaches that have worked in our institution have included the following:

- Emphasizing the important marketing and public relations role that high-quality preventive services can play. Our own surveys and national surveys

indicate that customers value prevention—that it is one of the top six indicators they examine when choosing a health plan and that it can decrease
disenrollment by 9 percent.[14]

- Emphasizing that our primary business is saving and improving the quality of
lives, not simply doing less, and that this applies to prevention as well as
treatment. We do require higher standards of proof both for effectiveness of
proposed prevention screenings and interventions, and for evidence that
harms have been quantified, because unlike therapeutic interventions where a
person in pain is seeking us out, we are usually asking asymptomatic people
to undergo preventive services.

The maxim *primum non nocere* is especially important for preventive services.[15] However, no one would require that a surgeon prove that operating on a
case of appendicitis is cheaper than watchful waiting, only that it improves the
probability of the patient surviving. We may work to control the costs associated
with treatment of appendicitis, by decreasing hospital length of stay and decreasing unnecessary operations for abdominal pain, but we don't require that the basic
intervention end up costing our system less than doing nothing. Our patients are
paying us as an insurer and deliverer of care to provide preventive services. Most
MCO planners initially want to apply the "it must end up saving us money" standard to prevention improvements. We have tried to move them toward the "there
must be evidence for cost-effectiveness" standard, where we are willing to spend
reasonable amounts of money to add years of quality life, based on an understanding that our patients are paying us to help prolong their life in a proactive fashion
where indicated, not just fix them when they break down.

GHC'S PUBLIC HEALTH EXPERIENCE

At Group Health, we have been involved in many areas that illustrate the rich
potential for large nongovernmental health systems to improve the public's health.
We present here a brief review of how we have structured this work, and some of
our experiences in one specific area for illustrative purposes: decreasing tobacco
use. Specific detailed information about our overall approach,[3] immunization programs,[16] breast cancer screening,[17] bicycle safety,[18] quality improvement infrastructure,[19] and prostate cancer screening[20] have been published previously.

Prevention structure

Twenty years ago a Department of Preventive Care (DPC) was formed within
our medical staff to provide an organizational focus for physician-led preventive
initiatives. This department brings an epidemiologic, population orientation to pri-

ority setting and uses an evidence-based approach for the analysis of issues. It also works to bring in external funding to help answer critical research questions that affect the delivery of preventive care. It cosponsors with our Center for Health Promotion a multidisciplinary Committee on Prevention with physicians, nurses, pharmacists, administrators, health educators, epidemiologists, and researchers that sponsors, prioritizes, and implements prevention improvement efforts, including critically reviewing prevention guidelines and screening schedules. The Center for Health Promotion is also charged with doing much of the implementation work that makes prevention guidelines and programs "come alive" in a systematic fashion. It also has a community services function that works closely with community organizations and governmental agencies to help improve the health of the entire community, and a health-at-work division that commercializes services such as our smoking cessation program in order to make them available to other health plans and employers.

The Center for Health Studies at GHC is a semiautonomous research unit supported by external grant dollars (approximately $9 million in 1995) involved in epidemiological and health services research, with particular interest in improvements of chronic disease management and population and clinic-based risk factor reduction.

The Division of Clinical Planning and Improvement, begun four years ago, oversees organized activity to improve and maintain the quality of clinical services at Group Health. It employs a "gaps" measurement quality improvement approach,[21] which systematically examines processes and outcomes of clinical care in order to focus improvement efforts on areas where there is a measurable, modifiable gap between what is currently happening in practice and what we are capable of achieving. Health status, satisfaction, and cost-effectiveness are the main outcomes of interest. Increasingly, its mission has overlapped with the other prevention players, particularly as its guideline development group has grown more systematic in the creation of processes for formal literature review and methods to integrate guidelines into clinical care. Recently, the DPC and this group have developed a coherent common approach to guideline development and implementation.

We have found that to be most effective, prevention improvement efforts need to start with an open mind as to what is the best venue to accomplish the desired outcome. We do not assume that every problem is best solved by a clinical intervention delivered in a physician's office. Indeed our most successful programs such as our breast cancer screening, immunizations, and tobacco cessation all use the entire "playing field" from the individual encounter in the primary care office through changing the office infrastructure and other organizational change, and including the external community.[3,11] In these latter areas, we become more similar to a public health agency.

Decreasing tobacco use: A case study

In 1991, a group of population-oriented planners began meeting regularly to develop a comprehensive strategy to decrease the prevalence of tobacco use at Group Health. Several years later, GHC formally adopted this goal as its number one prevention priority. A number of dramatic changes in how we approach tobacco use have resulted. The distinguishing characteristic of this effort was that it began from a population perspective: the planners did not ask how we could get more of the smokers who took part in our cessation program to quit; they asked how we can decrease the prevalence of tobacco use in our entire population. Improvement efforts focused on how we could get dramatically more smokers to participate in the program, how we could systematically get our doctors and nurses and pharmacists to provide brief, repetitive messages to smokers to quit, and change in public policy at the regulatory/legislative level.

Our major accomplishments include a profound retooling of our smoking cessation program[22] that has included making it available through telephone counseling in our Center for Health Promotion. We have completely removed all financial barriers to program participation, including coverage of nicotine replacement therapy for appropriate GHC program participants. As a result of these efforts, participation has increased tenfold, from 180 a year in 1991 to 1,500–2,000 a year since 1993. Our one-year cessation rate, which had been 22 percent, increased and has held steady at 30 percent (defined as no smoking, not even a puff, for at least a month prior to the call).[23,24] This program is also made available on a commercial basis to employers and other health plans.

We have also introduced a clinical guideline into our primary care system that is similar to the National Cancer Institute[25] and Agency for Health Care Policy and Research (AHCPR)[26] guideline, requiring clinical teams to routinely inquire and record smoking status, give brief advice, and offer assistance to all smokers. We have systematically measured multiple process outcomes over the past three years and fed results back to the teams, and have seen major progress, including an increase from less than 30 percent identification of smoking status to more than 85 percent in the medical records at all 29 of our primary care clinics (see Figure 1).

Documentation of advice to quit in identified smokers has doubled in the past year (see Figure 2), and 71 percent of our patients who smoke report in post-visit surveys that their doctor talked to them about smoking during their visit. This compares with national surveys reporting that half of smokers say smoking has never been discussed with them by any doctor.[27,28] In 1994, 45 percent of parents of children who are exposed to environmental tobacco smoke recalled being advised of its dangers. By 1996, this had increased to 68 percent ($p < 0.05$). Over the past decade, our smoking prevalence has declined from 25 percent to 15 percent, as

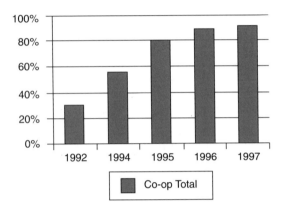

Figure 1. Group Health Cooperative of Puget Sound chart documentation of tobacco status.

measured by large surveys, while the state of Washington's prevalence has only declined from 25 percent to 23 percent (see Figure 3).

Group Health has also worked closely with the larger community, because clearly tobacco use is a community problem, not just a clinical problem. Our legislative lobbyist was instrumental in the passage of a state law that banned vending machines and established a merchant licensing fee to fund tobacco education programs at the local health department level and enforcement of the law prohibiting sales to minors. Because interventions in the schools and media have been shown to be effective[29] we have cosponsored a tobacco poster art contest in the schools that has been highly successful three years in a row. Other examples are outlined in the "governmental roles" section.

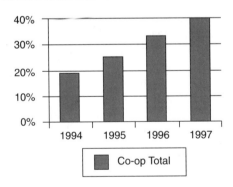

Figure 2. Group Health Cooperative of Puget Sound chart documentation of provider tobacco cessation intervention.

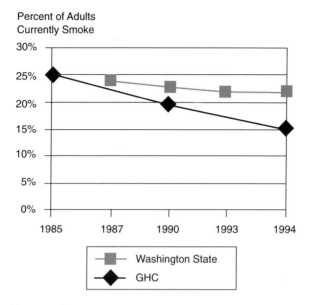

Figure 3. Smoking prevalence.

PREVENTIVE HEALTH IMPROVEMENT SYSTEM

Our sense is that the way of the future for the delivery of preventive services in MCOs lies not in the development of more isolated stand-alone programs for specific screening programs or specific risk factor reduction, but in building an integrated system that addresses all preventive issues from primary risk reduction to secondary screening to prevention of disability from existing chronic diseases within a cohesive, seamless framework. This ideal preventive care system will incorporate what is known about screening requirements[30] and changing individual behavior[31] with the incredible capacity of developing information systems to track and remind and directly intervene or refer individuals regarding all recommended prevention services. We envision a proactive interactive system that communicates regularly through multiple entry points with every health plan member, with real-time information about a member's prevention status available to clinical providers at the individual level during all patient encounters, as well as aggregate for population monitoring and local-level interventions. The system will blend centralized coordinated reminder systems and behavior change support utilizing personalized mail, on-line access, and telephonic capacity with local clinic-level efforts augmented by just-in-time information to providers and patient education support.

To our knowledge, no such comprehensive preventive health improvement system exists anywhere in the world, but many organizations and individuals are working on the development of different components of such a system.[32,33] We believe it is critical that both the governmental and academic public health systems and the not-for-profit private health systems work to help create this system. Many pharmaceutical companies are actively developing "disease-state management" subsidiaries that are increasingly getting into the business of managing and even delivering health care and preventive services for high-cost carve-out areas. If we don't influence or provide alternatives, the complex integrated health improvement system we envision will be created by the pharmaceutical industry and other for-profit health system players, whose motives and driving forces may include using it for the purpose of increasing sales of high-profit products, or otherwise increasing profitability rather than focusing on increasing health status.

GOVERNMENTAL ROLES IN IMPROVING MCOs' PREVENTION PERFORMANCE

As health departments continue to divest themselves of direct patient care responsibilities, they will continue to play several critical roles in regard to the delivery of direct patient care by MCOs (see box below). The following is a brief description of some of those roles.

Regulatory capacity

Especially in an era increasingly dominated by for-profit health care systems, it is appropriate and necessary that governmental health agencies be engaged in an oversight capacity. Although there has been a plethora of legislation that is primarily aimed at simply bashing MCOs,[34] there have also been thoughtful attempts both to limit excesses such as gag rules that do not allow physicians to discuss noncovered services, and to encourage more proactive delivery of preventive services. In the latter arena, however, health departments may be hampered by their

---

Governmental Roles in Improving MCOs' Prevention Performance

1. Rational regulator
2. Customer (i.e., Medicaid)
3. Provider of technical assistance and consultation
4. Underwriter of health services research
5. Partner for policy change
6. Leader and coordinator in community medicine

direct link to local/state legislative bodies that are more subject to lobbying by special interest groups. Examples of problems that can arise as a result have included attempts by special-interest groups to legislate requirements for coverage and even mandating specific care delivery patterns for questionable or controversial prevention screening procedures such as PSA testing and mammography under age 50. Another potential regulatory role for health departments would be to require that all MCOs devote a demonstrable fixed percent (i.e., 3–5%) of revenues to the development, implementation, and improvement of population-based prevention services for the members served. This would help counterbalance the difficult reality that the time period for beneficial program effects (either cost savings or avoiding negative health outcomes) is likely to be at least 3 to 5 years, not the standard 6- to 12-month result requirement under which MCOs currently operate.

A customer

Health departments are becoming a major purchaser of capitated health system services through their divestment of direct delivery of Medicaid services, developing Medicare managed care contracts, as well as other health service contracts. As a customer of these systems, they can exert powerful competitive pressure on health service deliverers to provide high-quality low-cost medical care, including preventive care. By requiring measurement and embedding into the bidding requirements key prevention services, they can help move health plans toward systematically providing and improving such services as childhood immunizations, Pap tests, mammography, and smoking cessation services to their populations. The Pacific Business Group and others have identified prevention targets such as immunization rates, with plans that do not meet the targets being at risk for decreased overall revenue.[35] Some of the keys to using this leverage point successfully are to:

- Choose key prevention interventions consistently recommended by evidence-based gold standard groups such as the U.S. Preventive Services Task Force. Examples of services not to require include eye exams in young adults, prostatic specific antigen (PSA) tests, or frequent general periodic health exams.
- Attempt to be consistent with other large purchasers wherever possible, such as the Health Plan Employer Data and Information Set (HEDIS) prevention measures of the National Commission for Quality Assurance (NCQA). As requiring measurement of processes and outcomes becomes increasingly popular among purchasers, MCOs are faced with growing noncomplementary requirements for measurement that can eat up scarce measurement and improvement resources.

- Require wherever possible population measures of effectiveness, rather than measures of care quality for those who have sought out care. For example, even if a plan is doing a good job of immunizing children receiving Medicaid who come in for a visit, they may have a poor rate of immunization for that population if they have no program for outreach to proactively encourage parents to bring in their children.
- Practice what you preach. An example of where this has not happened in our state is in the area of smoking cessation programs. Although our state and local health departments have been strong advocates for legislation to decrease tobacco use, our state has not yet included coverage of smoking cessation programs as part of the benefit package for either our Medicaid population or our "basic health plan," a state-sponsored insurance program funded by a tobacco tax, for those too poor to purchase insurance but not poor enough to be eligible for Medicaid. For several years, these were the only groups in our plan that had no coverage for smoking cessation programs, even though they have twice the smoking rate. At the same time that GHC's smoking cessation program participation rate was soaring tenfold, we had virtually no participation from this critical population. Our GHC solution eventually was to bypass the governmental public health arena, and bite the bullet by providing the service even though it is not required as part of the benefit package. Since doing this, Medicaid and Basic Health Plan participation have increased tenfold. In this way we are fulfilling a part of our community service mission.

Technical assistance and consultation

Particularly in the arena of disease surveillance, MCOs can benefit from the expertise in health departments, as well as university-based public health academics. Examples of how we have undertaken this role have included purchasing the expertise of state department of health surveyors who do the CDC-designed behavioral risk factor survey to survey our own membership, asking the same questions as well as some specific to our own institution. Another arena where health departments may have specific and valuable expertise important to MCOs is in the realm of outreach and behavior change for low-income populations.

Underwriter of health services research

MCOs have the capacity to deliver preventive care in new ways. Determining how best to do this, and how much more effective these ways are, requires further research. Ensuring that the most relevant and important questions are asked and answered with the most appropriate methodologies and sufficient funding will require continued dialogue and cooperation between MCOs, public health agencies such as the CDC, and academic research centers. The CDC is working actively to build such a partnership.[36]

MCOs, with their defined populations, often have utilization data including costs and diagnosis for members seen at all levels of care including primary care, emergency, specialty, and hospital. They can thus serve as mini population laboratories for disease surveillance,[37] for testing interventions directed to populations,[16,38] and for measuring the effects of community-based programs. We have been involved in numerous collaborative research projects with university-based public health researchers to help answer fundamental public health questions, such as: (1) Is chlamydia screening in younger women beneficial?[39] (2) Do community campaigns reduce head injuries?[35] (3) What interventions work to decrease falls in seniors?[40]

A partner for policy

We have worked with our state and local health departments to help champion anti-tobacco legislation. In fact, we have had the Washington state Department of Health Deputy Secretary/Health Officer sit on our tobacco steering committee, and the medical director sit on our Committee on Prevention. We have also worked in numerous partnerships both with health departments and other voluntary organizations such as the American Cancer Society, Heart Association, and Lung Association. At the national level, the CDC played a leadership role working with The HMO Group to call together a large group of MCOs to develop a strategy for tobacco policy work that led to a coalition of MCOs purchasing ad space to support FDA regulation of tobacco. At the local level, we have collaborated with our health departments and university researchers to develop a community-based campaign to increase bicycle helmet usage.[41]

A leader and coordinator in community medicine

Many MCOs will depend on leaders in public health to help identify the key issues that need to be addressed to improve the health of the entire community, to identify the strategies that can lead to solutions, and to recommend the specific roles that MCOs can play. Examples include the work our state health department has done to develop an immunization registry so that the immunization status of all children in the state is in a common database, a necessity given the rapid cycling of children from plan to plan. This example was a two-way street in that GHC investigators played a sizable technical role in developing the community registries because we had already developed one for our members.[33] The development of an evidence-based guide to community prevention services will be of considerable help in this arena.[42]

KEY FUTURE OPPORTUNITIES

Our most fundamental learning after working within a not-for-profit nongovernmental health improvement organization for 20 years is that this is a pioneer venue for public health activity. Following are some recommendations (see box below).

- Health departments should consider placement of public health workers in MCOs or at least having liaisons to help foster a public health approach to the populations served, and to learn more about the capacity of MCOs to deliver preventive care.
- Public health schools should develop training opportunities during public health and preventive medicine training programs within MCOs, as well as fostering research relationships.
- MCOs should invest a small but consistent portion of their resources in efforts that improve the health of the entire community, including supporting legislative and regulatory activity as well as community coalitions.
- MCOs should invest a portion of their resources in further development of their prevention delivery infrastructure. This tendency, which runs counter to the powerful force of treatment-oriented medicine, can be aided by external forces such as purchaser pressure requiring measurement of prevention processes and outcomes. If necessary, this should be legislatively mandated.
- Consult with and include MCO leaders in planning efforts, particularly around identification of measurement goals for populations historically served by public health departments.
- Any attempts by governmental public health agencies to influence how MCOs provide preventive care for the patients they are responsible for should only include measurement and accountability for key prevention interventions that have strong, established evidence both for importance and for capacity to intervene in a cost-effective manner.

Key Future Opportunities

1. Place public health workers within MCOs.
2. Develop training opportunities with MCOs.
3. MCOs invest resources into community health initiatives.
4. MCOs/governmental health agencies invest in developing prevention infrastructure.
5. Involve MCOs in public health planning efforts.
6. Emphasize areas where evidence is strong.
7. Consider financial structure of MCO as well as cost and short-term performance.

- When public health officials can influence which MCO plans will be made available to the poor or elderly, not-for-profit status should be taken into account along with cost and performance measures, because these plans spend in excess of 90 cents on the dollar on health care as opposed to the 70 cents by many publicly traded for-profit plans.[6] This might be done by, for instance, limiting the percentage of income that can go to profits or administration as opposed to patient care (including preventive care). Effects of different financial structures on quality of care is an important area for future research.

• • •

There is a major change occurring in the structure of health care delivery away from local fee-for-service toward large complex national health plans that provide both insurance and health care. This change will impact the delivery of preventive services profoundly. It is up to those of us who have training and commitment to improving the public health, whether we work in an academic setting, a governmental agency, or within an MCO, to work together to maximize the potential for benefit from this change, and minimize the potential harms.

REFERENCES

1. M.R. Greenlick. "The Emergence of Population-Based Medicine."*HMO Practice* 9 (1995): 120–122.

2. The Kaiser Commission of the Future of Medicaid. *Medicaid and Managed Care: Lessons from the Literature*. Menlo Park, Calif.: Henry J. Kaiser Family Foundation, 1995.

3. R.S. Thompson et al. "Primary and Secondary Prevention Services in Clinical Practice; Twenty Years of Experience in Development, Implementation, and Evaluation." *Journal of the American Medical Association* 273, no. 14 (1995): 1130–1135.

4. M. Von Korff et al. Self Management Training and Support: Requirements for Health Care Integration. Manuscript submitted to The Chronic Care Symposium, Seattle. June 1996.

5. D. Lawrence and I. Leverton. The Kaiser Quality Journal Address. Institute for Health Improvement Annual Meeting, Orlando, Fla., December 8, 1992.

6. P.M. Nudelman and L.M. Andrews. "The 'Value Added' of Not for Profit Health Plans." *New England Journal of Medicine* 16 (1996): 1057–1059.

7. J.P. Kassirer. "Is Managed Care Here to Stay?" *New England Journal of Medicine* 336, no. 14 (1997): 1013.

8. L. Laguado. "How Columbia Health Care Association Changed Health Care for Better or Worse." *The Wall Street Journal* 137, no. 23 (1997): 1.

9. A.L. Potosky et al. "Breast Cancer Survival and Treatment in HMO and Fee-for-Service Settings." *Journal of the National Cancer Institute* (1997): in press.

10. H.P. Greenwald and C.J. Henke. "HMO Membership, Treatment, and Mortality Risk Among Prostatic Cancer Patients." *American Journal of Public Health* 82 (1992): 1099–1104.

11. R.S. Thompson. "What Have HMOs Learned About Clinical Prevention Services? An Examination of the Experience at Group Health Cooperative of Puget Sound." *Milbank Quarterly* 74 (1996): 469–509.

12. R.H. Miller and H.S. Luft. "Managed Care Plan Performance Since 1980: A Literature Analysis." *Journal of the American Medical Association* 271 (1994): 1512–1519.

13. E.H. Wagner et al. "The Impact of Smoking and Quitting on Health Care Use." *Archives of Internal Medicine* 155 (1995): 1789–1795.

14. H. Schauffler and T. Rodriguez. "Exercising Purchasing Power for Preventive Care." *Health Affairs* 13 (1996): 1–2, 12.

15. H. Sox. "Preventive Health Services in Adults." *New England Journal of Medicine* 330 (1994): 1589–1595.

16. D.C. Pearson and R.S. Thompson. "Evaluation of Group Health Cooperative of Puget Sound's Senior Influenza Immunization Program." *Public Health Report* 109 (1994): 571–578.

17. S.H. Taplin et al. "Revisions in the Risk-Based Breast Cancer Screening Program at Group Health Cooperative." *Cancer* 66 (1990): 812–818.

18. D.C. Thompson et al. "Case Control Study of the Effectiveness of Bicycle Safety Helmets in Preventing Facial Injury." *American Journal of Public Health* 80 (1990): 1471–1474.

19. R. Johnson and D. Teeter. "The Roadmap for Clinical Quality." *HMO Practice* 8, no. 1 (1994): 5–9.

20. M.R. Handley and M.E. Stuart. "The Use of Prostate Specific Antigen for Prostate Cancer Screening; A Managed Care Perspective." *Journal of Urology* 152 (1994): 1689–1692.

21. M.R. Handley and M.E. Stuart. "An Evidence-Based Approach to Evaluating and Improving Clinical Practice; Guideline Development." *HMO Practice* 1 (1994): 10–19.

22. C.T. Orleans et al. "Self Help Quit Smoking Interventions; Effects of Self-Help Materials, Social Support Instructions, and Telephone Counseling." *Journal of Consulting and Clinical Psychology* 59, no. 3 (1991): 439–448.

23. T. McAfee et al. "Awakening the Sleeping Giant; Mainstreaming Efforts to Decrease Tobacco Use in an HMO." *HMO Practice* 9, no. 3 (1995): 138–146.

24. N.S. Sofian et al. "Telephone Smoking Cessation Intervention: The Free & Clear Program." *HMO Practice* 9, no. 3 (1995): 144–146.

25. T.J. Glynn and M.W. Manley. *How to Help Your Patients Stop Smoking. A National Cancer Institute Manual for Physicians.* Smoking and Tobacco Control Program, Division of Cancer Prevention and Control, National Cancer Institute and the U.S. Department of Health and Human Services, Public Health Service, National Institutes of Health; NIH Pub. No. 92-3064. Washington, D.C: Public Health Service, 1991.

26. Agency for Health Care Policy and Research Smoking Cessation Clinical Practice Guideline. *Journal of the American Medical Association* 275, no. 16 (1996): 1270–1280.

27. E. Frank et al. "Predictors of Physician's Smoking Cessation Advice." *Journal of the American Medical Association* 266 (1991): 3139–3143.

28. Centers for Disease Control and Prevention. "Physician and Other Health Care Professional Counseling of Smokers to Quit; United States, 1991." *Morbidity Mortality Weekly Report* 42 (1993): 854–857.

29. B.S. Flynn et al. "Prevention of Cigarette Smoking Through Mass Media Intervention and School Programs." *American Journal of Public Health* 82 (1992): 827–834.

30. U.S. Preventive Services Task Force. *Guideline to Clinical Preventive Services; Report of the U.S. Preventive Services Task Force*, 2nd ed. Baltimore: Williams & Wilkins, 1996.

31. C. Wiley et al. "Public Health and the Science of Behavior Change." *Current Issues in Public Health* 2 (1996): 18–25.

32. T. Payne et al. "Development and Validation of an Immunization Tracking System in a Large Health Maintenance Organization." *American Journal of Preventive Medicine* 9 (1993): 96–100.

33. T.H. Payne et al. "Practicing Population-Based Care in an HMO; Evaluation after 18 Months." *HMO Practice* 9, no. 3 (1995): 101–106.

34. J.P. Kisser. "Practicing Medicine Without a License—The New Intrusions by Congress." *New England Journal of Medicine* 336 (1997): 1747.

35. H. Schauffler and T. Rodriguez. "Exercising Purchasing Power for Preventive Care." *Health Affairs* 15 (1996): 73–85.

36. *Morbidity and Mortality Weekly Report*. 44, no. RR-14: 4–12.

37. R.T. Chen et al. "Vaccine Safety Datalink Project: A New Tool for Improving Vaccine Safety Monitoring in the United States The Vaccine Datalink Team." *Pediatrics* 99 (1997): 765–773.

38. J. Britt et al. "Implementation and Acceptance of Outreach Telephone Counseling for Smoking Cessation with Non-Volunteer Smokers." *Health Education Quarterly* 21 (1994): 55–68.

39. D. Scholes et al. "Prevention of Pelvic Inflammatory Disease by Screening for Cervical Chlamydial Infection." *New England Journal of Medicine* 334, no. 21(1996): 1362–1366.

40. E.H. Wagner et al. "Preventing Disability and Falls in Older Adults: A Population-Based Randomized Trial." *American Journal of Public Health* 84, no. 11 (1994): 1800–1806.

41. F.P. Rivara et al. "The Seattle Children's Bicycle Helmet Campaign; Changes in Helmet Use and Head Injury Admissions." *Pediatrics* 93 (1994): 567–569.

42. M. Pappaioanou and C. Evans. "Development of the *Guide to Community Preventive Services*: A U.S. Public Health Service Initiative." *Journal of Public Health Management and Practice* 4, no. 2 (1997): 48–54.

21

The Future of Cancer Control Research and Translation

Ross C. Brownson and Dileep G. Bal

"It is often necessary to make a decision on the basis of information sufficient for action but insufficient to satisfy the intellect."

—Immanuel Kant

As discussed in other chapters in this book, cancer is the second leading cause of death in the United States, accounting for more than 1.2 million new cases and 547,000 deaths in 1995.[1] The lifetime probability of developing cancer is now estimated at one in three, which is up from one in four 10 years ago.[2] Over the past 50 years, the death rate from cancer has increased steadily and has remained relatively stable in recent years. A sharp rise in lung cancer rates is the main reason for the long-term, upward trend.

One of the goals of public health is to provide preventive services and health care to disadvantaged segments of the population.[3,4] Within population subgroups, blacks have a higher overall cancer mortality rate than do any other major racial group. These rates are higher among blacks than among whites for both males and females. Excess cancer rates among blacks are largely attributed to factors associated with socioeconomic status.[5] Higher cancer incidence and mortality rates among the socioeconomically disadvantaged are the result of several factors. These include a higher prevalence of major cancer risk factors (e.g., cigarette smoking, poor diet), delays in cancer diagnosis, and lack of access to prompt and adequate treatment following diagnosis. Many of these factors are consequences of living in poverty.

To address cancer disparities and to improve the overall health of the population, this nation must place a greater emphasis on prevention. The annual U.S. health care budget is approaching $1 trillion.[6] Cancer accounts for a large part of the nation's health care expenditures, with an overall cost of more than $100 bil-

J Public Health Management Practice, 1996, 2(2), 70–78

lion annually.[7] Juxtaposed against these overall figures that largely relate to treatment costs, the percentage of resources spent on prevention is less than 5 percent.[8]

TYPES OF PREVENTION

A commonly used scheme classifies intervention activities as primary, secondary, and tertiary prevention, according to where it is applied along the disease continuum.[9] Primary prevention reduces disease incidence; secondary prevention shortens the duration of disease through early detection and treatment; and tertiary prevention reduces complications of the disease and limits disability by appropriate rehabilitation. It is important to note that these three levels of prevention are interrelated and frequently lack clear boundaries. For example, a measure such as hypertension screening is considered secondary prevention. Yet, identification of hypertension in an individual may motivate that person to increase physical activity, resulting in primary prevention benefits. Commonly, cancer *prevention* is considered primary prevention (e.g., smoking reduction); whereas cancer *control* is secondary prevention (e.g., mammography screening). For the sake of simplicity, we use cancer prevention and cancer control interchangeably in this chapter as they are so used elsewhere.

POTENTIAL FOR PREVENTION

In 1985, the National Cancer Institute (NCI) set a goal of reducing cancer mortality by up to 50 percent by the year 2000 through the systematic application of existing cancer control technologies.[10] Key elements in this effort include: (1) reducing the prevalence of smoking; (2) reducing the percentage of total calories in the diet from fat; (3) increasing the average daily consumption of fiber; (4) increasing the percentage of women who undergo annual breast cancer screening (mammography and physical breast exam); (5) increasing the percentage of women who have annual Papanicolaou (Pap) tests; and (6) increasing adoption of state-of-the-art cancer treatments. Although the 50 percent goal for the year 2000 will not be achieved, it has been beneficial in focusing cancer control efforts at all levels of public health practice. It is noteworthy, however, that even visionary goals cannot come to fruition without adequate allocation of targeted resources at federal, state, and local levels.[10]

Subsequent efforts at setting long-term goals, most notably *Healthy People 2000,*[4] have contributed to the public health discourse in cancer control by setting priorities for intervention activities. The *Healthy People 2000* goals are much more modest than the earlier NCI objectives.[4,10] In the most recent review of year 2000 objectives, some limited progress has been made toward achieving many cancer objectives although progress is minuscule in primary prevention areas.[11]

SCIENTIFIC PROGRESS IN CANCER CONTROL

Large strides have been made over the past several decades in understanding the causes of cancer. For example, the earliest studies of smoking and lung cancer led to larger and more detailed studies that have ascertained that smoking is responsible for nearly 90 percent of all lung cancers.[12] Research in applied epidemiology also has determined populations at highest risk for smoking and has evaluated the efficacy of various smoking control interventions.[13] Through a large body of epidemiologic and clinical research, we now know the causes of the majority of cancer cases.[14-16] Despite the great strides in etiologic research on cancer, there is a large lag time between elucidation of preventive options, application of these findings in applied research settings, and diffusion of technologies to the larger community (discussed in more detail later).[7,17]

PUBLIC HEALTH AGENCY PROGRESS IN CANCER CONTROL

As noted by Alciati and Marconi, public health agencies at the federal, state, and local levels are vital entities in translating cancer control technologies into practice.[18] The federal support for cancer control activities in state health agencies only began in 1986, when NCI initiated its Technical Development in Health Agencies Program.[19] More recent cancer control demonstration projects in the public health setting include the NCI-sponsored American Stop Smoking Intervention Study, and the Centers for Disease Control and Prevention (CDC)-funded Breast and Cervical Cancer Prevention Program.[20,21] Meissner et al. summarized internal and external factors contributing to success in controlling cancer in the public health setting.[19] Internal factors include (1) commitment of the organizations leadership to cancer control; (2) existence of appropriate data to monitor and evaluate programs; (3) appropriately trained staff, and (4) the ability to obtain funds for future activities. External factors include: (1) successful linkages and coalitions; (2) an established cancer control plan; (3) access to outside health experts; (4) an informed state legislature; and (5) diffusion of initially successful programs to other sites.

FUTURE PRIORITIES

Ten areas in cancer control considered of critical importance in the coming decade are summarized in Table 1 under the Institute of Medicine (IOM) rubric that describes the three core functions of public health.[3,22] The broad IOM categories are assessment, policy development, and assurance. Assessment refers to the concept of community diagnosis, including the tools of public health surveillance and

Table 1 Future cancer control priorities within the three core functions* of public health

Cancer Control Activity	Assessment	Policy Development	Assurance
1. Establishing long-term evaluation systems	✓		
2. Focusing on outcomes and using cost-effective analysis	✓	✓	
3. Applying new information technologies	✓	✓	
4. Integrating cancer prevention in managed care		✓	
5. Applying cancer control advances from molecular biology		✓	
6. Pursuing and evaluating cancer control policies		✓	✓
7. Training cancer control researchers and practitioners		✓	✓
8. Appying known primary prevention technologies		✓	✓
9. Developing and maintaining coalitions/partnerships		✓	✓
10. Obtaining and maintaining adequate cancer control resources		✓	✓

*The core functions of public health are described in reference 3 and in the text of this article.

epidemiologic research. Using the results of assessment as a basis, *policy development* is the process by which society makes decisions about health problems through planning, priority and goal setting, policy leadership and advocacy, and provision of public information. *Assurance* is the guarantor function of public health to ensure that health services and legislative mandates are met according to agreed-upon goals.[3] It is important to note that although our 10 priority cancer control areas are each assigned to one or more IOM categories, it is likely that many (if not all) of the 10 areas have some relevance to all three IOM categories.

The focus in the following section is on cancer control priorities that are likely to be important in the public health setting. This type of *applied* cancer control research uses etiologic findings from epidemiologic and clinical studies to address prevention on a population-wide basis. The list that follows is not meant to be an all-inclusive list, nor is the listing in order of priority. Rather, it is intended as a tool that public health agencies and cancer control researchers can use to help set priorities.

Establishing long-term evaluation systems

Public health surveillance systems support evaluation and have several key characteristics. These include the collection, analysis, and interpretation of health data essential to the planning, implementation, and evaluation of public health practice.[23] These activities must be closely integrated with the timely dissemination of these data to the appropriate audience(s).

Mainly through federally funded cancer control programs, states have enhanced surveillance and evaluation capacities in cancer control. The most comprehensive cancer data are collected by the NCI's Surveillance, Epidemiology, and End Results (SEER) Program, which was established in 1973.[24] The SEER Program collects incidence and survival information in five states and four metropolitan areas that comprise about 9.5 percent of the U.S. population. The recent CDC-implemented Cancer Registries Amendment Act (Public Law 10-515) will provide states additional resources to enhance population-based cancer reporting, although all states are not currently funded under this program. In addition, the CDC-sponsored Behavioral Risk Factor Surveillance System is now being conducted in all 50 states and the District of Columbia.[25] This system provides useful, state-level information on self-reported cancer risk factors and screening behaviors.

The wide array of cancer control data collected by health agencies generally have been underutilized in intervention planning and evaluation. In the future, comprehensive public health surveillance systems must be enhanced, maintained, and appropriately utilized in order to provide the tools necessary for evaluation of cancer control programs.

Focusing on outcomes and using cost-effectiveness analysis

Typically, our society has been willing to accept medical and surgical interventions to treat existing diseases with relatively little attention to cost-effectiveness; whereas, in many cases, prevention efforts have been held to a higher standard in needing to demonstrate cost-effectiveness prior to widespread application.[26] The public health model must be provided equal legitimacy with classic medical models in cancer control.

Cost-effectiveness and cost-benefit are similar analytic techniques that allow a comparison of the economic efficiencies of various cancer control technologies. *Cost-effectiveness* compares the net monetary costs of a preventive intervention with some measure of health outcome (e.g., years of life saved). Cost-effectiveness analysis is the most commonly conducted economic analysis for health program.[27] It is especially useful when the goal is to identify the most cost-effective prevention strategy among a number of options. *Cost-benefit* is assessed in the same way, except that health outcomes are converted to monetary units allowing comparison of the monies paid for an intervention with the monies saved. The cost-benefit analysis is considered the "gold standard" of economic evaluations because it allows calculation of the cost savings due to intervention.[27,28]

This priority also relates directly to the previous description of surveillance systems. As noted in the cancer-related objectives of *Healthy People 2000* and changes in the health care sector due to managed care, the importance of outcome-based program development is likely to increase.[4,29] These programs should include a stronger focus on cost-effectiveness analysis.

Applying new information technologies

With the recent advances in computer technology and exchange of information, public health professionals who have access to a personal computer can take advantage of numerous cancer control resources. The computer program CANTROL is useful for the development and analysis of cancer control programs.[30] CANTROL is flexible, interactive, and allows the user to input data specific to their geographic region and population(s) in order to plan cancer control programs.[31] The CDC-based system, Wide-Ranging Online Database (WONDER), allows access to numerous large databases useful in cancer control assessment and planning.[32] Many large health agencies and other providers of cancer control information are utilizing Internet and the World Wide Web to disseminate data in a timely and cost-efficient manner.

Information technology enhancements also are likely to improve delivery of specific cancer control interventions. For example, personal computer-based clinical interventions in the primary care setting have been shown to increase the likelihood of mammography screening, decrease smoking, and improve dietary practices.[33]

Integrating cancer prevention in managed care

The current changes in the health care system in the United States provide an opportunity for increasing cancer control interventions. Managed care organizations, specifically health maintenance organizations (HMOs), have grown from enrollments of 6 million people in 1976 to 50 million in 1994.[34] Among managed care providers, HMOs are likely to be the most amenable to prevention efforts.[29] The CDC recently summarized opportunities for public health prevention in the

HMO setting.[29] Issues relevant for cancer control efforts include prevention-related surveillance systems, "report cards" to measure quality-of-care, and private-public collaborations.[35]

Additional changes within the Medicare and Medicaid programs also are likely to influence cancer control opportunities among vulnerable populations. At the present time, it is unclear whether recent and pending changes will have overall positive or negative effects on cancer control efforts. However, there is concern, based upon current cost-cutting trends, that movement toward managed care may lessen access to clinical preventive services among indigent populations.[36]

Applying cancer control advances from molecular biology

Recent advances in molecular biology have contributed considerably to our understanding of the biological mechanisms underlying human cancer and potential mechanisms for enhanced prevention and early detection. Discoveries include the genetic structures responsible for inherited breast cancer and colorectal cancer.[37,38] These may lead to new opportunities in early detection and treatment. Other advances include the use of polymerase chain reaction as a sensitive detection mechanism for determining persons at high risk of certain cancers (e.g., human papillomavirus-related cervical cancer).[39]

Although these techniques are years away from application on a population-basis, public health practitioners should be aware of the major advance in molecular biology and need to be part of the dialogue when decisions are eventually made concerning the widespread application of new screening tests. Of paramount importance will be the ethical considerations in the use of new genetic markers—most notably: Would identification of a strong genetic predisposition toward a particular cancer affect a person's ability to be employed and/or insured?

Pursuing and evaluating cancer control policies

Public policies can have a considerable positive impact on controlling cancer.[26] Policies are defined as "those laws, regulations, formal and informal rules and understandings that are adopted on a collective basis to guide individual and collective behavior."[40] Perhaps the most widely evaluated cancer control policies are those related to tobacco control. For example, researchers estimate a 4 percent drop in the prevalence of adult smoking when the price of cigarettes is increased by 10 percent.[41,42] Policy interventions may be subject to political changes over which public health professionals have little control (e.g., the Congressional election of 1994).

Future efforts should focus on evaluation of public policies in cancer control with particular attention to effectiveness and cost-effectiveness. The policy intervention area is one that is ideally suited for public health agency–academic partnerships. Public health professionals are likely to have ready access to evaluation data and are likely to be more up-to-date on policy issues affecting public health practice. Academics may have more experience in evaluation methods and also may provide an independent, "objective" evaluation of a particular cancer control policy. To assist in evaluation, the NCI's State Cancer Legislative Database recently became available through the Internet.[43] This database tracks state-based legislation in cancer control back to 1963.

Training cancer control researchers and practitioners

As cancer control has become a key component of day-to-day public health practice, the need for researchers and practitioners knowledgeable in the science of cancer control has grown. Because cancer control activities were sparse in many health agencies until the mid-1980s, there has not been a large cadre of trained cancer control specialists as there is in a more established field such as communicable disease control. Therefore, other researchers and health agencies themselves have identified cancer control training as a high priority.[44,45] Weed and Husten have summarized the issues within two key questions: "Who should be trained?" and "What should be learned?"

The "who" answer for a public health agency is likely to include persons from each key discipline (i.e., epidemiology, health promotion, public information, and administration) who are involved in day-to-day cancer control programs. The "what" category should generally follow the model developed for the NCI's summer course.[44] The five modules of this course include: (1) principles of cancer statistics; (2) principles of epidemiology; (3) genetics and cancer biology; (4) cancer prevention and control (including health promotion and community intervention); and (5) grants, contracts, and administration.

For health agencies to take full advantage of training opportunities, future linkages should be enhanced with NCI CDC, and schools of public health.

Applying known primary prevention technologies

History teaches us that a long "latency period" exists between the scientific understanding of a viable cancer control method and its widespread application on a population basis. Three examples illuminate this point. First, the Pap test was perfected in 1943 but was not widely used until the early 1970s.[17] Second, the Surgeon General first warned about the link between smoking and cancer in 1964, yet it was not until the late 1980s that comprehensive, population-based interventions to control tobacco use were implemented.[46,47] Finally, the first study linking diet with cancer was published in 1913.[7] There are now hundreds of studies linking dietary practices to various cancer types, and experts have called for specific dietary change strategies.[48,49] However, as yet there is no action plan in place to systematically transfer dietary change technology into practice and there are few dedicated resources for diet intervention and cancer.[7] Shrinking this latency period must be a top priority of cancer control researchers and advocates in the future.

Developing and maintaining coalitions/ partnerships

Nearly all of the other nine priorities in this section are influenced by the development of partnerships and coalitions. Simply put, a coalition is a group of people representing diverse organizations and/or interests who are working together for a common goal. An effective coalition has the power to influence cancer control policies and community-level actions much beyond the influence of any single member. Coalitions can generally be described as "grassroots" or "professional." Grassroots coalitions are frequently organized by people who volunteer their time to support a public health issue. Professional coalitions tend to include significant staff time from member agencies such as state and local health agencies or the American Cancer Society (ACS). The grassroots versus professional designation is often not distinct.

Over the past decade, public health professionals have learned a great deal about the attributes that contribute to successful coalition development and maintenance.[50-52] Because the community-based trials to prevent cardiovascular disease have been in the field much longer than most cancer control interventions, public health practitioners should review the cardiovascular disease trials to determine lessons useful for cancer control applications, including methods involving measurement and evaluation.[52-56]

An issue that cancer control practitioners will face in the coming decade is the proliferation of risk factor- and disease-specific coalitions. In many areas of the United States, coalitions exist for control of tobacco, drug abuse, physical inactivity, cancer, cardiovascular disease, diabetes, human immunodeficiency virus (HIV)/acquired immunodeficiency syndrome (AIDS), and child health. At the local level, the same individuals may be called upon to serve on grassroots coalitions on numerous issues, making their contributions to any single issue more limited. Practitioners may need to reexamine the roles of multiple coalitions versus development of overall "prevention coalitions" that address several complementary issues.

Partnerships in cancer control research and intervention, with clear definitions of roles, must be enhanced at the federal, state, and local levels. At the *federal* level, close cooperation and clear role delineation are essential between the two major agencies (i.e., the NCI and the CDC) that are mainly responsible for translating preventive practices to large populations. At the *state* level, cancer control programs must be viewed as essential to the health of the public as are infectious disease control programs. States need to clearly define the role(s) for which they are best suited. For example, a large state health agency might be well suited for conducting research as well as translating findings; whereas, a small state agency may be ill-suited for research but ideally positioned for program delivery. At the *local* level, perhaps the largest payoff will come from active involvement in prevention coalitions that will change local cancer control policies.

Obtaining and maintaining adequate cancer control resources

Without adequate resources, the previous nine priorities cannot be adequately addressed. As described in earlier chapters in this issue, public health resources to control cancer have increased significantly over the past decade. Despite these increases, many states currently lack resources for comprehensive cancer control programs to address both primary prevention (i.e., tobacco control and dietary enhancement) and secondary prevention (i.e., breast and cervical cancer screening). Many states continue to lack the core disciplines needed to establish an effective cancer control program. For example, in a 1994 survey of state health agencies, 10 states and the District of Columbia did not have at least one full-time equivalent chronic disease epidemiologist on staff (personal communication, Leonard Palozzi, CDC, August 31, 1995).

Recent changes in the U.S. Congress and the possibility of merging many categorical programs into block grants are likely to lessen resources for cancer control in some states.[57] Public health practitioners must continually remind policy makers that resources have not been allocated in proportion to the morbidity and mortality patterns in today's society—re-allocations may be necessary in the current era of level funding. To put it bluntly, in some health agencies, current resource allocations reflect the priorities of the early twentieth century rather than current disease burdens. If resource allocation decisions are shifted more toward the states, vigilance and focused advocacy efforts will be necessary to ensure adequate cancer control resources. Public health advocates can learn from entities that have been successful in recent years (e.g., HIV/AIDS coalitions, breast cancer research coalitions) to plan future efforts. Alliances between public health agencies and voluntary health agencies (e.g., the American Cancer Society) will become even more critical.

CONCLUSION

In many respects, public health efforts in cancer control are at a crossroads. A decade ago, the first federally funded activities in cancer control were initiated by public health agencies.[19] These efforts began to revolutionize cancer control research by moving it beyond etiologic studies to intervention trials.[10] The potential of this paradigm shift has been largely unrealized—overall cancer mortality rates remain level and many public health agencies face threats to their cancer prevention programs. We can expect little progress or even backsliding on limited successes without a renewed commitment to cancer control at all levels of public health.

To maximize the public health potential in cancer control, 10 future priorities for public health practitioners have been outlined. Since the "war on cancer" began in 1971 with the passage of the National Cancer Act, the mythical and much-sought-after single, "magic bullet" cure has eluded researchers. Many in the public health arena have argued that our collective failure has been our inability to widely implement existing cancer control technologies at the population-level. Unless we meet this challenge, we will be guilty of dereliction in our public health duty.

REFERENCES

1. American Cancer Society. "Cancer Facts and Figures—1995." Atlanta, Ga.: ACS, 1995.

2. Boring, C.C., et al. "Cancer Statistics, 1994." *CA Cancer Journal for Clinicians* 44 (1994): 7-26.

3. Institute of Medicine. *The Future of Public Health.* Washington, D.C.: National Academy Press, 1988.

4. U.S. Department of Health and Human Services. *Healthy People 2000: National Health Promotion and Disease Prevention, Objectives.* DHHS Pub. No. (PHS) 91-50212. Washington, D.C.: Government Printing Office, 1990.

5. Baquet, C.R., et al. "Socio-economic Factors and Cancer Incidence among Blacks and Whites." *Journal of the National Cancer Institute* 83 (1991): 551–557.

6. Burner, S.T., Waldo, D.R., and McKusick, D.R. "National Health Expenditures Projections through 2030." *Health Care Finance* 14 (1992): 1–15.

7. Bal, D.G., et al. "Cancer Prevention." In *American Cancer Society Textbook of Clinical Oncology,* edited by G.P. Murphy, W. Lawrence Jr., and R.E. Lenhard Jr. 2nd ed. Atlanta, Ga.: American Cancer Society, 1995.

8. Centers for Disease Control and Prevention. "Estimated National Spendingon Prevention—United States, 1988." *Morbidity and Mortality Weekly Report* 41 (1992): 529–531.

9. Taylor, W.R., et al. "Current Issues and Challenges in Chronic Disease Control." In *Chronic Disease Epidemiology and Control,* edited by R.C. Brownson, P.L. Remington, and J.R. Davis. Washington, D.C.: American Public Health Association, 1993.

10. Greenwald, P., and Sondik, E.J., eds. "Cancer Control Objectives for the Nation: 1985–2000." *National Cancer Institute Monographs,* No. 2, DHHS Pub. No. 862880. Washington D.C.: Government Printing Office, 1986.

11. U.S. Department of Health and Human Services. *Healthy People 2000 Review, FY 1994.* Pub. No. (PHS) 951256-1. Washington, D.C.: Government Printing Office, 1995.

12. Wynder, E.L., and Graham, E.A. "Tobacco Smoking as a Possible Etiologic Factor in Bronchiogenic Carcinoma. A Study of Six Hundred and Eighty-four Proved Cases." *Journal of the American Medical Association* 143 (1950): 329–336.

13. Giovino, G.A., et al. "Epidemiology of Tobacco Use and Dependence." *Epidemiologic Reviews* 17, no. 1 (1995): 48–65.

14. Doll, R., and Peto, R. "The Causes of Cancer. Quantitative Estimates of Avoidable Risks of Cancer in the United States Today." New York: Oxford University Press, 1981.

15. Miller, A.B. "Planning Cancer Control Strategies." In *Chronic Diseases in Canada,* 13, no. 1. Toronto, Ontario: Health and Welfare, 1992.

16. Brownson, R.C., et al. "Cancer." In *Chronic Disease Epidemiology and Control,* edited by R.C. Brownson, P.I. Remington, and J.R. Davis. Washington, D.C.: American Public Health Association, 1993: 137–167.

17. Breslow, L., et al. "Cancer Control: Implications from Its History." *Journal of the National Cancer Institute* 59, suppl. 2 (1977): 671–686.

18. Alciati, M.H., and Marconi, K.M. "The Public Health Potential for Cancer Prevention and Control." In *Cancer Prevention and Control,* edited by P. Greenwald, B.S. Kramer, and D.L. Weed. New York: Marcel Dekker, 1995: 435–449.

19. Meissner, H., Bergner, L. and Marconi, K. "Developing Cancer Control Capacity in State and Local Public Health Agencies." *Public Health Report* 107 (1992): 15–23.

20. Siegfried, J. "Largest Tobacco-Control Program Begins." *Journal of the National Cancer Institute* 83 (1991): 1446–1447.

21. Reynolds, T. "States Begin CDC-Sponsored Breast and Cervical Cancer Screening." *Journal of the National Cancer Institute* 84 (1992): 7–9.

22. Miller, C.A., et al. "Validation of a Screening Survey to Assess Local Public Health Performance." *Journal of Public Health Management and Practice* 1, no. 1 (1995): 63–71.

23. Thacker, S.B., and Berkelman, R.L. "Public Health Surveillance in the United States." *Epidemiologic Reviews* 10 (1988): 164–190.

24. U.S. Department of Health and Human Services, Public Health Service. *Cancer Statistics Review, FY 1973–88.* National Cancer Institute NIH Pub. No. 91-2789. Bethesda, Md.: Government Printing Office, 1991.

25. Remington, P.L., et al. "Design, Characteristics, and Usefulness of State-Based Behavioral Risk Factor Surveillance: 1981–1987." *Public Health Reports* 103 (1988): 366–375.

26. Warner, K.E. "Public Policy Issues." In *Cancer Prevention and Control,* edited by P. Greenwald, B.S. Kramer, and D.L. Weed, New York: Marcel Dekker, 1995.

27. Centers for Disease Control and Prevention. "A Practical Guide to Prevention Effectiveness: Decision and Economic Analyses." Atlanta, Ga.: CDC, 1994.

28. Centers for Disease Control and Prevention. "Assessing the Effectiveness of Disease and Injury Prevention Programs: Costs and Consequences." *Morbidity and Mortality Weekly Reports* 44 (1995): RR-10.

29. Centers for Disease Control and Prevention. "Prevention and Managed Care: Opportunities for Managed Care Organizations, Purchasers of Health Care, and Public Health Agencies." *Morbidity and Mortality Weekly Reports* 44 (1995): RR-14.

30. Eddy, D.M. "A Computer-Based Model for Designing Cancer Control Strategies." In *Cancer Control Objectives for the Nation 1985–2000,* edited by P. Greenwald and E.J. Sondik, NCI Mono. No. 2 (NIH Pub. No. 86-2880), 1986.

31. Habbema, J.D.F., and Sondik, E.J. "Cancer Control Modeling." In *Cancer Prevention and Control,* edited by P. Greenwald, B.S. Kramer, and D.L. Weed. New York: Marcel Dekker, 1995.

32. Friede, A., Reid, J.A., and Ory, H.W. "CDC WONDER: A Comprehensive On-Line Public Health Information System of the Centers for Disease Control and Prevention." *American Journal of Public Health* 83 (1993): 1289–1294.

33. Skinner, C.S., et al. "The Potential of Computers in Patient Education." *Patient Education and Counseling* 22 (1993): 27–34.

34. Group Health Association of America. "1994 National Directory of HMOs." Washington, D.C.: GHAA, June 1994.

35. Baker, E.L., et al. "Health Reform and the Health of the Public: Forging Community Health Partnerships." *Journal of the American Medical Association* 272 (1994): 1276–1282.

36. Lipsman, J. "Editorial: The Impact of Health Care Reform on Local Health Departments." *Journal of Public Health Management and Practice* 1, no. 1 (1995): 1–2.

37. Miki, Y., et al. "A Strong Candidate for the Breast and Ovarian Cancer Susceptibility Gene BRCA1." *Science* 266 (1994): 66–71.

38. Peltom_ki, P., et al. "Genetic Mapping of a Locos Predisposing to Human Colorectal Cancer." *Science* 260 (1993): 810–812.

39. Palefsky, J.M. "Serologic Detection of Human Papillomavirus-Related Anogenital Disease: New Opportunities and Challenges." *Journal of the National Cancer Institute* 87 (1995): 401–402.

40. Schmid, T.L., Pratt, M., and Howze, E. "Policy as Intervention: Environmental and Policy Approaches to the Prevention of Cardiovascular Disease." *American Journal of Public Health* 85 (1995): 1207–1211.

41. Warner, K.E. "Smoking and Health Implications of a Change in the Federal Cigarette Excise Tax." *Journal of the American Medical Association* 255 (1986): 1028–1032.

42. National Cancer Institute. "The Impact of Cigarette Excise Taxes on Smoking among Children and Adults. Summary Report of a National Cancer Institute Expert Panel." Bethesda, Md.: NCI, August 1993.

43. National Cancer Institute. "State Cancer Legislative Database Program." Bethesda, Md.: NCI, August 1994.

44. Weed, D.L., and Husten, C.G. "Training in Cancer Prevention and Control." In *Cancer Prevention and Control,* edited by P. Greenwald, B.S. Kramer, and D.L. Weed. New York: Marcel Dekker, 1995.

45. Association of State and Territorial Chronic Disease Program Directors. "Reducing the Burden of Chronic Disease: Needs of the States." Washington, D.C.: Public Health Foundation, 1991.

46. U.S. Department of Health, Education, and Welfare, Public Health Service. *Smoking and Health. Report of the Advisory Committee to the Surgeon General of the Public Health Service.* CDC, DHEW Pub. No. (PHS) 1103. Washington, D.C.: Government Printing Office, 1964.

47. National Cancer Institute. "Strategies to Control Tobacco Use in the United States: A Blueprint for Public Health Action in the 1990s." Smoking and Tobacco Control Monographs 1 (NIH Pub. No. 92-3316). Bethesda, Md.: NCI, 1991.

48. Thomas, P.R., ed. *Institute of Medicine (US), Committee on Dietary Guidelines Implementation, Food and Nutrition Board. Improving America's Diet and Health: From Recommendations to Action.* Washington, D.C.: National Academy Press, 1991.

49. Ames, B.N., Gold, L.S., and Willett, W.C. "The Causes and Prevention of Cancer." *Proceedings of the National Academy of Sciences* 92 (1995): 5258–5265.

50. Bracht, N., and Kingsbury, L. "Community Organization Principles in Health Promotion. A Five-stage Model." In Bracht, N. *Health Promotion at the Community Level.* Newbury Park, Calif.: Sage Publications, 1990, 66–88.

51. Butterfoss, F.D., et al. "Community Coalitions for Prevention and Health Promotion." *Health Education Resource* 8 (1993): 315–330.

52. Goodman, R.M., Wheeler, F.C. and Lee, P.R. "Evaluation of the Heart to Heart Project: Lessons Learned from a Community-based Chronic Disease Prevention Project." *American Journal of Health Promotion* 9 (1995): 443–455.

53. Farquhar, J.W., et al. "Effects of Communitywide Education on Cardiovascular Disease Risk Factors. The Stanford Five-City Project." *Journal of the American Medical Association* 264 (1990): 359–365.

54. Carleton, R.A., et al. "The Pawtucket Heart Health Program: Community Changes in Cardiovascular Risk Factors and Projected Disease Risk." *American Journal of Public Health* 85 (1995): 777–785.

55. Luepker, R.V., et al. "Community Education for Cardiovascular Disease Prevention: Risk Factor Changes in the Minnesota Heart Health Program." *American Journal of Public Health* 84 (1994): 1383–1393.

56. Brownson, R.C., et al. "Preventing Cardiovascular Disease Through Community-Based Risk Reduction: Five-Year Results of the Bootheel Heart Health Project." *American Journal of Public Health* February 1996.

57. American Public Health Association. "Public Health Threatened." *The Nations Health* March 1995.

Index

A

Accountability, North Carolina Community-Based Public Health Initiative, 192–193

African American women, physical activity, 156

Age, mammogram, 135, 136

Aggregated data, 218

American Indian women, physical activity, 156

Antismoking policy development, 28–35

Avon Products, Inc.
  breast cancer, 134
  Centers for Disease Control and Prevention, 134

B

Basic science, applications, 4

Behavioral change
  action, 12
  community-based health promotion program, 12
  contemplation, 12
  maintenance, 12
  precontemplation, 12
  preparation, 12
  stages, 12

Behavioral Risk Factor Surveillance system, cancer control, 290

Bias, 217–218

Bootheel Heart Health Project, cardiovascular disease control, 68–75
  background, 68–69
  baseline survey, 69–71
  changes in knowledge and attitudes, 70, 71–72
  follow-up survey, 69–71
  methods, 68–71
  results, 71–72

Breast and Cervical Cancer Mortality Prevention Act, 124
  new legislation, 127–128

Breast cancer
  Avon Products, Inc., 134
  incidence, 122
  legislation, 124–126
  national strategic plan, 126–127
  New York, 173
  risk factors, 135
  screening, 140–149

health care provider sites
recruitment, 232
identification of children, 232–233
immunization of children, 232–233
implementing documentation, 230
methods, 229–231
parent survey findings, 233–234
planning, 231–232, 235–237
planning documentation, 230
results, 231–235
Human immunodeficiency virus.
See HIV

I

Immunization. *See* Children's
immunization program
Individual behavior change, xiii
Individual risk factor, xiii
Information, policy development,
34–35
formats, 34–35
sources, 34–35
Information technology, 3
Injury prevention
E-code data reporting, 56–65
emergency department, 56–65
Injury surveillance, 56
International Classification of
Diseases, 9th Revision, Clinical
Modification, 56
Intervention development, 105–107
Intervention implementation, 105–107

K

Kansas Department of Health and
Environment, Behavioral Risk
Factor Surveillance Unit, 78–80
Kellogg Community-Based Public
Health Initiative, 157–163
coalition building, 183–184

future directions, 162–163
Maryland consortium, 161
Michigan consortium, 161–162
North Carolina consortium, 162,
183–184
program history, 158
programmatic framework, 157–158
sites, 159–160
theoretical framework, 157–158

L

Legislation, breast cancer, 124–126
Local health agency, Centers for
Disease Control and Prevention, 124
Local health department
cardiovascular disease control, 67–
75
characteristics, 73
Logic model, 213–216, 214

M

Maine, chronic disease, causes of
death, 47–54
Mammography, 122–123, 135, 136
age, 135, 136
ethnic group, 135–138
National Breast and Cervical
Cancer Early Detection Program,
technical guidelines, 133
racial group, 135–138
state health agency, 133
Managed care organization, 269–283
changing marketplace, 22–23
integrating cancer prevention in
managed care, 291–292
nongovernmental but public-health
oriented, 270–271
prevention
economic factors, 271–273
future opportunities, 282–283